# Biomathematics

Volume 23

*Managing Editor*
S. A. Levin

*Editorial Board*
C. DeLisi  M. Feldman  J. Keller  R. M. May  J. D. Murray
A. Perelson  L. A. Segel

Stavros Busenberg
Kenneth Cooke

# Vertically Transmitted Diseases

## Models and Dynamics

With 35 Figures

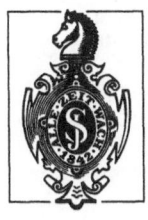
Springer-Verlag
Berlin Heidelberg New York
London Paris Tokyo
Hong Kong Barcelona
Budapest

Stavros Busenberg

Department of Mathematics
Harvey Mudd College
Claremont, CA 91711, USA

Kenneth Cooke

Department of Mathematics
Pomona College
Claremont, CA 91711, USA

ISBN-13: 978-3-642-75303-9     e-ISBN-13: 978-3-642-75301-5
DOI: 10.1007/ 978-3-642-75301-5

© Springer-Verlag Berlin Heidelberg 1993
**Softcover reprint of the hardcover 1st edition 1993**

Typesetting: Camera-ready by authors
41/3140 – 5 4 3 2 1 0 – Printed on acid-free paper

# Preface

More human lives are taken each year by infectious diseases such as malaria, AIDS, Chagas' disease, cholera and dengue fever than by any other single cause. In the past there was little hope of controlling the course of epidemics caused by these diseases, but modern scientific advances are now providing a variety of means for combatting many of the infections that afflict human populations. The spread of a communicable disease is a dynamic population process that cannot be truly understood unless methods are developed for measuring and reliably quantifying the pertinent parameters that govern these dynamics. However, measurements in themselves provide no more than a record of past epidemics. In order to design control strategies and assess their efficacy, reliable procedures need to be developed for simulating and predicting the future courses of diseases when various control strategies are applied. The central goal of mathematical epidemiology is to provide these crucial predictive tools.

The purpose of this book is to describe a class of predictive tools and their application to diseases whose modes of transmission include vertical transmission, that is, the passing of the infection from a parent to an unborn or newborn offspring. The predictive methods that we describe are currently undergoing rapid development. However, these methods follow a typical sequence of steps. They start with the formulation of mathematical models of the dynamics of the disease transmission, proceed to the analysis of these models via mathematical methods and computer simulations, and then use the analytical and numerical results to make predictions about the possible courses of diseases. These predictions, which forecast the rate of spread of the disease under a variety of possible conditions and control measures, form the basis for developing rational strategies for controlling and preventing the spread of these diseases.

We have concentrated on the study of vertically transmitted diseases because there is no single source where the work in this recently developed area of modeling and analysis can be found. About ten years ago, we observed that there were few papers in mathematical and scientific journals that dealt with models of diseases

that are transmitted directly from parent to offspring (called vertical transmission). There are several books which describe mathematical models of disease transmission. However, for the most part,
they do not include vertical transmission. In view of the widespread
occurrence and biological significance of this mode of disease transmission, we determined to gather together and extend the existing
literature on the dynamics of models that include vertical transmission. The result is this book.

The mathematical study of the transmission of infectious diseases may be regarded as a part of the study of population dynamics. For example, one of the objects of study is the variation over
time of the incidence (number of new cases reported per unit time)
of a particular disease within a specified host population. As with
other parts of population dynamics, a mathematical model must
be formulated which takes into account the most important factors
which influence the results. During the present century, mathematicians and biologists have devoted increasing attention to these models, and there are now several books that describe them. Among
the books that are devoted in whole or in part to this subject
are the following: Anderson and May [1991], Bailey[1975], Bartlett
[1960], Edelstein-Keshet [1988], Hethcote and Yorke [1984], Hoppensteadt [1975], Macdonald [1957], Muench [1959], Murray [1989],
Ross [1911], and Waltman [1974].

There are three basic objectives of this book. The first is to show
the reader how to formulate a set of mathematical equations that
capture the essentials of a given epidemiological situation. Thus
the book treats the modeling process within the context of disease
transmission dynamics. We endeavor to do this by presenting and
discussing many models, which may differ in the types of questions
addressed or types of mathematical equations employed. A second
objective is to demonstrate the mathematical analysis by which
the implications from a model may be derived. We feel that it is
desirable to have as complete and rigorous a mathematical understanding of a model as can be obtained. For the benefit of readers
who may be unfamiliar with some of the mathematical techniques
and principles that are employed, we have included at the end of
Chapters 2, 3, and 4 short explanations of those techniques and
principles. It is our hope that the book may therefore be useful not
only to persons who have worked actively in this field, but also to
biologists and mathematicians who wish to gain sufficient familiar-
ity with it to be able to follow its research literature and perhaps
also contribute to its development.

The mathematical prerequisites for reading most of the book
consist of a working knowledge of calculus and an acquaintance
with differential equations and linear algebra. However, parts of the
book, and in particular the latter sections of Chapter 5, require fur-

ther mathematical background for their full understanding. Thus, the book is addressed to modelers, to biologists and epidemiologists who are interested in general principles, and to applied mathematicians who would like to contribute to the development of this field.

A third objective is to show how the mathematical analysis of models yields epidemiological inferences which cannot be easily detected from either the statistical analysis of data or from qualitative logical inferences. For example, it may provide a framework for comparing models with available data, for identifying key parameters, for suggesting future possible trends, or for evaluating proposed strategies for control or eradication of a disease.

We have organized the book along mathematical lines partly in order to present the most widely accessible material in the early chapters, but also because the mathematical descriptions are often closely tied with specific epidemiological and population dynamics hypotheses. Thus, after a short introductory chapter, we begin with models framed in terms of ordinary differential equations. Then we take up, in the order listed, models using difference equations, delay differential equations, and partial differential equations.

The book contains a number of features which we believe deserve special attention. These include the emphasis on non-constant population size, which is in contrast with most of the classical epidemic models; the use of a systematic approach in modeling the force of infection terms; and the derivation of several key parameters relating demographics and epidemics. Special models are constructed for several important diseases, but we have included very little in the way of statistical analysis or parameter identification.

There remains much work to be done in the modeling and analysis of vertically transmitted diseases. In several places in the book we have pointed out problems which have been only partially modeled or analyzed. The direction of ongoing work with which we are acquainted is also discussed. Our main hope is that by collecting and ordering the current state of knowledge of this active interdisciplinary research field, the book can serve as one of the bases for its future development.

We have been helped in our work on this book by many colleagues and students who have stimulated us with their questions, inspired us with their original contributions and encouraged us with their comments. In particular, we want to express our gratitude to Carlos Castillo-Chavez, Eric Funasaki, David Grabiner, Mimmo Iannelli, Simon Levin, Pauline van den Driessche, Horst Thieme, Jorge Velasco-Hernandez, and David Williamson. The contributions to this book of all these friends and colleagues, both named and unnamed, through their comments, their criticism, their joint work with us, and their sharing of ideas which influenced our thinking, are deeply appreciated. We also express our gratitude to the

National Science Foundation for its financial support over the years which helped sustain and encourage our work in this area. Finally, we thank our wives, Bonnie and Margaret, for their support and for their cheerful tolerance of the long working hours that were needed to complete this book. We hope that some of their exemplary patience and loyalty has been vertically transmitted to our offspring.

Claremont, California       *Stavros Busenberg and Kenneth Cooke*
July 1992

# Contents

# 1 Introduction

## 1.1 What Is Vertical Transmission?

Vertical transmission is the direct transfer of a disease from an infective parent to an unborn or newly born offspring. Several of the scourges that currently afflict humanity, AIDS, Chagas' disease, Hepatitis B, are vertically transmitted. Efforts to control the spread of such diseases require quantitative predictions of the future trends of these infections, and consequently, lead to the construction and analysis of appropriate predictive models that take into account the distinctive aspects of vertical transmission. The purpose of this book is to describe the results that have been obtained to date in the formulation and use of such models, and to lay a foundation for future work in this area.

Infectious diseases are caused by organisms such as bacteria, viruses, protozoa, and fungi, which enter and infect a host organism. These infecting organisms are passed from one individual host to another, in this way spreading the infection throughout the host population. This passing of the infection may be accomplished either directly or indirectly via one or more intermediate host species. There are many mechanisms, some quite intricate, by which this passage of the infection is physically accomplished. In this book we shall not concentrate on the biological details of these mechanisms, but will be primarily concerned with modeling and describing the dynamics of the spread of diseases in host and vector populations. Biologically, we will be distinguishing between two broad categories of disease transmission, called horizontal transmission and vertical transmission.

Horizontal transmission refers to the passage of the infection from one host individual to another, for example by inhalation or ingestion of infective material, or else by direct physical contact. Vertical transmission, on the other hand, occurs through a variety of other mechanisms. In rinderpest, a disease of cattle and other animals, the transmission is transplacental, that is, through the placenta to the embryo. Transplacental transfer also occurs in several diseases affecting humans, including congenital rubella and AIDS. In some insects, a virus may be passed through the infected eggs. A few plant diseases, such as bean and lettuce mosaic, are transmitted through the seed. A number of examples of vertically transmitted diseases will be discussed throughout this book.

From the prevalence of vertical transmission, it may be inferred that this must be an important biological mechanism. This leads to several questions.

What role does it play in the perpetuation of the disease or infection? How important is vertical transmission in comparison to horizontal transmission? How did this mode of disease transmission evolve? What effect does it have on the possibility or methods of control of the disease? How does it affect the age distribution of the infected part of the population? To give one example of its importance, we mention that for some diseases for which mosquitoes, or other arthropods, are carriers, and for which the vector population is reduced to virtually zero during winter, the disease may be carried into the next generation through infected eggs, which successfully survive the winter (over-winter). A model of this type, applicable to such diseases as Rocky Mountain Spotted Fever, will be discussed in Chapter 3.

The epidemiological role of vertical transmission can be seen as a quantitative problem, involving its rates of transfer relative to transfer rates by other mechanisms. Therefore, the construction and analysis of mathematical models that include vertical transmission should be helpful in addressing such questions as those in the preceding paragraph. It is our purpose in this book to gather together a wide collection of such models, to provide their mathematical analysis, and to show the significance of the vertical transmission mechanism in the epidemiology of these diseases. We have attempted to refer to most such models that have appeared in print and that include a mathematical treatment. In many cases, we have formulated and analyzed new models ourselves. We hope that some readers will be stimulated to fill in the many gaps that this book will leave in this area of modeling and analysis, both in a general theoretical way and in connection with specific diseases that have not yet been studied.

## 1.2 Methodology, Terminology and Notation

In translating a biological population problem into a mathematical model, certain constitutive assumptions need to be made concerning the type of mathematical equations that are chosen to describe the actual situation. A model, of course, involves simplifications of the real situation and a judicious exclusion of details which may be interesting and important in certain individual cases, but are not the dominant factors determining the dynamics of the population. On the other hand, mathematical models, by their very nature, make clear statements of the assumptions concerning the biological and population mechanisms that influence the propagation of the disease. Consequently, predictions based on such models, when compared to actual epidemiological data, can be used to test the validity of these assumptions. Similarly, models can be used as tools for the estimation of various parameters which cannot be directly measured. This is particularly important in the case of human diseases where controlled laboratory experiments are often not possible due to sociological or ethical reasons. It is important to note that the range of validity of a particular model is always limited, yet that need not detract from its value when restricted to situations where it applies. This should not be a source of distrust of modeling in epidemics, nor should it be a reason to regard epidemic models as less worthwhile than models in the physical sciences. In fact, this limitation of the range of validity of mathematical models is ubiquitous to all of the sciences, even though in certain fields, such as physics, older mathematical models which have well known limitations to their range of applicability are traditionally presented as if they were the true description of physical phenomena. Such an example is the Newtonian mathematical model of dynamics that is taught in introductory physics courses. Similar questions on the appropriate degrees of simplification occur in biological models (see Black and Singer [1987], Levin [1991]).

All of the models that we present here will be limited to the case of large populations and will not be an appropriate description of epidemics in small populations where stochastic fluctuations tend to dominate, and hence, probabilistic and statistical models would be more appropriate. We shall not deal with such probabilistic models of epidemics, partly because we are not aware of any major theoretical work on such models which deals with vertical transmission, and partly because our own work has been mainly in the area of deterministic models.

Most of the models of transmission of infection in a population take as their starting point the assumption that the entire population can be divided into subpopulations of epidemiologic significance. In the simplest models, these are the subpopulations of susceptibles, infectives, and removed. An individual who is at first susceptible may have contact with an infective, thus receiving the infection. Furthermore, an infective individual may in due course be removed from the infective class because of recovery, isolation, or death. Thus, the progression of an individual can be from susceptible, $S$, to infectious, $I$, to removed, $R$. Such a model has been called an $SIR$ model, and often has been symbolized by the diagram $S \rightarrow I \rightarrow R$. Some infections do not give rise to acquired immunity in the host. In this case, if the disease is non-lethal, an individual who has recovered from the infection will again be susceptible. Then the disease is said to be of the $S \rightarrow I \rightarrow S$ type. In order to take account of other features and to achieve more realism, additional stages of the infection may be distinguished. For example, there may be a *latent period* between the time that an individual is infected and the time that the individual is infectious to others. It has been common to introduce a class of such individuals, usually called the exposed class and denoted by the letter $E$. Thus, there are models of type $S \rightarrow E \rightarrow I \rightarrow R$ and $S \rightarrow E \rightarrow I \rightarrow S$. It may be remarked that epidemiologists often make a distinction between the latent period and the *incubation period*, which is the time between receiving an infection and first exhibiting symptoms of illness.

Early work on models of infectious diseases was directed at epidemic diseases, in which there is a sudden rise in incidence and then a fall-off to low or zero incidence. Since the course of such an epidemic, for example, of a childhood disease or of influenza, occurs rapidly, it was customary to ignore the vital dynamics of births and deaths. In recent years, attention has also been devoted to *endemic* diseases, which are constantly prevalent, though perhaps at varying intensities. In such cases, it is important to include the vital dynamics of the population. For example, an $S \to I \to S$ model in which births to individuals are included, and in which all newborn individuals are considered to be susceptible, can be symbolized by the diagram that follows.

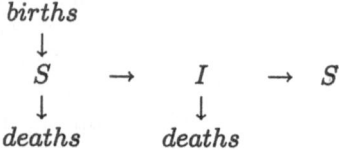

For vertically transmitted diseases, it is obviously necessary to account for births and deaths. Because the dynamical relationships can now become considerably more complicated, we have found it useful to extend the familiar schematic diagrams in the following way. Suppose that the population is separated into four basic epidemiological classes: the susceptibles, the exposed, the infective, and the removed. In Chapter 5, where we consider the age structure of the population, we have to deal with densities per unit age rather than numbers. We denote the proportion or age-specific density of individuals in these classes by the symbols $s, e, i$, and $r$, respectively, reserving the corresponding upper case letters for the total number of individuals in these epidemiological classes. In using graphs to depict the dynamics of the disease, we employ horizontal arrows to denote transfers among classes that are caused by horizontal transmission mechanisms, and vertical arrows to denote vertical transmission. Vertical transmission clearly affects only the newborn. Transfers between classes due to recovery or to the lapse of an incubation or immunity period are denoted by horizontal arrows also, while changes due to births and deaths are denoted by vertical arrows.

Let us give a few examples of this notation. The following diagram is for a model with only $s$ and $i$ classes.

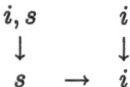

The horizontal arrow indicates horizontal transmission. The vertical arrows indicate that new susceptibles are brought in by birth from both the $i$ and $s$ classes, and new infectives by vertical transmission from the infective $i$ class. This diagram, therefore, represents the simplest situation in which all offspring of susceptibles are susceptible, but some offspring of infectives are susceptible and some are infectious. Diseases, such as AIDS, from which there is no recovery and which are vertically transmitted may be described by such a model. Age dependent models of this type have been analyzed by El Doma [1985, 1987] and by Busenberg, Cooke and Iannelli [1988, 1989] and are described in Chapter 5.

The diagram that follows is for an $s \to i \to r$ model that is similar to the above model, except for the inclusion of a removed or immune class $r$ that is not fertile.

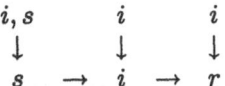

The next diagram indicates an $s \to e \to i \to r$ model where susceptibles can become exposed via horizontal transmission, then move to the $i$ class, and finally to the immune or removed class. Vertical transmission brings in newborn susceptibles from the exposed, infective, and susceptible classes; and newborn exposed and infectives from the infective class only. The infective class is structured by an internal variable which takes the values 0, 1, and 2. This internal variable might denote the level of pathogen load in the individual. Individuals with the lowest load of pathogen are those who have just come into the infective class from the exposed class via horizontal transmission, and those with the highest load are individuals who are newborn infectives from a parent with a high pathogen load. The internal structure of the class $i$ is denoted by underlining $\underline{i}$ and then detailing in a separate diagram the dynamics within that class.

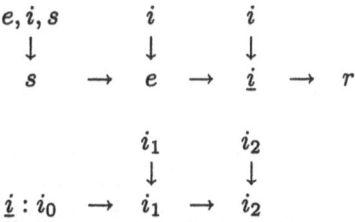

In the above diagrams, removals due to deaths have not been depicted explicitly. If desired, vertical arrows below the several classes can be used to depict such removals. We shall have occasion to do this in certain cases later on.

## 1.3 Examples of Vertically Transmitted Diseases

We have already mentioned a few infections that are vertically transmitted. In this section, we shall give brief descriptions of a few more, in order to give the reader a better idea of the widespread nature of this phenomenon and of the severe impact of these diseases. Throughout this monograph, we give examples of vertically transmitted diseases, describing those features of each which can affect the dynamics of the disease transmission process. The following partial list indicates the diversity of these diseases. The rubella virus and the herpes simplex virus in man, the protozoan *Nosema plodiae* infecting the insect *Plodia interpunctella*, a cytoplasmic polyhedrosis virus infecting the silkworm *Bombyx mori*, the protozoan *Amblyospora* infecting the mosquito *Culex salinarius*.

One of the vertically transmitted viruses for which a specific model exists is the Keystone virus. The model will be given in detail in Chapter 3, but here we merely wish to point out some of the important biological facts. Keystone (KEY) virus is one of the California group of arboviruses. The word arbovirus has been introduced to indicate that the infection is carried by arthropods, and the word arthropod refers to invertebrates such as spiders, mites, ticks, and mosquitoes. In this case, it is the *Aedes atlanticus* mosquito. This disease is prevalent in the Eastern United States among small mammals such as rabbits or squirrels. It is transmitted from an infected mosquito to a susceptible mammal, or from an infected mammal to a susceptible mosquito, when the mosquito takes a blood meal from the mammal. The vertical transmission occurs through the eggs laid by an infected female mosquito and plays a role in the maintenance of the infection. Although Keystone virus has not been shown to cause human illness (so far as we know), several other viruses of the California group are transmitted vertically and are known to cause human diseases. It is likely that the Keystone virus model could serve as a prototype for models of these other California group viruses. Another example of vertical transmission in mosquitoes is the Dengue virus which causes a serious human illness. The vertical transmission of this virus by the mosquitoes of the *Aedes scutullaris* group has been reported by Freier and Rosen [1987] as a likely mechanism for the survival of the virus during the absence of vertebrate hosts or in unfavorable climatic conditions.

Vertical transmission of pathogenic agents is common in insect vectors but it also occurs in mammals. Two examples of vertical transmission of diseases in humans are Hepatitis B and Chagas' disease (American trypanosomiasis.) In both these cases, even asymptomatic mothers can transmit the disease to their offspring. Chagas' disease is related to African sleeping sickness and is caused by parasitic protozoa which enter the body through an insect bite contaminated by insect feces. This disease is characterized by fever, enlarged lymph nodes, and various serious long-term complications including permanent cardiac damage. In its acute form, it can be fatal but it frequently has only mild subclinical symptoms over a multi-year period. It occurs mainly in Central and South America where up to twenty million cases have been estimated (Ponce and Zeledon [1973]), however, there are reports of its occurrence and possible spread in North America as well, Theis *et al.* [1987]. It is vertically transmitted across the placenta from the mother to the fetus, Loke [1982].

A somewhat different example is Rocky Mountain Spotted Fever which is transmitted to humans mainly by the tick vectors *Dermacentor andersoni* and *Dermacentor variabilis*. This disease has high fever and rash symptoms that are similar to those caused by typhoid, and is caused by the organism *Rickettsia rickettsi*. In this case, the vertical transmission of the disease occurs in the tick vector population, and is one of the primary mechanisms for its maintenance at endemic levels, Burgdorfer [1975].

Plasmids are extrachromosomal elements in the cell which are vertically transmitted and which determine phenotypic characteristics even though they are not part of the cell genome. There are many interesting and important consequences of the presence of certain plasmids in cells, such as the development of drug resistence in bacteria (Falkow [1975]), and the production of toxic agents by the Paramecium aurelia (Preer, Preer and Jurand [1974]). We do not treat models of vertical transmission that have been specifically motivated by plasmids. However, this is an area where there are many fascinating questions which possibly could be elucidated by the formulation and analysis of appropriate mathematical models. One of these is the question of how plasmids co-evolved with the cells that act as their hosts. In fact, the general question of the interaction between disease transmission and genetics is an aspect of vertical transmission that has not been modeled and analyzed to our knowledge. The paper by Levin and Lenski [1983] treats a model of coevolution in bacteria and their viruses and plasmids, that of Longini [1983] treats a model for a population undergoing genetic selection due to infection by a disease, while that of Novick and Hoppensteadt [1978] treats the question of how the replication and partition of plasmids can be governed to ensure their hereditary stability. These papers can provide starting points for further work in this area.

When we refer to vertical transmission in this book, we do not intend to include the so-called genetic diseases that are due to parental genes and are transmitted to offspring according to Mendelian laws. We do not include these because of the absence of horizontal transmission in these cases, and because there is already an extensive literature dealing with them. On the other hand, some of our models may well be applicable to the passage of extrachromosomal material from mother cells to daughter cells. We also have not included models of cultural inheritance, which are similar in that one may distinguish between the influence of parents and of other individuals on a child. This interesting area has been addressed in a book by Cavalli-Sforza and Feldman [1981].

## 1.4 Organization and Principal Results

The most commonly used deterministic dynamical models of epidemics employ ordinary differential equations and the methods of analyzing such equations have become fairly well known to students of this field. However, the need to include a number of biologically significant effects, such as incubation periods and age-specific effects, has led to models that employ more involved formulations which use delay differential equations and partial differential equations. Since the increase in the mathematical complexity of the models is almost invariably due to specific biological considerations, it has been possible to organize the book on parallel modeling and mathematical considerations. Each of the next four chapters concentrates on models that use a particular general mathematical formulation. Each of Chapters 2, 3 and 4 concludes with a section where the mathematical techniques that are used in the analysis of these models are outlined. These concluding sections can be skipped by those familiar with the requisite mathematical tools, but can serve others as a convenient source of these results, without cluttering the rest of our treatment with side excursions into the development of the necessary mathematical methods.

The main body of the book begins in Chapter 2, where we discuss models that can be expressed by ordinary differential equations. In this chapter, we begin by formulating the basic $S \to I \to R$ model with vertical transmission. Then, after a discussion of some biological properties of microorganisms, we consider a much simplified model with only $S$ and $I$ classes. This permits us to give rigorous global mathematical results. That is, we can completely describe all qualitative behavior that may occur, for any possible values of the transmission parameters. The concepts of basic reproductive number (or reproductive coefficient) and effective reproductive number (or coefficient) for the infection are introduced, and it is shown how these provide important, but not complete, information about the spread and maintenance of infections. Reference is made to the literature for most of the details of the proofs. After a thorough discussion of this model, we proceed to the $S \to I \to R$ model and to models with latency or maturation time, where only local or partial results have been proved. In the next section, we discuss the problem of parameter estimation in the context of a study of the rice dwarf virus. We then discuss a simple model of Chagas' disease which yields a number of interesting conclusions concerning the dynamics of the propagation of this disease. We then proceed to another general $S \to I \to R \to S$ model with vertical transmission in a population that is undergoing demographic changes. A complete analysis of this model is given and the fine structure of the new basic reproductive numbers which occur when the population is undergoing demographic changes is discussed. In the next section we consider a model which explores the role of vertical transmission in the evolution of viruses.

Chapter 3 is devoted to situations where the models are formulated in terms of difference equations. Two particular models are treated in detail. The first is a model for the transmission of Keystone virus. Difference equations appear to be a suitable *genre* for this virus, because seasonal variations introduce a generation-by-generation structure. Next, we discuss a model for Rocky Mountain Spotted Fever. This again has a generation structure due to several effects, but has an additional interesting feature. It is necessary to keep track of the pathogen load which tends to increase with successive transmissions from one generation to the next. We study the epidemiological effects of different forms of the force of infection terms within the context of this model and discuss in some detail the possibility that the total population size may be controlled by the disease. We next describe a model by Régnière [1984] for vertical transmission in insect pests. We then proceed to the discussion of a discrete-continuous model, that is, a model using a combination of ordinary differential equations to describe one aspect of the dynamics and difference equations to describe another. This is one of a very few models of a vertically transmitted disease using this type of mathematical form. This model includes a logistic control on the total population, and we show the differences in dynamic behaviors that occur between the case when the logistic control acts on the birth rate and when it affects the death rate. In this chapter we also encounter one of the striking phenomena that occur in difference equations models, which is the possibility of chaotic dynamic behavior. We discuss the implications that this type of dynamic behavior has on both the understanding of the significance of data on the incidence rates of diseases, and on the interpretation of the predictions based on models. We also give an example of the phenomenon of the occurrence of long term transient states which are not stable but which can describe the dynamics of the disease for very long periods of time.

In Chapter 4, we treat models with delays which can occur because of long incubation periods, fixed periods of infectivity and a variety of other mechanisms where a transfer between classes does not occur instantaneously. The presence of delays can introduce new dynamic phenomena, and in particular, we shall see how periodic oscillations can be caused by these latency periods. We also consider a model which includes both delays and population migration in a spatial domain. We then discuss vertical transmission of diseases which have long subclinical periods during which the disease may be transmitted yet does not cause detectable symptoms. We derive a model with a time delay which can be used to study the effects of such subclinical periods.

In Chapter 5, we turn our attention to models that explicitly include age structure within the host population. Not many such models with vertical transmission have appeared in the literature and the methods for their mathematical analysis are still being actively developed. However, it is clear that age may play an important role in the dynamics of disease transmission. For example, the degree of susceptibility of an individual to a pathogen may depend on age, and contact rates between individuals may depend on the ages of those individuals. Also, it is only the newborn, that is, individuals of age zero, that are susceptible to vertical transmission of infections. In addition, it may be necessary to include other internal structure variables to describe the state of the population. For example, the length of time that an individual has been infected may be an important parameter. Therefore, in this chapter, we describe some basic methods for including age and other internal structure variables to describe the state of the population. The literature in this area is very recent and many open questions remain for investigation. However, some very interesting results have been obtained using analytical as well as numerical methods. Many of these methods of analysis have been developed only in the past few years, and we describe them and also provide a guide to the literature where they are treated in greater detail. In this chapter, we outline the current state of knowledge in this field, present some of the significant results that have been obtained and point out a number of open questions which are of current interest.

We have not attempted to provide a catalog of known vertically transmitted diseases. The paper by Fine [1975] provides a good starting point for such a catalog and a classification scheme which facilitates understanding of the basic dynamics of vertical transmission. Throughout this monograph, we give examples of a number of vertically transmitted diseases which have either been modeled and analyzed or seem amenable to such a theoretical treatment. This includes many instances that have come to our attention, but is not meant to be a complete catalog. For each disease, we point out those salient features which play a role in the model and in the dynamics of its transmission. These include one or more of the following list: the host species, the species of the infecting organism, the geographical location of prevalence, immunity status, and in a few cases estimates of transmission parameter values. We also indicate references to detailed descriptions of the diseases, and to specific mathematical models when any exist. From this we hope that the reader can obtain an overview of the similarities between different vertically transmitted diseases and, hence, some initial direction in constructing appropriate mathematical models that describe their dynamics.

# 2 Differential Equations Models

## 2.1 A Classical Model Extended

A natural way to begin the treatment of models of vertical transmission is to extend the classical epidemic models as contained, for example, in the book of Bailey [1975]. In order to provide a baseline for understanding the effects of vertical transmission and to introduce some of the standard terminology we briefly describe the classical Kermack-McKendrick [1927] model of an $S \rightarrow I \rightarrow R$ epidemic. This has the form

$$dS/dt = \dot{S} = -kSI,$$

$$dI/dt = \dot{I} = kSI - cI,$$

$$dR/dt = \dot{R} = cI.$$

Here, $S$ is the number of susceptible individuals, $I$ is the number of infected individuals, and $R$ is the number of recovered or immune individuals in the host population, at time $t$. The dot denotes differentiation with respect to time $t$. The constant $k$ is the "contact rate" and $c$ is the removal rate or recovery rate of infectives. A mass-action term $kSI$ is assumed for the rate at which susceptible individuals are infected through contact with infectives. This form of the term describing the rate of transmission of the disease is based on the assumption that the affected population is homogeneously mixing and is often used when the total population size is constant. Other forms of the transmission rate are also used and will be discussed later. The infectives are assumed to be cured at a constant rate $cI$, at which point they enter the removed or immune class. This implies that the average time of infectivity is $1/c$ because the probability of remaining infected for a time interval $t$ is $e^{-ct}$. Since the model which we shall treat below includes the above equations as a special case, we shall not give the analysis of these equations at this point but will only provide a short description of their consequences.

The above equations are only appropriate in cases in which the epidemic is fast-acting so that the host population can be considered to be of constant size. In particular, births in the host population are not considered. In dealing with vertical transmission, however, births are an essential element, especially since vertically transmitted infections may affect host survival or fecundity. Consequently, births and deaths must be explicitly included in the models we consider.

The basic predictions of the Kermack-McKendrick model are most easily explained via reference to Figure 2.1 which shows the possible relationship between the subpopulation sizes $S(t)$ and $I(t)$. Since $R = P - S - I$, where $P$ is the constant total population size (it is normalized to $P = 1$ in the figure), this graph gives a complete description of the behavior of this model. Letting $S_0$, $I_0$, denote the initial sizes of the subpopulations $S$ and $I$, and defining the dimensionless *basic reproductive coefficient* $R_0 = S_0(k/c)$, the behavior of this model can be described as follows. If $R_0 \leq 1$, then the number of infectives $I(t)$ decreases to zero as $t \to \infty$, while if $R_0 > 1$, then $I(t)$ first increases to a maximum value $I_m$, and then decreases to zero as $t \to \infty$. The number of susceptibles $S(t)$ decreases with $t$ and has the limiting value $S_\infty$. Both $I_m$ and $S_\infty$ depend on the threshold value $R_0$, and $I_m$ is given by

$$I_m = S_0 + I_0 + \frac{c}{k}\left[\ln\left(\frac{c}{kS_0}\right) - 1\right],$$

and $S_\infty$ is the the unique solution that lies in the interval $(0, S_0)$ of the equation

$$S_0 + I_0 - S_\infty + \frac{c}{k}\ln\left(\frac{S_\infty}{S_0}\right) = 0.$$

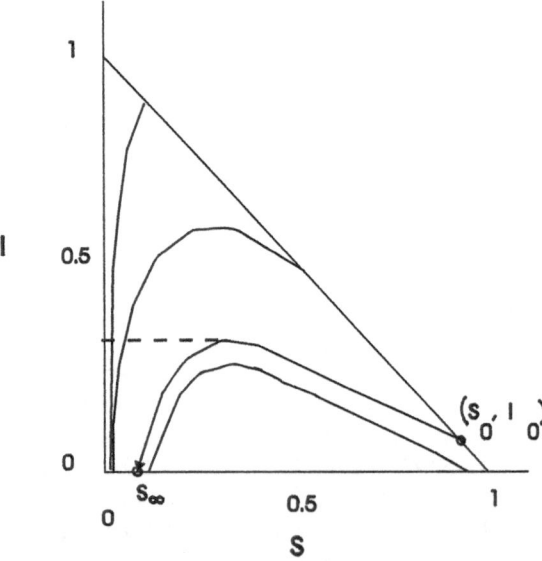

**Fig. 2.1.** Dynamic behavior of the Kermack-McKendrick model

It is important to understand the significance of the threshold parameter $R_0$. The ratio $k/c$ is the *effective contact number* and is the product of the expected period of infectiousness $1/c$ and the horizontal per capita contact rate $k$. Thus, it represents the expected number of per capita contacts that one infective will have over the entire period of infectivity. Consequently, $R_0$

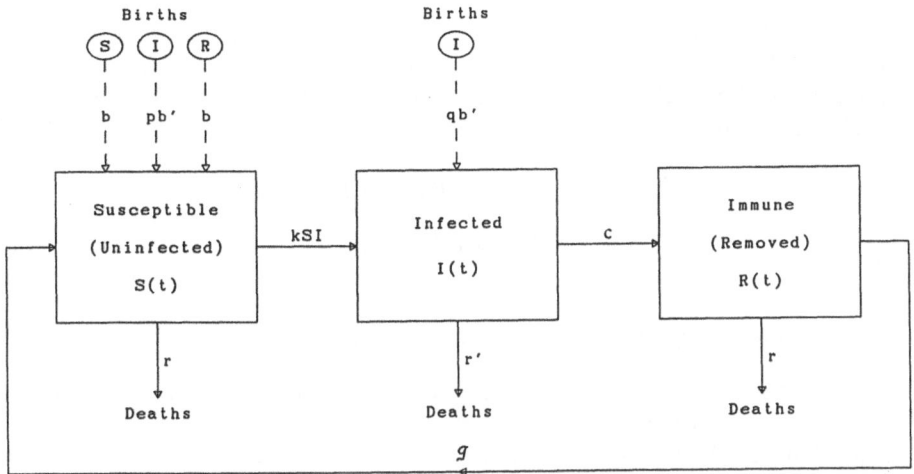

**Fig. 2.2.** Structure of $S \to I \to R \to S$ model

is the expected total number of new infections caused by each infective in the initial population. The results on this model say that an epidemic will occur only when each infective introduced in the initial population, on the average, causes more than one new infection. Of course, the contact rate depends on both the horizontal transfer rate $k$ and the cure rate $c$, and these two parameters are the ones that need to be estimated in order to predict the course of such an infection. It should also be noted that the basic reproductive coefficient $R_0 = (S_0/P)(Pk/c)$ is directly proportional to the proportion $S_0/P$ of susceptibles in the initial population and to $Pk/c$, the total number of contacts with the entire population by one infective during the expected duration of the infection. This model does not take vertical transmission or vital dynamics into account and we now proceed to study appropriate generalizations which remedy this situation.

We begin with a model formulated in a special case by Anderson and May [1979, 1981] and independently in a more general form by Busenberg, Cooke and Pozio [1983] who also provided a complete analysis which is the basis of our discussion. This model extends that of Kermack-McKendrick by taking account of births and deaths and by allowing the possibility that some new-born individuals may be infected. The general structure of the model is suggested in Figure 2.2. This model is for a *directly transmitted* infectious agent. This means that there is only one host for the infectious organism. The organism is transmitted from one host individual to another by some direct contact between hosts or by transmission stages of the organism which pass into the habitat of the host and are then acquired by the host. A special case of direct transmission, already discussed in Chapter I, is *vertical transmission* in which the agent is conveyed by a parent to its offspring. The term *horizontal transmission* refers to modes of direct transmission that are not vertical.

In this model, it is assumed that the host population is asexual, or at any rate, that it suffices to keep track of only one sex (female). Let $S(t)$, $I(t)$ and $R(t)$ denote the numbers of susceptible, infectious, and immune or removed host organisms, respectively. The following extension of the Kermack-McKendrick model is proposed:

$$\dot{S} = -kSI + b(S + R) + pb'I - rS + gR,$$
$$\dot{I} = kSI + qb'I - r'I - cI, \qquad (2.1)$$
$$\dot{R} = cI - rR - gR.$$

The assumptions underlying this model are listed as follows:

(i) Horizontal transmission of infection may be expressed by a mass-action term $kSI$ where $k$ is a constant.

(ii) The birth rate $b$ is constant and is the same for the susceptible and immune classes. The birth rate $b'$ for infectives may be different from $b$.

(iii) Progeny of susceptible and immune individuals are all susceptible at birth. Of the total offspring of infected individuals, $b'I$, a fraction $p$ are susceptible and a fraction $q$ are infected at birth. Here $p + q = 1$.

(iv) The death rate $r$ is constant and is the same for the susceptible and immune classes, but the rate $r'$ for the infected class may be different from $r$.

(v) Infectives recover with immunity at a rate $c$.

(vi) Immune individuals lose immunity and again become susceptible at the rate $g$.

(vii) The incubation time for infection is zero. The incubation time is the length of time from the moment of infection until either symptoms appear or else asymptomatic infectiousness starts.

(viii) The gestation time is zero and newborns are instantly fertile.

In addition, it is assumed, as is customary with deterministic population models, that the population sizes are sufficiently large that we can treat $S$, $I$, and $R$ as real-valued continuous quantities.

It is clear that several of these assumptions may be unrealistic. The assumption (i) requires some discussion and is taken up in detail in the next section. In this model we choose the mass-action form $kSI$, since it is the simplest. Further on in this chapter we shall treat models with other forms of the force of infection term.

Assumptions (vii) and (viii) are questionable, but may be acceptable approximations if the incubation and gestation times are short. The model is also unrealistic in that it does not include density-dependent regulation of the size of the host population. Models incorporating various modifications will be formulated subsequently. A reason for at first not including density-dependent regulation is to show that disease-induced mortality may in itself suffice to check population growth. This point has also been emphasized by Anderson and May [1979, 1981] and will be further discussed below. It is easy to see that the Kermack-McKendrick model is obtained as a special case of (2.1) by setting $b = b' = r = r' = g = 0$.

## 2.2 Some Biological and Modeling Considerations

Before commencing a mathematical analysis of the model (2.1), we give a preliminary discussion of infectious diseases for which it might be an appropriate description. In Chapter 1, we have already mentioned a number of diseases that are transmitted vertically. These, and others, are diverse in the type of host, the type of pathogen or agent, the mode of transmission, and also in such factors as the degree and duration of infectiousness of the pathogen and of the incubation period. Equation (2.1) is sufficiently general to account for considerable diversity, but modifications may be required in particular cases.

There is an important distinction between vertebrate and invertebrate hosts. Both may be able to mount a defensive response of one sort or another to invasion by a pathogen. However, vertebrates may develop acquired immunity, whereas invertebrates apparently do not. That is, if an invertebrate recovers from infection, it will be susceptible to reinfection. A vertebrate may retain immunity for some period of time, possibly for life. For example, the viral infections rubella and herpes simplex confer lifelong immunity to those who recover from the disease. Equations (2.1) can, in a sense, simulate both possibilities. For, by taking $g$ extremely large, we obtain a model in which the average time spent in the immune state is very small; by taking $g$ to be zero, we obtain a model in which immunity is lifelong. The general model (2.1) is often called an SIRS model, since an individual may pass from susceptible to infective to immune (removed) and back to the susceptible state. When $g = 0$, it reduces to an SIR model. In the next section, we shall also discuss an SIS model in which there is no $R$ state ($g = \infty$, symbolically).

Another distinction, made by Anderson and May [1979, 1981], is between *microparasites* and *macroparasites*. By microparasites they mean pathogens, such as viruses, bacteria, protozoans, and fungi, that are small in size, have short generation time, and have a rapid rate of direct reproduction within the host. For such pathogens, simple models like (2.1) afford a good description. On the other hand, macroparasites such as helminths typically do not reproduce within the host, and the effect of the infection upon the host depends on the number present. A different kind of mathematical model is required in this case. We shall concentrate on the microparasitic type here.

An important term in the models that we will be considering which requires some explanation is the force of horizontal infection. In assumption (i) of the previous section we used the form $kSI$ for this term. This is justified as follows. Suppose that we let $N$ denote the number of encounters that an individual susceptible has with other individuals, per unit of time. If $P = S+I+R$ is the total population size, then on the average, the number of encounters by one susceptible with infectious individuals will be $NI/P$, and the total rate of new infections will be proportional to $SNI/P$. If one assumes that the encounter rate $N$ is proportional to the total population size $P$, then $N = \alpha P$ and the rate of new infections is $kSI$ as in (2.1). This assumption appears to be a reasonably good approximation in some cases, for example, for populations with rapid homogeneous mixing. In some other cases, it may be better to assume that $N$ is a constant. For example, for sexually transmitted human diseases, the number of sexual contacts by an individual is perhaps more or less independent of $P$, at least for $P$ above some value. For discussions of this term see Nold [1980] and the early work of Wilson and Worcester [1945a,b]. Another form that has been suggested is $N = kI/(1 + k'I)$ where $k$ and $k'$ are constants, so that $N$ increases linearly with $I$ at low densities but reaches a saturation level when $I$ is large. Some models of this kind (without vertical transmission) have been studied recently by Liu, Levin, and Iwasa [1986] and Liu, Hethcote, and Levin [1987], and Huang [1990].

In a population which is composed of only susceptible and infective individuals, the two main types of such terms that we shall meet here have the forms $kSI$ and $k\frac{SI}{S+I}$. These are commonly called the *mass-action* and *proportional mixing* rate of infection terms, respectively. When the sum $S + I$ =constant, then these two types of terms are equivalent, except for a change of the constant $k$. This is not the case when $S + I$ is not constant, and we need to look at the reasoning that leads to these terms.

First, let us consider the case of an infection whose transmission requires direct contact between individual infectives and susceptibles. Also, suppose that the fact that an individual is infected or not does not affect the probability of having direct contacts with others, and that the rate at which an individual comes into contact with others in the population is a constant $\kappa$. Then, one reasons that, of all the contacts that a single susceptible has, a proportion equal to $\frac{I}{I+S}$ is with infective individuals. Thus, the rate at which contacts between infectives and susceptibles is occurring is equal to $\kappa S \frac{I}{I+S}$. If $\rho$ is the probability that a contact between a susceptible and an infective will lead to the transfer of the infection then, setting $k = \kappa\rho$, we obtain the form $k\frac{SI}{S+I}$ for the force of horizontal transmission. However, if the infection is not transmitted via direct contacts between infective and susceptible individuals, but rather via the level of contamination of some common resource, say the water or a food item, then this type of reasoning would be inappropriate and the resulting term would not accurately model the force of infection. In this latter case, one reasons that the degree of contamination of the resource is proportional to the total number of infectives present in the population. Hence, if $\kappa$ now represents the contact rate of the susceptible population with this resource, and $\rho$ is the probability that a contact will lead to an infection, then setting $k = \kappa\rho$, as before, we obtain the other type of force of infection, namely, $kSI$. Note that it is not appropriate to think of $\kappa$ as also representing the rate at which the infectives may be contaminating the resource, since the use of the resource is invariably different from the way in which it gets contaminated. An example would be a man-environment disease such as cholera which can be transmitted via drinking water which, in turn, is contaminated from improper treatment of sewage. In such cases, it is often important to note that, when the degree of infectivity becomes high enough, then sociological or other mechanisms often come into play which tend to saturate the effect that a large number of infectives may have. Then it is more appropriate to use a modification of this term which takes the form $kS\frac{I}{1+k'I}$, which, for small $k'$, starts out being a close approximation of the term $kSI$, and approaches the form $\frac{k}{k'}S$ when $I$ becomes very large.

We shall be encountering variants of all these types of terms in this monograph. At times, we shall analyze a particular model with one form of the force of infection term and will not proceed to the treatment of the same model with a different form. This is often the case because the predictions of otherwise identical models, except for a change in the form of the force of infection, can be very different. Hence, in using such models to explain epidemiological data, it is important that a determination of the appropriate form of force of infection be made. In the model of the previous section we used the term $kSI$, while in Section 2.13, when we discuss some recent models of Chagas' disease, we shall be using force of infection terms of the form $k\frac{SI}{S+I}$. We shall return to the general issue of constructing appropriate mathematical forms for the force of infection in Chapter 5, where we will describe recent work on an axiomatic approach to the derivation and classification of such terms.

Much of the classical work on epidemiological models has been restricted to situations where the affected population is of constant size. This assumption is relatively valid for diseases of short duration with limited effects on mortality. However, it fails to hold for diseases that are endemic in communities with changing populations, and for diseases which raise the mortality rate substantially. Well known examples of such diseases are malaria in developing countries with growing populations, and the current AIDS pandemic. In such situations, the effects of the disease induced mortality and of the change in population size are far from negligible, and in fact, may have a crucial influence on whether or not the disease can reach epidemic levels. Consequently, we treat a variety of models where the population size is not assumed to be constant and where there are interactions between the demography and the disease transmission dynamics.

## 2.3 Model Without Immune Class

When there is no immunity, equations (2.1) may be replaced by

$$\dot{S} = -kSI + bS + pb'I - rS + gI,$$
$$\dot{I} = kSI + qb'I - r'I - gI,$$

(2.2)

where $p + q = 1$ and where we now interpret $g$ as the rate at which infected individuals recover and again become (instantly) susceptible to reinfection. This is now an $S \to I \to S$ model. Since the system (2.2) is mathematically easier to treat than (2.1), we shall discuss it first and show the kinds of mathematical and biological inferences that may be drawn. Our discussion is based on the detailed analysis of Busenberg, Cooke and Pozio [1983]. Equation (2.1) is discussed in Section 2.7 below.[1]

Along with (2.2), we shall use the equation for $\dot{P}$ where $P(t) = S(t) + I(t)$ is the total population. Using (2.2), we easily find the system

$$
\begin{aligned}
\dot{I} &= (qb' - r' - g)I + k(P - I)I, \\
\dot{P} &= (b' - r')I + (b - r)(P - I) = (b - r)P - \alpha I,
\end{aligned}
\tag{2.3}
$$

where $\alpha = (b - r) - (b' - r')$. We may now work with either (2.2) or (2.3). Given an initial condition for (2.2), $S(0) = S_0$, $I(0) = I_0$, $S_0 \geq 0$, $I_0 \geq 0$, a unique solution will exist, at least in a neighborhood of $t = 0$. Given an initial condition $I(0) = I_0$, $P(0) = P_0$, $0 \leq I_0 \leq P_0$, the same is true for (2.3).

It will also be useful and convenient to introduce a variable given by the ratio

$$
y = \frac{I}{P}
\tag{2.4}
$$

which represents the *prevalence* of infection in the host population. Then

$$
\dot{y} = \frac{P\dot{I} - I\dot{P}}{P^2} = \frac{\dot{I} - y\dot{P}}{P}.
$$

A calculation using (2.3) leads to the equations

$$
\begin{aligned}
\dot{y} &= y[kP(1 - y) + qb' - r' - g - b + r + \alpha y] \\
&= y[kP(1 - y) - \alpha(1 - y) - pb' - g], \\
\dot{P} &= (b - r - \alpha y)P.
\end{aligned}
\tag{2.5}
$$

In order that the above equations may be said to constitute a biologically reasonable model, it is necessary that their solutions exist for all $t \geq 0$, that is, they should not "blow up" to infinity in finite time. Also, they should remain nonnegative, $y(t) \leq 1$, and for (2.3) one should have $I(t) \leq P(t)$ if $I_0 \leq P_0$. These properties will be proved in Section 2.5. For now, we want to analyze the existence and local stability of equilibrium solutions, and to introduce the useful notion of the basic reproductive coefficient.

To find all possible equilibrium solutions of (2.2), we set the right hand sides of the differential equations to zero. One equilibrium is given by $S = 0$, $I = 0$, $P = 0$. If $I \neq 0$, then from (2.2) we find $S = (r' + g - qb')/k$ and

$$
(b' - r')I = (r - b)S.
$$

---

[1] Defining $r'' = r' + g - qb'$, and $b'' = g + pb'$, we may write (2.2) in the form $\dot{S} = -kSI + (b - r)S + b''I$ , $\dot{I} = kSI - r''I$. In this form, we have a system that may be formally regarded as a model in which there is no vertical transmission, births of infectives are at the rate $b''$ and all are susceptible, and deaths of infectives are at the rate $r''$. However, this interpretation fails if $r'' < 0$, and in any case there is no treatment of the latter system, in full generality, available for quotation. Therefore, we shall give a full analysis of (2.2) here.

If $b' \neq r'$, we thus find a unique nontrivial equilibrium solution

$$S^* = \frac{r' + g - qb'}{k}, \qquad I^* = \frac{(b-r)(r' + g - qb')}{k(r' - b')},$$

$$P^* = \frac{\alpha(r' + g - qb')}{k(r' - b')}, \qquad y^* = \frac{(b-r)}{\alpha}, \tag{2.6}$$

where $\alpha = (b - r) - (b' - r')$. However, if $b' = r'$, then there is no nontrivial equilibrium unless $b = r$ and then $\dot{P} = 0$ and (2.3) yields

$$P(t) \equiv P(0), \qquad I(t) \equiv P(0) - (pb' + g)/k. \tag{2.7}$$

It is also useful to ask whether the prevalence $y$ can approach a constant while $I$ and $P$ do not tend to constants. If $y(t) = I(t)/P(t)$ tends to a constant other than one or zero, while $P$ does not, the limiting form of (2.5) leads to a contradiction because the term $kPy(1 - y)$ would then vary in time, and $\dot{y}$ could not be zero. However, if $y(t)$ tends to one then (2.5) yields $pb' + g = 0$ and $\dot{P}/P$ is asymptotically $b - r - \alpha = b' - r'$. If $y(t)$ tends to zero, then $\dot{P}/P$ is asymptotically $b - r$. Thus, if $y(t)$ tends to 0 or 1, $P(t)$ asymptotically has exponential growth at the respective rates $b - r$ and $b' - r'$. For the moment, let us set aside the special case $b' = r'$ and the situations in which the prevalence tends to zero or one, reserving discussion of these possibilities for later.

Throughout the rest of the discussion, we shall also assume that $r' \geq r$, on the grounds that an infection, almost by definition of the word, is very unlikely to decrease the death rate of the host population. We can now begin to address questions such as the following:

(i) Under what conditions will the population become extinct? Approach the nonzero equilibrium? Grow unboundedly?

(ii) Under what conditions can an infection be introduced into a population and persist in it? What will the limiting prevalence be?

(iii) Under what conditions will disease-induced excess mortality cause a limitation of a population which otherwise would grow unboundedly?

In this section we introduce some basic concepts and derive partial answers to these questions. The next section contains a more complete analysis. A very important and useful parameter in the discussion of disease models is the basic *reproductive coefficient* of the infecting agent. This is denoted by $R_0$ and defined to be the number of secondary cases produced, on the average, when one infected individual is introduced into a population in which all individuals are susceptible. The use of this parameter in modeling has been emphasized by Dietz [1975, 1976], and Anderson and May [1981] among others. We have assumed that the number of new infections per unit time is $kSI + qb'I$. Thus, one infective produces $kS + qb'$ infections per unit time, or taking $S = P$, $kP + qb'$ infectives. Since the removal rate of infectives is $(r' + g)$, the mean length of infectiousness is $1/(r' + g)$. Thus, one infective during its expected period of infectiousness will produce $(kP + qb')/(r' + g)$ new (secondary) infectives. Based on this reasoning, we define the *basic reproductive coefficient*

$$R_0(t) = \frac{kP(t) + qb'}{r' + g}.$$ (2.8)

When the number of susceptibles is $S(t) \neq P(t)$, the *effective reproductive coefficient* $R(t)$ is

$$R(t) = \frac{kS(t) + qb'}{r' + g}.$$ (2.9)

We note from (2.6) and (2.9) that if the equilibrium $S^*$ is achieved, then $R^* = 1$ but $R_0^* \geq 1$. This is intuitively reasonable, since at equilibrium each infective must, on the average, produce one new infective to replace itself. One sees that if an endemic infection is to be achieved, the total population and the susceptible population must adjust themselves until $R$ approaches one.

The quantity $R_0$ depends on the basic biology of the infectious organism and on ecological, environmental, and social factors that influence transmission and recovery rates. In Anderson and May [1981], one may find a discussion of factors which affect the value of $R_0$, tables of values for certain cases, and discussion of the extent to which $R_0$ may be said to characterize particular host-parasite associations.

Anderson and May [1981] give tables in which they indicate, for a variety of models, two quantities, called the *threshold host population*, $P_T$, and the *growth characteristic*. We now give a preliminary discussion of what they may have had in mind when they considered the first of these quantities. Imagine that a small proportion of infectives is introduced into a wholly susceptible population. Will the infection grow and spread or will it die out? From (2.2),

$$dI/dt = I(kS + qb' - r' - g)$$

and $dI/dt$ will be positive if and only if $kS > r' + g - qb'$. Since $S \approx P$, Anderson and May define

$$P_T = \frac{r' + g - qb'}{k}$$

and observe that if $P(0)$ is less than $P_T$, the number of infectives will initially decrease, whereas if $P(0)$ is greater than $P_T$, it will increase. As one sees from (2.8), this criterion is the same as $R_0(0) < 1$ versus $R_0(0) > 1$. However, we will prove below that in some situations (see Case i of Theorem 2.1 in the next section) the infection will persist even though $P(0) < P_T$ ($R_0(0) < 1$). In these situations, the number of infectives decreases at first but then increases, and the population grows with the disease persisting until its equilibrium $P^*$ exceeds $P_T$.

We note that the concept of a threshold host population size has been widely used in discussions of diseases such as measles. For measles, there is no vertical transmission, the total population is considered to be constant, and typically it is assumed that $b = b' = r = r'$. A pathogen is said to "regulate the population" if its presence makes the population approach an equilibrium rather than continue to grow. Note that for (2.2), with $b > r$, the population would grow exponentially in the absence of infection. A quick, intuitive criterion for regulation in this sense can be obtained by finding when the quantities in (2.6) are positive and $I^* \leq P^*$. The conditions for this are

$$r' + g - qb' > 0 \quad \text{and} \quad \frac{b-r}{r'-b'} > 0. \tag{2.10}$$

When (2.10) holds, we say that $S^*$, $I^*$, $P^*$ is a *feasible* equilibrium.

More information can be gleaned from a local stability analysis of the equilibria. We continue to assume $b' \neq r'$ and $r' \geq r$. The linearization of (2.2) near $S = I = 0$ is

$$\dot{S} = (b-r)S + (pb' + g)I,$$
$$\dot{I} = (qb' - r' - g)I. \tag{2.11}$$

The eigenvalues of the matrix of coefficients are $b - r$ and $qb' - r' - g$, and this equilibrium point is (locally) asymptotically stable if and only if $b - r < 0$ and $qb' - r' - g < 0$. Of course, this does not guarantee that all solutions are attracted to zero. In the next section, we shall find the region of attraction, that is, the set of initial values for which the corresponding solutions tend to $(0,0)$.

So far, we have shown the following:

(a) If $b < r$ and $r' + g - qb' > 0$, then $(0,0)$ is asymptotically stable. If $r' > b'$, then $(S^*, I^*)$ is not feasible, but if $r' < b'$ then $(S^*, I^*)$ is another feasible equilibrium.

(b) If $b < r$ and $r' + g - qb' < 0$, $(0,0)$ is unstable and $(S^*, I^*)$ is not feasible. In fact, system (2.11) has one positive and one negative eigenvalue and $(0,0)$ is a saddle point.

(c) If $b > r$, then $(0,0)$ is unstable, and is an unstable node if also $qb' - r' - g > 0$. If $qb' - r' - g < 0$, $(S^*, I^*)$ is feasible, since (2.10) is satisfied.

More information can be obtained from the stability analysis of $(S^*, I^*)$, when it is feasible. We let $S = S^* + u$, $I = I^* + v$, and from (2.2) obtain the linearized system

$$\dot{u} = (b - r - kI^*)u + (pb' + g - kS^*)v,$$

$$\dot{v} = kI^*u + (kS^* + qb' - r' - g)v,$$

with corresponding matrix

$$\begin{bmatrix} b - r - kI^* & pb' + g - kS^* \\ kI^* & kS^* + qb' - r' - g \end{bmatrix}.$$

The trace of this matrix is

$$b - r - kI^* + kS^* + qb' - r' - g = b - r - kI^* = (b - r)\left[1 - \frac{r' + g - qb'}{r' - b'}\right].$$

Since $kS^* = g + r' - qb'$, the determinant of this matrix is

$$-kI^*(pb' + g - r' - g + qb') = -kI^*(b' - r').$$

As is well-known, the eigenvalues of this $2 \times 2$ matrix will have negative real parts if, and only if, the trace is negative and the determinant is positive. Thus, we have $(S^*, I^*)$ asymptotically stable if and only if

$$I^* > \frac{b - r}{k} \quad \text{and} \quad I^*(b' - r') < 0.$$

Assuming $I^* > 0$, we thus require $b' - r' < 0$. From (2.6) we conclude that when $(S^*, I^*)$ is feasible (and $r' \neq b'$), it is asymptotically stable provided $b > r$, $b' < r'$.

Of course, this local stability analysis guarantees nothing about the size of the region of attraction of the equilibrium. It is conceivable that for many initial conditions, the solution might approach some periodic solution or become unbounded as $t \to \infty$. In order to provide a definitive answer to the above questions (i), (ii) and (iii), a complete global analysis is required. For the system under consideration, this is possible. In the next section, we will state the complete result, with discussion, and in the following section outlines of proofs will be provided.

Finally, let us take a look at the special case when $b' = r'$. First, suppose that $b = r$. Then $\alpha = 0$ and from (2.3) we get $\dot{P} = 0$. Hence, $P(t)$ is constant, $P(t) = P_0$. Moreover, $\dot{I}/I = qb' - r' - g + k(P_0 - I) = -pb' - g + k(P_0 - I)$. The behavior of $I(t)$ depends on whether $P_0$ is above or below the threshold $P_T$, as will be described in detail in the next section. If $b' = r'$ and $b \neq r$, then $\dot{P} = (b-r)(P-I)$ and at an equilibrium we have $P = I$ and $\dot{I} = (qb' - r' - g)I \neq 0$. Thus, $(0,0)$ is the only equilibrium in this case, and this is the only case in which there is a threshold value of the population below which $(S, I) \to (0, 0)$.

## 2.4 Discussion of the Global Result

Because of the many parameters in (2.2), it is somewhat complicated to state the full results on qualitative behavior of solutions. We have divided the discussion into a number of cases. Figures 2.3(a), and 2.3(b) illustrate the regions of parameter space for these parameters. As previously stated, we restrict attention to the case $r' \geq r$. However, the case $r' < r$ was also treated in Busenberg, Cooke, and Pozio [1983] and the theorem stated below is valid in that case also. We discuss this case in Section 2.7.1 where we show that it can be used to analyze the corresponding $S \to I \to R$ model. In each case, we state the mathematical results, interpret these biologically, and relate them to the ideas of reproductive coefficient and the threshold population as previously introduced. Proofs of all results are sketched in the next section. The cases are as follows:

Case i $b/r > 1$ and $b'/r' < 1$.
Case ii $b/r \leq 1$ and $b'/r' \leq 1$, and at least one of these inequalities is strict.

Case iii $b/r = 1$ and $b'/r' = 1$.
Case iv $b/r > 1$ and $b'/r' \geq 1$, or else $b/r \leq 1$ and $1 \leq (qb' - g)/r' < b'/r'$.
Case v $b/r \leq 1$ and $(qb' - g)/r' < 1 < b'/r'$.

As seen from Figures 2.3(a) and 2.3(b), if $b' < b$, only Cases i, ii and iv may occur; if we also have $b' = b$, Case iii may occur; and if $b' > b$, all cases may occur[2]. It is most likely that $b' \leq b$ in real biological situations. However, we have included the case $b' > b$ so that the results will be available in any systems fitting that condition. We now state our results for each case.

**Theorem 2.1** *The following hold for system (2.2) if $q < 1$, $k > 0$ and $g \geq 0$ or $q = 1$, $k > 0$ and $g > 0$. Either $P(t) = S(t) + I(t) \rightarrow \infty$ as $t \rightarrow \infty$, or the solution $(S(t), I(t))$ approaches a constant limit $(S^+, I^+)$ as $t \rightarrow \infty$. Nontrivial periodic solutions cannot occur. More explicitly, the following occurs in the five cases defined above.*

**Case i.** *$(S^*, I^*)$ is feasible and, whenever $S_0 \geq 0$, $I_0 > 0$, $(S^+, I^+) = (S^*, I^*)$. If $I_0 = 0$ we have either $(S, I) \equiv (0, 0)$ or $(S^+, I^+) = (\infty, 0)$. The equilibrium $(S^*, I^*)$ is globally asymptotically stable within the class of solutions having initial data $S_0 \geq 0$, $I_0 > 0$.*

**Case ii.** *If $b/r < 1$, then the equilibrium $(S^*, I^*)$ is not feasible and $(S^+, I^+) = (0, 0)$. If $b/r = 1$, $(S^+, I^+) = (S_0 + I_0 + (b' - r')\beta, 0)$ where $\beta$ is the unique non-negative root of the equation*

$$S_0 + I_0 - (pb' + g)/k + (b' - r')\beta = [S_0 - (pb' + g)/k]e^{-k\beta}.$$

**Case iii.** *Let $P_0 = S_0 + I_0$. If $I_0 = 0$ or if $kP_0/(pb' + g) < 1$ then $(S^+, I^+) = (P_0, 0)$. If $I_0 > 0$ and $kP_0/(pb' + g) \geq 1$ then $(S^+, I^+) = ((pb' + g)/k, P_0 - (pb' + g)/k)$.*

**Case iv.** *In this case, either $(S, I) \equiv (0, 0)$ or else $I^+ = P^+ = \infty$ and $S^+ = (pb' + g)/k$. Moreover, $y(t) = I(t)/P(t) \rightarrow 1$.*

**Case v.** *$(S^*, I^*)$ is feasible and unstable. Moreover, there exists $\tilde{I}_0 > 0$ and a monotone decreasing continuous function $\phi$, defined on $(0, \tilde{I}_0)$ with values in $(\tilde{I}_0, \infty)$, such that $\phi(I^*) = I^* + S^* = P^*$ and the following holds:*
*(i) If $I_0 > \tilde{I}_0$ or else if $I_0 \in (0, \tilde{I}_0]$ and $P_0 > \phi(I_0)$, then $(I^+, P^+) = (\infty, \infty)$.*
*(ii) If $\phi(I_0) = P_0$, $I_0 \in (0, \tilde{I}_0]$, then $(I^+, P^+) = (I^*, P^*)$.*
*(iii) If neither (i) nor (ii) holds, then $(I^+, P^+) = (0, 0)$.*

**Discussion:** We note first of all that the condition $k > 0$ in the hypothesis of the theorem means that there is some horizontal transmission occurring. The case $k = 0$ will be dealt with below. The condition $q < 1$ and $g \geq 0$ or $q = 1$ and $g > 0$ will be satisfied if vertical transmission is not complete ($q < 1$), or even if it is complete provided there is some recovery of infectives back to the susceptible class.

---

[2] In Anderson and May [1981], it is assumed that $b = b'$, and Case iii is not considered.

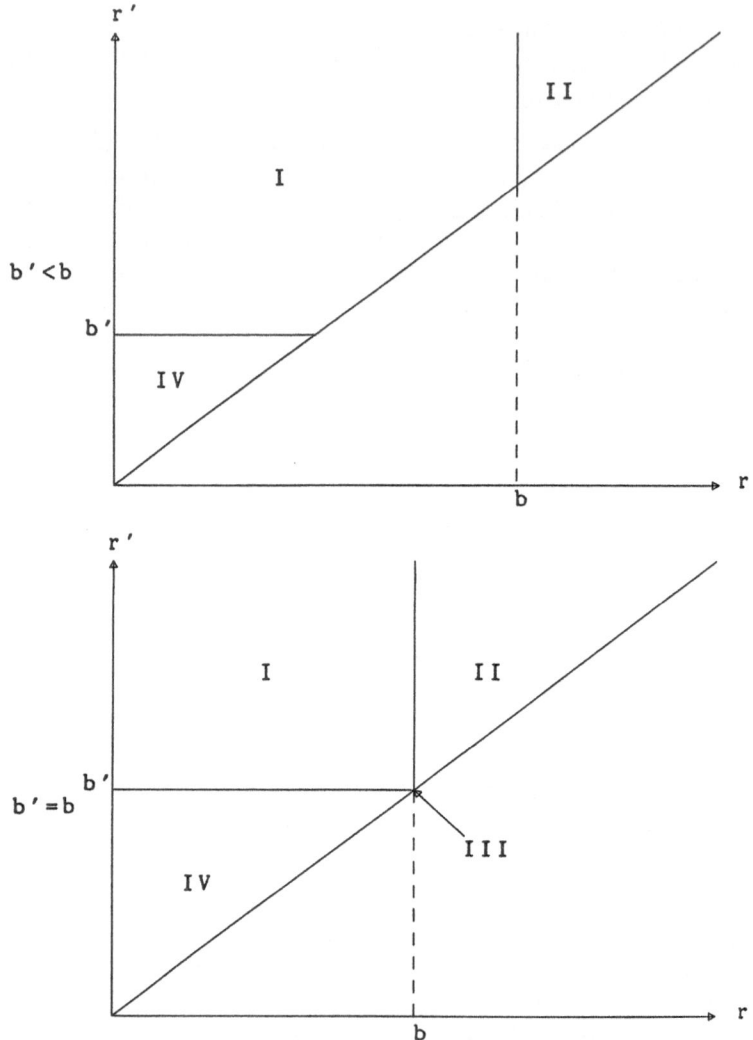

**Fig. 2.3(a).** Parameter regions for the various cases when $b' < b$ or $b' = b$

It may be worth emphasizing that the stated theorem is global. That is, within the range of parameters, $b$, $b'$, $r$, $r'$, $g$, $q$ specified, it gives the behavior of all possible solutions for any initial conditions $S_0 \geq 0$, $I_0 \geq 0$. Complete results of this sort are much harder to obtain and to prove for more complicated systems such as those to be encountered later in this book. From the biological and modeling point of view, the following questions about the above model seem to be important.

(a) Under what conditions will the infection regulate or restrict the population to a finite size?

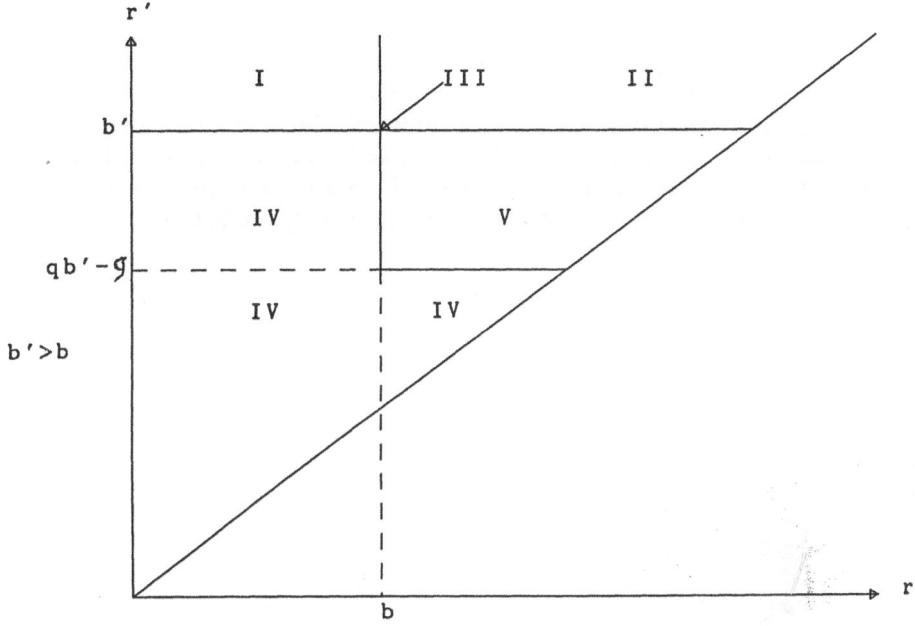

**Fig. 2.3(b).** Parameter regions for the cases in Theorem 2.1 when $b' > b$

(b) In this model, how important is vertical transmission in assuring persistence of the disease, and what is its effect on the prevalence ratio?

(c) Does the basic reproductive coefficient provide a useful guide to the behavior of the model?

(d) What are the interactions between demographic changes and the dynamics of the disease?

Let us begin our discussion with the question of regulation of the population by the infection. We must then suppose that $b/r > 1$, so that the host population would grow indefinitely in the absence of the infectious agent. Thus we need to consider Cases i and iv. The dynamic behavior of the model in these cases is illustrated in Figs. 2.4(a)-2.4(d). From the theorem we see that in Case i, where $b'/r' < 1$, an equilibrium is achieved with $S = S^*$, $I = I^*$, independent of the initial values $S_0$ and $I_0$. In Case iv, with $b/r > 1$ and $b'/r' \geq 1$, we have $P(t) \to \infty$ as $t \to \infty$. We conclude that the population is regulated to a finite level if and only if $b'/r' < 1$. That is, the infection must either depress the host fertility, or increase the host death rate, or both, until $b'/r' < 1$. We note that this conclusion is independent of the magnitude of the horizontal and vertical transmission rates.

In this connection, we also ask under what circumstances the entire population will tend to extinction. We see that this is true if $b/r < 1$ and $b'/r' \leq 1$ (Case ii). Also, if $b/r \leq 1$ and $(qb' - g)/r' < 1 < b'/r'$ (Case v), then this may be true, depending on the initial conditions. In this case, there is a separatrix $P = \phi(I)$ in the $(I, P)$ phase plane. This separatrix is a curve such that, for initial conditions lying below it, $I(t)$ and $P(t)$ tend to zero as $t \to \infty$, but for initial conditions above the curve, $I(t)$ and $P(t)$ tend to $\infty$. For initial conditions exactly on the curve, the saddle point $(I^*, P^*)$ is approached. The behavior of solution orbits in this case is illustrated in Figure 2.4(e). This case can only occur in biological situations in which the infectious agent improves the viability of the host so that $b'/r' > 1$, and also $(qb' - g)/r' < 1$. There is an interplay here between $r'$, $b'$, $g$ and $q$ because if $1 \leq (qb' - g)/r' < b'/r'$ then we are in Case iv and, as observed above, $P(t)$ tends to $\infty$.

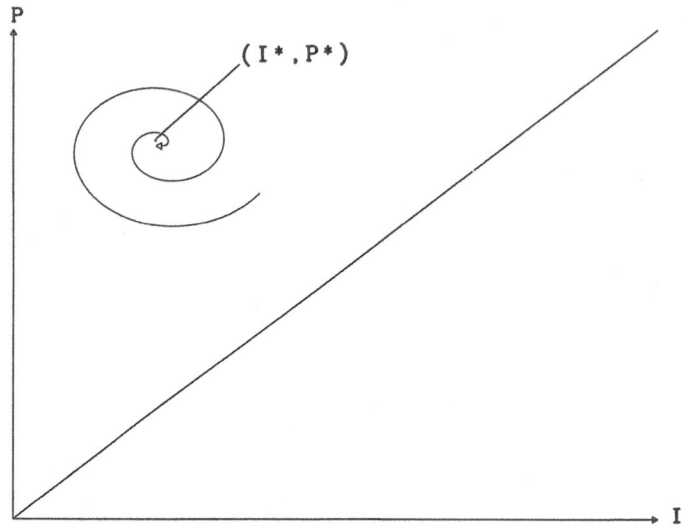

**Fig. 2.4(a).** Case i:  $r < b$ and $b' < r'$

We next examine the conditions for persistence of the infection in the host. In Case i, $I(t)$ tends to $I^*$. In Case ii, $I(t)$ tends to zero. In Case iii, $I(t)$ tends to zero if $P_0 \leq (pb' + g)/k$ and tends to a positive limit if $P_0 > (pb' + g)/k$. In Case iv, $I(t)$ tends to $\infty$, and in Case v this is also true if the initial condition lies above the separatrix. Examining Case i in more detail, we note that there is no threshold population size $P(0)$ for validity of the conclusion. Moreover, the conclusion holds for any value of $q$, hence vertical transmission is not essential to persistence of the disease. However, the values of $S^*$, $I^*$, $P^*$, and the relative prevalence $y^* = I^*/P^*$ and relative incidence depend on $k$, $g$ and $q$ in the manner indicated in Table 1. By the relative incidence, $RI^*$, we mean

$$RI^* = (kS^* + qb')\frac{I^*}{P^*} = (r' + g)y^*,$$

which is the rate of new infections $(kS^* + qb')I^*$ divided by the total population $P^*$, at equilibrium. Notice that the prevalence rate $y^*$ is independent of $k$, $q$ and $g$, and hence, the percentage of infectives is insensitive to variations in these parameters.

**Table 1.** Effect of Parameters on Equilibria in Case i

| When: | $k$ increases | $q$ increases | $g$ increases |
|-------|---------------|---------------|---------------|
| $S^*$ | decreases | decreases | increases |
| $I^*$ | decreases | decreases | increases |
| $P^*$ | decreases | decreases | increases |
| $y^*$ | no change | no change | no change |
| $RI^*$ | no change | no change | increases |

In Case iii, there is a threshold population size $P_T = (pb'+g)/k$ in the sense that if $P_0 < P_T$ the infection dies out. This is the same as $P_T = (r'+g-qb')/k$, the expression given in Section 2.3, in the case in which $r' = b'$. We note that vertical transmission may play a crucial role in maintaining the infection in this case. Indeed, $P_T$ decreases as $q$ increases, and the infection persists only if

$$q > 1 - \frac{kP_0 - g}{b'}$$

For fixed values of $P_0$, $b'$, and $g$, this condition implies that, in circumstances where the horizontal transmission rate is small, a large vertical transmission coefficient $q$ is needed for the survival of the pathogen species. We also note that the equilibrium in this case is $S^+ = (pb' + g)/k$, $I^+ = P_0 - (pb' + g)/k$. An increase in $k$ or $q$ or a decrease in $g$ results in a decrease in $S^+$ and an increase in $I^+$. The behavior of solution orbits in the $(I, P)$ phase plane is depicted in Figure 2.4(c).

In Case iv, there is no threshold population size, $I(t)$ and $P(t)$ tend to $\infty$, and the relative prevalence $y(t)$ tends to 1. In Case v, there is a threshold of a different sort, provided by the separatrix. With all parameters fixed, the separatrix is fixed, and the threshold condition for persistence is that $(I_0, P_0)$ lie above the separatrix. This is a condition on both $I_0$ and $P_0$, not just on the total population size $P_0$. It may also be worth commenting that as $q$ increases, the point $(I^*, P^*)$ and the separatrix drop. If $q$ can increase sufficiently to achieve $r' \leq qb' - g$, then we have switched from Case v to Case iv and the separatrix no longer plays a role.

Case iii occurs when $b = r$ and $b' = r'$, that is, the birth and death rates of the host, both infected and not infected, are exactly equal. There are some experimental data (see for example, Burgdorfer [1975]) reporting that in some situations the pathogen does not change the fecundity or survival rate of the host, so $b' = b$, and $r' = r$. Still, one may doubt whether the exact equalities $b = r$, and $b' = r'$ could persist for long in a real population. In practice, perhaps the rates might fluctuate in a narrow range around mean values with $b = r$, and $b' = r'$. It might be useful to simulate such a situation to see whether there is a threshold population size.

In Section 2.3, we defined the basic reproductive coefficient

$$R_0(t) = \frac{kP(t) + qb'}{r' + g}$$

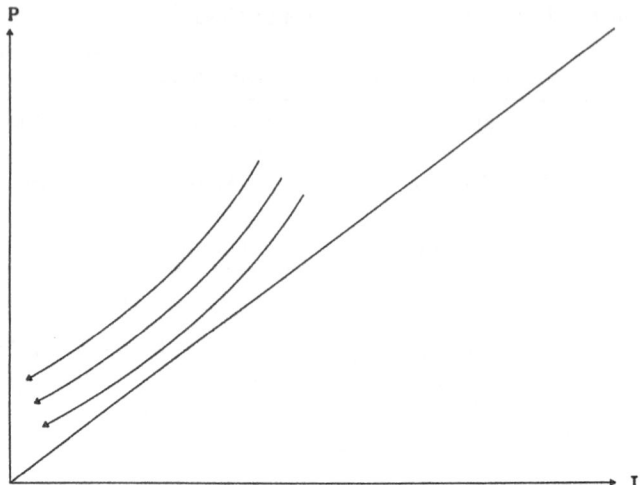

**Fig. 2.4(b).** Case ii:   $b < r$ and $b' < r'$

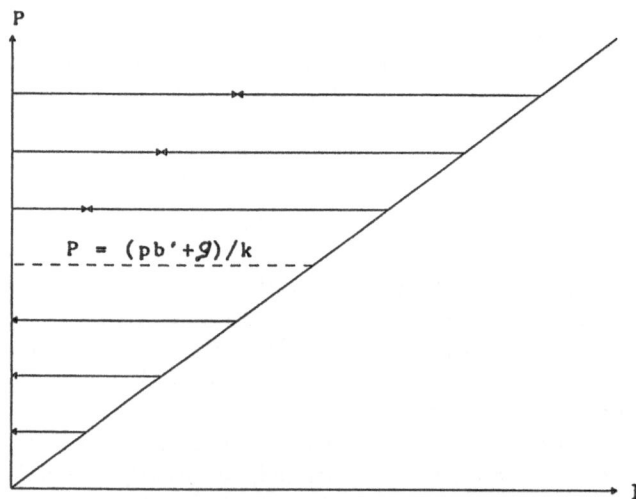

**Fig. 2.4(c).** Case iii:   $b = r$ and $b' = r'$

and the effective reproductive coefficient

$$R(t) = \frac{kS(t) + qb'}{r' + g}.$$

If the equilibrium of (2.6) is approached, the effective reproduction coefficient approaches 1, which agrees with the intuition that each infective must be exactly replaced. In Case iii, if the equilibrium $S^+ = (pb' + g)/k$ is approached,

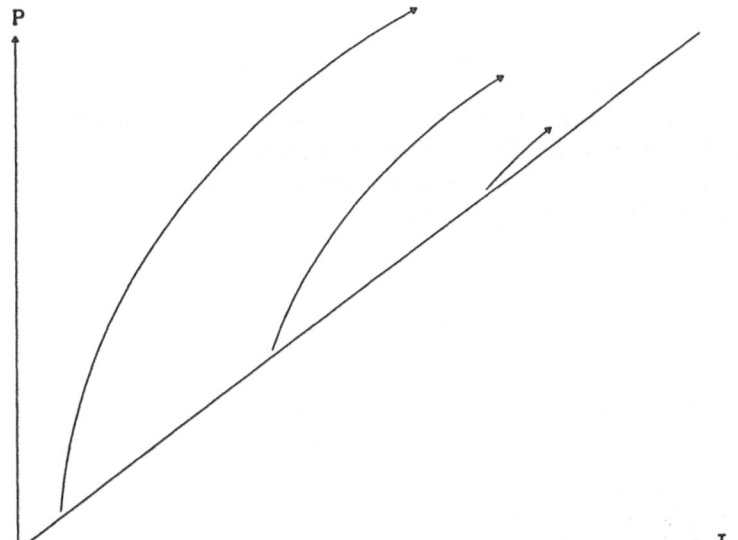

**Fig. 2.4(d).** Case iv:    $r < b$ and $r' \leq b'$ or $b \leq r$ and $r' \leq qb' - g < b'$

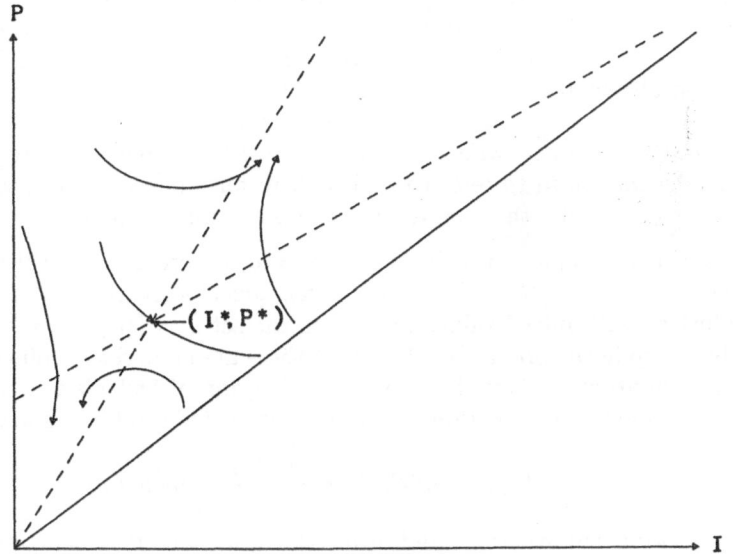

**Fig. 2.4(e).** Case v:  $b \leq r$ and $qb' - g < r' < b'$

then also $R(t)$ tends to one, since $b' = r'$. In Case iii, $R(t)$ is monotone; in Case i, $R(t)$ may tend to one monotonely or in an oscillatory way, since the equilibrium can be either a node or a spiral point (in Figure 2.4 (a), only the spiral case is shown). In Case iv, in which $P(t) \to \infty$, we note that $S(t)$ has a finite limit and $R(t)$ tends to one. However, in Case ii with $b = r$, $S(t) \to S^+$ and the limiting value of $R(t)$ is not one.

We conclude this section by noting that Anderson and May [1981, Tables 1 and 2] give estimated values of mortality rates and reproductive rates for a number of host-pathogen situations. For example, for non-inclusion virus in *Panonychus citri*, the estimates are $r = 0.34$, $r' = 1.25$, $b = 1.8$, $b' = 0.93$ individuals per week. The corresponding figures for the protozoan *Nosema stegomyiae* in *Anopheles albimanus* are $r = 0.23$, $r' = 0.64$ and $b = 2.4$, $b' = 2.3$ per first gonotrophic cycle.

## 2.5 Proofs of the Results

We observe that (2.2) can be written in the form

$$\dot{S} = -kSI + bS + p_1 b'I - rS,$$
$$\dot{I} = kSI + q_1 b'I - r'I,$$
(2.12)

where

$$q_1 = q - g/b', \quad p_1 = p + g/b', \quad p_1 + q_1 = 1. \tag{2.13}$$

System (2.12) is identical in form to the system considered in Busenberg, Cooke and Pozio [1983], and complete proofs are given there. Here, we shall merely outline the proofs and refer the reader to the paper cited for details. Note that although $q \geq 0$, $q_1$ may be positive, zero, or negative, but certainly $q_1 < 1$ if either $q = 1$ and $g > 0$ or $q < 1$ and $g \geq 0$. We point out that the proofs in the reference, when transferred to (2.12), depend on having $q_1 < 1$. The reader may need to refer to Section 2.16 for a description of some of the mathematical results that are used in the proof that follows.

**Case i.** ($b > r$, $b' < r'$). If $S_0 \geq 0$, $I_0 = 0$, we see from (2.12) that $I \equiv 0$ and hence $\dot{S} = (b-r)S$, so $S(t) \to \infty$. It remains to show that $(S^*, I^*)$ attracts all solutions with initial values $(S_0, I_0)$ in the set $J = \{(S, I) : S \geq 0, I > 0\}$. The first step in the proof is to show that there are no periodic solutions in the positive quadrant. This is done by an application of Dulac's Criterion. That is, a certain auxiliary function $\rho(S, I)$ is constructed, and it is shown that

$$\frac{\partial}{\partial S}[F_1(S, I)\rho(S, I)] + \frac{\partial}{\partial I}[F_2(S, I)\rho(S, I)]$$

has a constant sign, where $F_1$ and $F_2$ are the right-hand members, respectively, of the two equations (2.12). By the criterion, the existence of periodic solutions in the positive quadrant is impossible.

The next step in the proof is facilitated by considering the equations

$$\dot{P} = (b - r)P - \alpha I = (b' - r')I + (b - r)(P - I),$$
$$\dot{I} = (q_1 b' - r')I + k(P - I)I.$$
(2.14)

It is then possible to construct an invariant set in the $(I, P)$-plane containing the feasible equilibrium point $(I^*, P^*)$. This is done by using properties and estimates of the direction field. The proof in the cited paper applies directly to (2.14), once it is noted that $q_1 < 1$ and $r' - q_1 b' = r' - qb' + g$ is positive. It can be shown that every trajectory with $S_0 \geq 0$, $I_0 > 0$ enters this invariant set or tends to $(I^*, P^*)$. But since the invariant set contains no closed orbit, it follows from the Poincaré-Bendixson Theorem that every trajectory tends to $(I^*, P^*)$.

**Case ii.** ($b < r$ and $b' \leq r'$, or else, $b \leq r$ and $b' < r'$.) First, suppose that $b < r$ and $b' < r'$. Then $I^* < 0$ since $r' + g - qb' = r' - q_1 b' > 0$. Also, from (2.14), $\dot{P} < 0$ whenever $P \geq I > 0$. Now, $\dot{I} = 0$ on the boundary $I = 0$, and on $P = I$,

$$\frac{d}{dt}(P - I) = p_1 b' I,$$

so we see that a trajectory cannot leave the region $P \geq I \geq 0$. Therefore $P(t)$ tends monotonically to zero and $I(t)$ tends to zero. If $b < r$ and $b' = r'$, the equilibrium (2.6) does not exist; moreover, $\dot{P} = 0$ on $P = I$ and

$$d^2 P/dt^2 = (b - r)(\dot{P} - \dot{I}) = -(b - r)\dot{I} = -(b - r)(q_1 b' - r')I < 0,$$

so again $P(t)$ is strictly decreasing to zero. If $b = r$ and $b' < r'$, we note that for any constant $C$, $S = C$, $I = 0$ is an equilibrium (or $P = C$, $I = 0$). Again, $\dot{P} = (b' - r')I < 0$ and $P$ is decreasing. It is impossible for the trajectory to reach $I = P = 0$ in finite time since $\dot{I}/I \geq (q_1 b' - r')I$. Hence, the trajectory must tend to some point $I = 0$, $P = P^+ > 0$. It is then not very difficult to show that $P^+ = S^+$ has the value stated in the theorem. Using the fact that from $\dot{S} = (p_1 b' - kS)I$ we obtain

$$S(t) = \left(S_0 - \frac{p_1 b'}{k}\right) \exp\left[-k \int_0^t I(y)dy\right] + \frac{p_1 b'}{k}.$$

See the reference for details.

**Case iii.** ($b = r$, $b' = r'$). In this case, also, the equilibrium in (2.6) does not exist. We have $\dot{P} = 0$ and $\dot{S} = (p_1 b' - kS)I$. Thus $P(t) = P_0$ is constant and

$$\dot{S} = (p_1 b' - kS)(P_0 - S) = (pb' + g - kS)(P_0 - S).$$

If $S_0 = P_0$, $I_0 = 0$, then $S(t) = S_0$ and $I(t) = 0$ is the solution. If $kP_0 < pb' + g$, then since $S_0 \leq P_0$ we see that $S(t)$ is increasing and approaches $P_0$. If $kP_0 > pb' + g$, then $S(t)$ is decreasing if $kS_0 > pb' + g$ and increasing if $kS_0 < pb' + g$, and therefore $S(t)$ tends to $(pb' + g)/k$.

**Case iv.** ($S^*, I^*$) is not feasible. The proof again consists of estimates and monotonicity arguments of a detailed kind.

**Case v.** ($b \leq r$ and $q_1 b' < r' < b'$). In this case, $(I^*, P^*)$ is feasible. From a simple computation, it is seen that $(I^*, P^*)$ is a saddle point with one stable and one unstable manifold intersecting at the saddle point. The flow induced by (2.14) in this case is shown in Figure 2.5 and the conclusions follow from the topological situation depicted. To show the existence of the function $\phi$, one has to show that there is a one-dimensional invariant manifold that separates the region $K = \{(I, P) : 0 < I \leq P\}$ into two parts: one which consists of those initial values for which the solution tends to $(0, 0)$ and the other of those initial values for which the solution tends to $(\infty, \infty)$. See the reference for this construction and Section 2.16 for the definitions of the notions of invariant, stable and unstable manifolds.

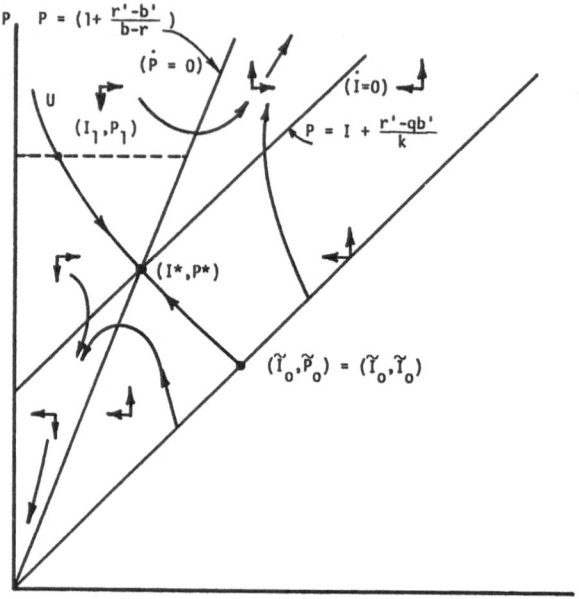

**Fig. 2.5.** The flow in the I-P plane

## 2.6 No Horizontal Transmission

It has been suggested by Fine [1975] that certain species of microparasites are perpetuated by vertical transmission alone, with horizontal transmission completely absent or negligible. In our model, this corresponds to taking $k = 0$, so that the equations (2.2) reduce to the linear system

$$\dot{S} = (b - r)S + (pb' + g)I,$$
$$\dot{I} = (qb' - r' - g)I, \tag{2.15}$$

Also, we have

$$\dot{P} = (b - r)P - \alpha I,$$
$$\dot{y} = -y(\alpha + g + pb' - \alpha y), \tag{2.16}$$

where $\alpha = (b - r) - (b' - r')$, $P = S + I$, and $y = I/P$. This system can be solved explicitly, yielding

$$I(t) = I_0 e^{\beta t}, \quad \beta = qb' - r' - g < b' - r',$$

$$P(t) = P_0 e^{(b-r)t} - \frac{\alpha I_0 (e^{\beta t} - e^{(b-r)t})}{\beta - b + r},$$

provided $\beta - b + r \neq 0$. If $\beta < b - r$, then $P(t)$ has asymptotic order

$$P(t) \sim \left( P_0 + \frac{\alpha I_0}{\beta - b + r} \right) e^{(b-r)t}, \quad \text{as } t \to \infty$$

and $I(t)/P(t)$ has asymptotic order $\exp(\beta - b + r)t$. Thus, the relative prevalence $y(t)$ tends to zero. This is the case normally to be expected since we expect $b' \leq b$, $r' \geq r$. Note, in addition, that $I(t) \to 0$ if $\beta < 0$, and $I(t) \to \infty$ if $\beta > 0$.

If $\beta > b - r$, then

$$\frac{I(t)}{P(t)} \sim \frac{I_0 e^{\beta t}}{\alpha I_0 e^{\beta t}/(b - r - \beta)} = \frac{b - r - \beta}{\alpha}$$

and the prevalence $y(t)$ tends to a constant. Since $qb' - r' - g > b - r$, it follows that $\alpha = (b - r) - (b' - r') < b - r - \beta < 0$ and the constant limit is positive and less than one. This shows that microparasites can possibly be maintained by vertical transmission alone, but only in case $qb' - r' - g > b - r$. In particular, the net growth rate $b' - r'$ of the infected host must be greater than the net growth rate $b - r$ of the uninfected host.

We leave it to the reader to show that if $\beta = b - r$, then $\alpha$ is negative, and $y(t) \to 0$ as $t \to \infty$.

In all cases, $I(t) = I_0 e^{\beta t}$ grows exponentially if $\beta > 0$ and decays exponentially if $\beta < 0$. The better measure of whether the parasite "dies out" is, however, the relative prevalence $y(t)$.

Equations (2.15) have an equilibrium solution if and only if $qb' - r' - g = \beta = 0$. In that case, there is a family of equilibria given by

$$S^* = -\frac{pb' + g}{b - r} I^*, \quad P^* = \frac{\alpha}{b - r} I^*$$

where $I^*$ is arbitrary. This is feasible if $b - r < 0$ and $\alpha < 0$ or equivalently, $b - r < \min\{0, b' - r'\}$. In this case, the uninfected host would become extinct, but the parasite confers an advantage sufficient to sustain the population. An interesting example of this type of situation occurs in grasses infected with system fungal endophytes which make them toxic to domestic mammals and increase their resistance to insect herbivores. Many of these endophytes are vertically transmitted through the seeds of their grass hosts, Schneider [1965] and Clay [1988].

## 2.7 The Model with Immune Class

We now return to the full $SIRS$ model formulated in (2.1), which includes a removed or immune class. For convenience, we repeat the equations

$$\dot{S} = -kSI + b(S + R) + pb'I - rS + gR,$$
$$\dot{I} = kSI + qb'I - r'I - cI, \tag{2.17}$$
$$\dot{R} = cI - (r + g)R.$$

In Section 2.7.1 we will treat the $SIR$ model when individuals in the removed class do not relapse or give birth into the susceptible or infected classes.

Here $q$ is the vertical transmission coefficient and $p = 1 - q$. The question to be investigated is whether this system exhibits any behavior distinctly different from that of the simpler system treated in the previous sections.

It is not hard to see that the non-negative orthant $\{(S, I, R) : S \geq 0, I \geq 0, R \geq 0\}$ is an invariant set for (2.17), so we begin by computing the equilibria. One is $S = I = R = 0$. If $I \neq 0$, then we get $kS^* = r' + c - qb'$. Then by writing $R^* = cI^*/(r + g)$ and substituting into the equation $\dot{S} = 0$, we finally find the unique nontrivial equilibrium

$$S^* = \frac{r' + c - qb'}{k},$$
$$I^* = \frac{(b - r)(r' + c - qb')(r + g)}{k[(r + g)(r' - b') - c(b - r)]}, \tag{2.18}$$
$$R^* = \frac{cI^*}{r + g}.$$

From now on, we shall restrict attention to the special case

$$b' = b, \quad r' > r, \quad b > r. \tag{2.19}$$

The assumption $b > r$ means that the population would not die out in the absence of infection. The other assumptions correspond to a case in which the infection increases the death rate, but does not affect the birth rate. These assumptions are appropriate for some infections, and the analysis is similar in other cases. We shall find that even with the assumptions (2.19), the mathematical analysis is algebraically complicated. We now look for conditions on the parameters under which $S^* > 0$, $I^* > 0$ (feasibility conditions).

**Case 1.** $r' > b$. In this case, $S^*$ is positive, since $0 \leq q \leq 1$. $I^*$ is positive if and only if

$$\frac{r - b}{(r + g)(b - r') + c(b - r)} > 0,$$

and since $b > r$ this is equivalent to

$$c(b - r) < (r + g)(r' - b). \tag{2.20}$$

This condition can also be written in the form

$$r' - r > (b - r)\left(1 + \frac{c}{r + g}\right),\tag{2.21}$$

which has the interpretation that the excess mortality due to the disease must be large enough to control the growth of population. If this condition is not satisfied, the whole population will grow unboundedly. Observe that $q$ does not enter into condition (2.21).

**Case 2.** $r' \leq b$. In this case, $S^*$ is positive if and only if $r' + c - qb > 0$, and then the sign of $I^*$ is that of

$$\frac{b - r}{(r + g)(r' - b) - c(b - r)},$$

or of

$$(r + g)(r' - b) - c(b - r).$$

But this is negative, so a nontrivial equilibrium cannot exist when $r' \leq b$.

The local stability of the equilibria can be determined from the linearization of (2.17). When $b' = b$ the Jacobian matrix of (2.17) is

$$J = \begin{bmatrix} -kI + b - r & -kS + pb & b + g \\ kI & kS + qb - r' - c & 0 \\ 0 & c & -(r + g) \end{bmatrix}$$

At the trivial equilibrium $S = I = R = 0$, this is

$$\begin{bmatrix} b - r & pb & b + g \\ 0 & qb - r' - c & 0 \\ 0 & c & -(r + g) \end{bmatrix}$$

The eigenvalues of this matrix are $b - r$, $qb - r' - c$, and $-(r + g)$. Since $b > r$, the trivial equilibrium is unstable. It has a one dimensional unstable manifold when $qb - r' - c < 0$ and a two dimensional unstable manifold when $qb - r' - c > 0$.

At the nontrivial equilibrium, since $kS^* + qb - r' - c = 0$, and $pb - kS^* = b - r' - c$, we have

$$J = \begin{bmatrix} -kI^* + b - r & b - r' - c & b + g \\ kI^* & 0 & 0 \\ 0 & c & -(r + g) \end{bmatrix}$$

The equation for the eigenvalues therefore is

$$\lambda^3 + A\lambda^2 + B\lambda + C = 0,$$

where

$$A = 2r + g - b + kI^*,$$
$$B = (r + g)(kI^* - b + r) + kI^*(r' + c - b),$$
$$C = kI^*[(r + g)(r' - b) - c(b - r)].$$

According to the Routh-Hurwitz conditions, the equilibrium will be asymptotically stable provided $A$, $B$, $C$ are positive and $AB > C$. We first note that when $I^* > 0$, the condition (2.20) holds, and therefore $C > 0$. When (2.20) ceases to hold, we have $C \leq 0$. Thus, when $I^*$ becomes negative, its stability is lost.

It can be shown by direct but tedious computation that $A > 0$ and $B > 0$. The following demonstration that $A > 0$, $B > 0$, and $AB > C$ has been provided by Dr. Wei-min Liu. Introduce the quantities

$$x = b - r, \qquad y = r' - b - \frac{cx}{r+g},$$

which are positive by (2.19) and (2.20). Then

$$b - r' - c = -y - \frac{c(r+g+x)}{r+g},$$

$$kI^* = \frac{x}{y}\left(y + \frac{c(r+g+x)}{r+g} + pb\right),$$

$$-kI^* + b - r = -\frac{x}{y}\left[\frac{c(r+g+x)}{r+g} + pb\right].$$

Therefore

$$J = \begin{bmatrix} -\frac{x}{y}\left[\frac{c(r+g+x)}{r+g} + pb\right] & -y - \frac{c(r+g+x)}{r+g} & r+g+x \\ \frac{x}{y}\left[y + \frac{c(r+g+x)}{r+g} + pb\right] & 0 & 0 \\ 0 & c & -(r+g) \end{bmatrix}$$

Instead of proving that $J$ is stable, the matrix $\hat{J} = y(r+g)J$ will be proved stable.

The characteristic polynomial of $\hat{J}$ was obtained using the symbolic manipulation program MACSYMA. The program expresses the coefficients in the polynomial in expanded form, as sums of products of the type

$$r^{n_1} g^{n_2} x^{n_3} y^{n_4} c^{n_5} p^{n_6},$$

where the $n_j$ are integers. It turns out that all the terms have positive signs. Since $r$, $g$, $x$, $y$, $c$, and $p$ are positive, all the coefficients in the characteristic polynomial are positive. Moreover, the expression corresponding to $AB - C$ also consists entirely of positive terms (almost 200 of them!). Therefore, the matrix $J$ has all its eigenvalues with negative real parts, and thus the endemic equilibrium is locally asymptotically stable whenever conditions (2.19) and (2.20) hold. If $r'$ is so small that (2.20) is not satisfied, the population size will not be controlled by disease deaths. Of course, other density-dependent factors, not included in the model (2.17), would come into play as the population's size grows. See Section 2.11 for a brief discussion.

### 2.7.1 The SIR Model with Vaccination

The analysis of the $SIRS$ model of the previous section is restricted to the description of the existence and the local stability of the disease free and endemic equilibria. In this section we show how the global stability results of Section 2.3 can be re-interpreted to yield a complete analysis of the following SIR model with vertical transmission and vaccination.

$$
\begin{aligned}
\dot{S} &= -kSI + bS + p_1\bar{b}I - rS + g_1I, \\
\dot{I} &= kSI + q_1\bar{b}I - \bar{r}'I - gI, \qquad\qquad (2.22) \\
\dot{R} &= \tilde{b}R - \tilde{r}R + q_2\bar{b}I + g_2I + g_3S,
\end{aligned}
$$

Here, we assume that the offspring of susceptible individuals are all susceptible, and that all progeny of the immune individuals acquire immunity. The proportions $0 \leq q_1, q_2, p_1 \leq 1$ obey $p_1 = 1 - q_1 - q_2$, and $q_1$ denotes the vertical transmission probability, $q_2$ the probability of vertically transmitted immunity, and $p_1$ the probability that the offspring of an infected be born in the susceptible class. The vaccination rate at which susceptibles acquire immunity is $g_3$, hence, $r - g_3$ is the death rate of the suceptibles. The cure rate of the infected who do not acquire immunity is $g_1$, the rate at which infected individuals are cured and acquire immunity to future infection is $g_2$, hence, $g = g_1 + g_2$. $\bar{r}'$ is the death rate of the infectives. Finally, $\tilde{b}$ and $\tilde{r}$ are the birth and death rates of the removed (immune) individuals. In Section 2.9, we consider a different model with vaccination.

In order to reinterpret the global stability results of Section 2.3 in the context of this more general model, we only need to choose the parameters in (2.2) in order to make the following identification:

$$
q_1\bar{b} - \bar{r}' = qb' - r', \quad p_1\bar{b} + g_1 = pb' + g,
$$

where $b', r', g, p$ and $q$ are the parameters in (2.2). The endemic proportion $I^*$ now becomes

$$
I^* = \frac{(b - r)(\bar{r}' - q_1\bar{b} + g)}{k(\bar{r}' - (p_1 + q_1)\bar{b} + g - g_1)}.
$$

Theorem 2.1 can thus be reinterpreted in the context of this $SIR$ model, and in particular, the thresholds that are shown to govern the global behavior of the disease and demographic processes are expressible in terms of the parameters entering in (2.22). This type of reinterpretation of the epidemiological implications of general mathematical results on model equations occurs frequently and is a valuable byproduct of the analytical approach to the study of epidemic processes.

## 2.8 The Case of Constant Population

In the above section, we have not treated the variety of cases that were examined in Section 2.4 for the model without immunity, since the mathematical analysis is now more difficult because of the higher dimensionality of the system. The reader may try to resolve some of the cases we have not discussed. However, the case $b = r$, $b' = r'$ is of some interest since then the total population is fixed, $P(t) \equiv P(0) = P_0$, and we can again reduce the system to two dimensions. The condition for existence of a nontrivial endemic equilibrium is that

$$P_0 > \frac{b'(1-q)+c}{k},$$

or equivalently,

$$q > 1 - \frac{kP_0 - c}{b'}.$$

We may interpret the first inequality as saying that there is a minimum population size for the disease to be sustained, and the second inequality as saying that the vertical transmission rate must be above a certain threshold to sustain the disease. In this case a complete stability analysis is possible using a method due to Beretta and Capasso [1986] which relies on the special structure of the equations of epidemic models and yields global stability conclusions under certain special conditions. We will describe this method in the mathematical sections at the end of this chapter. Here we will describe how it can be used to complete the analysis of this case. The details of the analysis in this and the next section are due to Grabiner [1988].

Since the total population $P$ is constant, we can let $R = P - S - I$, use the conditions $b = r$, $b' = r'$, and eliminate $R$ from equations (2.17) to obtain

$$\frac{dS}{dt} = -kSI + pb'I + (b+g)(P - S - I),$$
$$\frac{dI}{dt} = kSI - pb'I - cI, \tag{2.23}$$

When $P > (pb' + c)/k$ an endemic equilibrium, $(S^*, I^*)$, exists with

$$S^* = (pb' + c)/k, \quad \text{and} \quad I^* = \frac{(b+g)(Pk - pb' - c)}{(c+b+g)k}.$$

Letting $z$ denote the vector

$$\mathbf{z} = \begin{bmatrix} S \\ I \end{bmatrix},$$

the system (2.23) can be expressed in the form

$$\frac{d\mathbf{z}}{dt} = \operatorname{diag}(\mathbf{z})(\mathbf{e} + Az) + \mathbf{c} + B\mathbf{z}. \tag{2.24}$$

with $\operatorname{diag}(\mathbf{z})$ denoting the $2 \times 2$ matrix

$$\text{diag}(\mathbf{z}) = \begin{bmatrix} S & 0 \\ 0 & I \end{bmatrix},$$

$$A = \begin{bmatrix} 0 & -k \\ k & 0 \end{bmatrix}, \quad B = \begin{bmatrix} 0 & pb' - b - g \\ 0 & 0 \end{bmatrix}, \tag{2.25a}$$

$$\mathbf{e} = \begin{bmatrix} -b - g \\ -pb' - c \end{bmatrix}, \quad \mathbf{c} = \begin{bmatrix} (b + g)P \\ 0 \end{bmatrix}. \tag{2.25b}$$

Denoting by $\mathbf{z}^*$ the endemic equilibrium value of $z$, the matrix $\tilde{A} = A + \text{diag}(\mathbf{z}^*)^{-1}B$ is given by

$$\begin{bmatrix} 0 & k\frac{pb'-b-g-pb'-c}{pb'+c} \\ k & 0 \end{bmatrix} = \begin{bmatrix} 0 & k\frac{-b-g-c}{pb'+c} \\ k & 0 \end{bmatrix}, \tag{2.26}$$

which is, in the terminology of Section 2.16.5, $W$-skew-symmetrizable. The associated graph of matrix (2.26) is such that the stability criterion of Beretta and Capasso implies that the equilibrium $z^*$ is globally asymptotically stable within the set of feasible solutions.

Thus, when the total population size is constant, the endemic equilibrium is globally asymptotically stable whenever it is feasible. The threshold criterion shows that if the birth rate and horizontal and vertical transmission rates are held constant, then the total population acts as the critical parameter determining whether or not the disease will reach endemic conditions.

## 2.9  A Model with Vaccination

One important reason for studying epidemic models is to provide a means for estimating the consequences of immunization. Here we consider a simple case that is based on the model (2.17). We assume that immunity is permanent, so we take $g = 0$, and we assume that immunization occurs just after birth. Let $m$, with $0 < m < 1$, be a measure of the effectiveness of vaccination, which takes into account both the percentage of newborn who receive vaccination and the effectiveness of the vaccine itself. Thus $mb(S + R)$ is the number of newborn who go into the immune class and $(1 - m)b(S + R)$ is the number who remain susceptible. We assume that the vaccine does not create immunity in those born of infected parents. This seems to be true in some cases, since the short-lived immunity derived from the parents seems to interfere with the action of the vaccine. These assumptions lead to the following equations.

$$\begin{aligned} \dot{S} &= -kSI + (1 - m)b(S + R) + pb'I - rS, \\ \dot{I} &= kSI + (qb' - r' - c)I, \\ \dot{R} &= cI - rR + mb(S + R). \end{aligned} \tag{2.27}$$

It should be remarked that more sophisticated models for immunization for diseases such as measles and rubella, taking account of the age structure in the population, have been formulated and analyzed by several authors; see Schenzle [1984], Fine and Clarkson [1982] and Hethcote and Van Ark [1987], for example.

We are now interested in the effect of vaccination in suppressing the infection in a steady population. We therefore assume that $b = r$ and $b' = r'$. If $P = S + I + R$, we then have

$$\dot{P} = (b - r)P + [(b' - r') - (b - r)]I = 0,$$

so that $P(t) \equiv P_0$ is constant. Replacing $R$ by $P_0 - (S + I)$ in the first two equations of (2.27), we now obtain the system

$$\dot{S} = -kSI + (1 - m)b(P_0 - I) + pb'I - bS,$$
$$\dot{I} = kSI + (qb' - b' - c)I = kSI - (pb' + c)I. \qquad (2.28)$$

One equilibrium is $S^+ = (1 - m)P_0$, $I^+ = 0$, and another is

$$S^* = \frac{pb' + c}{k},$$

$$I^* = \frac{1}{c + (1 - m)b}\left\{(1 - m)bP_0 - \frac{b(pb' + c)}{k}\right\}.$$

The Jacobian of (2.28) is

$$\begin{bmatrix} -kI - b & -kS - (1 - m)b + pb' \\ kI & kS - pb' - c \end{bmatrix}.$$

At $(S^+, I^+)$ this is

$$\begin{bmatrix} -b & -kS^+ - (1 - m)b + pb' \\ 0 & kS^+ - pb' - c \end{bmatrix}$$

and the eigenvalues are $-b$ and $kS^+ - pb' - c = k(1 - m)P_0 - pb' - c$. Thus, the condition for stability of $(S^+, I^+)$ is

$$k(1 - m)P_0 - pb' - c < 0.$$

This can be written as

$$m > 1 - \frac{pb' + c}{kP_0}. \qquad (2.29)$$

That is, if the vaccinated fraction $m$ is large enough, the disease-free state is stable. Note that condition (2.29) is equivalent to the condition $I^* < 0$. Note also that the necessary fraction $m$ for the stability of the disease-free equilibrium increases as $P_0$ increases and decreases as $p$ increases.

The global asymptotic stability of the endemic equilibrium can be obtained, in the case of constant population, by again using the method of Beretta and Capasso, even when the relapse rate $g$ is not zero. The model equations when $b = r$ and $b' = r'$ now are

$$\dot{S} = -kSI + (1-m)b(P-I) + pb'I - bS + g(P-S-I),$$
$$\dot{I} = kSI - (pb'+c)I.$$

(2.30)

The endemic equilibrium is

$$S^* = \frac{pb'+c}{k}, \quad I^* = \frac{[(1-m)b+g]kP - (b+g)(pb'+c)}{(c+(1-m)b+g)k}.$$

Thus $I^* > 0$ if $m < (b+g)(kP - pb' - c)/bkP$. If this condition holds, let

$$z = \begin{bmatrix} S \\ I \end{bmatrix},$$

and write (2.30) in the form (2.24) with

$$A = \begin{bmatrix} 0 & -k \\ k & 0 \end{bmatrix}, \quad B = \begin{bmatrix} 0 & (m-1)b + pb' - g \\ 0 & 0 \end{bmatrix},$$

$$e = \begin{pmatrix} -b-g \\ -pb'-c \end{pmatrix}, \quad c = \begin{pmatrix} (1-m)bP + gP \\ 0 \end{pmatrix},$$

$$\tilde{A} = \begin{pmatrix} 0 & k\left(\frac{(m-1)b-g-c}{pb'+c}\right) \\ k & 0 \end{pmatrix}.$$

Since $0 < m < 1$ and $b > 0, g \geq 0, c \geq 0$, $(m-1)b - g - c$ is negative, $\tilde{A}$ is $W$-skew-symmetrizable, and its graph is such that the equilibrium is globally asymptotically stable whenever it is feasible.

## 2.10 Models with Latency or Maturation Time

Various extensions of the previous model can be constructed, in order to include more realistic features. For example, one may include a latent or exposed class, consisting of individuals who are infected but not yet infectious. We let $E(t)$ denote the number of individuals in this class at time $t$. For the model with no immune class, the structure is

$$\downarrow \qquad \downarrow \qquad \downarrow$$
$$S \ \rightarrow \ E \ \rightarrow \ I \ \rightarrow \ S$$

and for the model with immune class, it is

$$\downarrow \qquad \downarrow \qquad \downarrow$$
$$S \ \rightarrow \ E \ \rightarrow \ I \ \rightarrow \ R \ \rightarrow \ S$$

We assume that the progeny of those in the latent class are all susceptible, since the parasite density within an individual host in this class may not have reached a level at which offspring are likely to be much affected. Of the progeny of infectious individuals, we may suppose that a fraction $p$ are susceptible, a fraction $q_1$ are exposed but latent, and a fraction $q_2$ are infectious, where $p + q_1 + q_2 = 1$.

The equations for the model without immune class may be taken to be of the form

$$\dot{S} = -kSI + b(S + E) - rS + pb'I + gI,$$
$$\dot{E} = kSI - rE + q_1 b'I - vE, \qquad (2.31)$$
$$\dot{I} = vE - r'I + q_2 b'I - gI.$$

Here, $b$ and $r$ are the birth and death rates of the $S$ and $E$ classes, $b'$ and $r'$ are the birth and death rates of infectives, $v$ is the rate at which individuals pass from the latent to the infectious class, and $g$ is the rate at which individuals recover back to the susceptible class.

The assumption that individuals move from $E$ to $I$ at a rate $v$ is, in probabilistic terms, equivalent to the assumption that the chance that an individual makes this transition in a time interval $\Delta t$ is independent of how long the host has been in the latent class. The latent period is more often of fixed length, or is distributed over a narrow band of lengths. Models that take this into account lead to delay-differential or integral equations, and examples are given in Chapter 4.

The system (2.31) is difficult to analyze fully, for it is not reducible to a system of two equations and phase plane methods cannot be used. However, it is possible to find the equilibria. Anderson and May [1981] have done this and have given a partial analysis of local (linearized) stability. Since the mean time of residence in state $E$ is $v^{-1}$, the system implicitly involves a delay. Moreover, there is a feedback of individuals from state $I$ to state $S$, by virtue of the term $gI$ as well as the birth term $pb'I$. This suggests the possibility that steady-state oscillations may occur, and indeed Anderson and May found that they do occur in certain parameter ranges. Interesting reviews of oscillatory behavior in epidemic models, albeit without vertical transmission, are provided by Hethcote, Stech and van den Driessche [1981, 1983], and Hethcote and Levin [1989]. However, under certain conditions we can show that the endemic equilibrium is globally asymptotically stable whenever it is feasible. In particular, assuming constant total population size, that is, $b = r$ and $b' = r'$, then $E = P - S - I$, so (2.31) becomes

$$\dot{S} = -kSI + b(P - I) - bS + pb'I + gI,$$
$$\dot{I} = v(P - S - I) - b'I + q_2 b'I - gI. \qquad (2.32)$$

It can be shown that if the endemic equilibrium $(S^*, I^*)$ is feasible, then it is globally asymptotically stable. In fact, we first note that the region $\mathcal{R} = \{(S, I) : 0 \leq S + I \leq P\}$ is invariant since the direction field defined by the right hand side of (2.32) points towards the interior of $\mathcal{R}$ when evaluated at its boundary. Now, the condition for the stability of the disease free equilibrium $(S, I) = (P, 0)$ is easily computed to be

$$R_0 = \frac{vkP}{bb' + vg + bg - q_2 bb' + vpb'} < 1, \qquad (2.33)$$

and the condition $R_0 \leq 1$ implies that the only equilibrium in $\mathcal{R}$ is $(P, 0)$. Thus, by the Poincaré-Bendixson theorem (see Section 2.16.3) this equilibrium attracts all solutions with initial data in the feasibility region $\mathcal{R}$ if $R_0 \leq 1$, and is also locally asymptotically stable if $R_0 < 1$. When $R_0 > 1$, there exists a unique endemic equilibrium in $\mathcal{R}$, namely

$$(S^*, I^*) = \left( \frac{p_2 bb' + vg + bg + pb'v}{kv}, \frac{vkP - (p_2 bb' + vg + bg + pb'v)}{k(v + p_2 b' + g)} \right),$$

where $p_2 = 1 - q_2$. Moreover, computing the gradient

$$\nabla \cdot \left( \frac{\dot{S}}{IS}, \frac{\dot{I}}{IS} \right) = -\frac{b(P - I) + pb'I + gI}{IS^2} - \frac{v(P - S)}{I^2 S} < 0,$$

we conclude by applying Dulac's criterion (see Section 2.16.3) that there are no periodic solutions in $\mathcal{R}$. Thus, again by the Poincaré-Bendixson theorem, all solutions with feasible initial data that differ from the disease free equilibrium $(P, 0)$ approach $(S^*, I^*)$.

Another way in which more realism can be introduced into the model is to introduce a maturation time for newborn host individuals. We formulate a model with zero latent time (no class $E$) and no immunity (no class $R$), but in which we distinguish mature and immature hosts of classes $S$ and $I$. Let $S$ and $I$ denote mature hosts and let $X$ and $Y$ denote immature hosts, susceptible and infective, respectively. The structure of the model is

$$\begin{array}{ccccccc} S \downarrow\downarrow I & & & & & & \\ X & \rightarrow & S & \rightarrow & I & \rightarrow & S \\ & & & & \uparrow\downarrow & & \\ & & & & Y & \rightarrow & X \end{array}$$

Thus, individuals in class $S$ give birth to immature susceptibles, whereas individuals in class $I$ give birth to immature susceptibles and infectives. Immature individuals do not give birth. We assume maturation rates $m$ and $m'$ from $X$ to $S$ and $Y$ to $I$, respectively, and we assume recovery rates $g$ and $g'$ from $I$ to $S$ and $Y$ to $X$, respectively. Assume that horizontal transmission occurs only among mature hosts, for simplicity. If $b$, $b'$ are birth rates and $r$, $r'$ are death rates, as before, we may write the equations

$$\dot{S} = -kSI + mX - rS + gI,$$
$$\dot{I} = kSI + m'Y - r'I - gI,$$
$$\dot{X} = bS + pb'I - mX + g'Y,$$
$$\dot{Y} = qb'I - m'Y - g'Y.$$

A more realistic model would involve a fixed time in the immature class, or some distribution of length of the immature period (different from the implied exponential distribution in the above equation). Such a model is presented in Chapter 4.

## 2.11 Models with Density Dependent Death Rate

We may modify the basic SI model of (2.2) by supposing that the birth and death rates are not constant, but rather depend on population sizes. That is, $b$, $b'$, $r$, $r'$ are functions of $S$ and $I$. Of many possible assumptions about this dependence, we first mention one proposed by Anderson and May [1981]. In their model, density dependence was assumed to act only on death rates, not birth rates. Therefore, they postulated

$$r = r_0 + sP, \quad r' = r_0 + sP + \delta \quad (s > 0),$$

where $P = S + I$ is the total population and $\delta$ is the excess mortality in infectives ($\delta \geq 0$). Anderson and May did not consider vertical transmission, but we include it here. Our model is thus

$$\begin{aligned}
\dot{S} &= -kSI + bS + pb'I - (r_0 + sP)S + gI, \\
\dot{I} &= kSI + qb'I - (r_0 + sP + \delta)I - gI,
\end{aligned} \tag{2.34}$$

or

$$\begin{aligned}
\dot{I} &= [qb' - (r_0 + sP) - \delta - g]I + k(P - I)I, \\
\dot{P} &= [b - (r_0 + sP)]P + (b' - \delta - b)I.
\end{aligned} \tag{2.35}$$

The relative prevalence $y = I/P$ satisfies

$$\dot{y} = y[kP(1 - y) + qb' - \delta - b - g - y(b' - \delta - b)], \tag{2.36}$$

and we may also write

$$\dot{P} = P[b - (r_0 + sP) + (b' - \delta - b)y]. \tag{2.37}$$

We now report the results obtained by Anderson and May (in the case $q = 0$, $p = 1$). Afterward, we make some comments about changes needed when $q > 0$. Assume that $b' = b > r_0$. From (2.34) and (2.35), one finds the following equilibria:

(i) $S = I = 0$

(ii) $I = 0$, $S = K$ where $K = m/s$, $m = b - r_0$

(iii) $P^*$, $I^*$, with

$$P^* = \frac{K}{2}\{1 - \zeta + [(1 - \zeta)^2 + 4\zeta\xi]^{1/2}\}, \tag{2.38a}$$

$$\begin{aligned}
I^* &= k^{-1}\{(k - s)P^* - G\} \\
&= K\frac{k - s}{2k}\{1 - \zeta - 2\xi + [(1 - \zeta)^2 + 4\zeta\xi]^{1/2}\},
\end{aligned} \tag{2.38b}$$

where

$$G = \delta + r_0 + g,$$

$$\zeta = \frac{\delta}{m}\left(1 - \frac{s}{k}\right),$$

$$\xi = \frac{G}{m}\left(\frac{s}{k-s}\right),$$

(2.39)

The number $K = m/s$ is the carrying capacity for the population in the absence of disease. In the case $q = 0$, equilibrium (i) is a saddle point (and, of course, is unstable). If $k < s$, then the equilibrium (2.38) does not lie in the positive quadrant, and it can be shown that the equilibrium (ii) is locally asymptotically stable, because the eigenvalues of the linearization at this point are $-m$ and $-G + (k-s)(m/s)$, both being negative.

Now consider the case $k > s$. The equilibrium (ii) now becomes unstable when $-G + (k-s)(m/s) > 0$, or equivalently, $\xi < 1$. Furthermore, it can be shown that the equilibrium (iii) lies in the positive quadrant if and only if $\xi < 1$, and Anderson and May demonstrate that (iii) is asymptotically stable when $\xi < 1$. Thus, there is a transfer of stability from (ii) to (iii) at $\xi = 1$ (given that $k > s$). Phase plane portraits suggest, according to Anderson and May, that these local stability properties are also global properties.

One may now ask whether these same results hold when $q > 0$. Relations (2.38) and (2.39) remain valid except that we must redefine $G$ by

$$G = \delta + r_0 + g - qb.$$

The equilibrium (i) has eigenvalues $m$ and $-G$, and is unstable. (If $G < 0$, both eigenvalues are now positive.) The eigenvalues of (ii) are $-m$ and $-G + (k-s)(m/s)$, as before, and the condition for stability is

$$\frac{(k-s)m}{sG} = \frac{1}{\xi} < 1.$$

Now if $k < s$ and $G > 0$, this is satisfied, and $I^*$ also is negative, so that the situation is just as before. But if $k < s$ and $G < 0$, then the condition for stability of (ii) is $\xi > 1$, as before. Is it now possible to have $I^* > 0$? In fact, $I^* > 0$ implies

$$1 - \zeta - 2\xi + [(1-\zeta)^2 + 4\zeta\xi]^{1/2} < 0,$$

hence, $0 < \xi(\xi - 1)$. Since $\xi > 0$, this implies $\xi > 1$ and we have stability. The case $k > s$ is handled in a similar way.

A global asymptotic stability analysis of this model, which we now present, has been given by Grabiner [1988]. We again start by writing the dynamical system (2.35) in the form (2.24) with the vector $z$ defined as before and with

$$A = \begin{bmatrix} -k & k-s \\ 0 & -s \end{bmatrix}, \quad B = \begin{bmatrix} 0 & 0 \\ b' - \delta - b & 0 \end{bmatrix},$$

$$e = \begin{bmatrix} qb' - r_0 - \delta - g \\ b - r_0 \end{bmatrix}, \quad c = \begin{bmatrix} 0 \\ 0 \end{bmatrix}.$$

Thus

$$\tilde{A} = \begin{pmatrix} -k & k-s \\ \frac{b'-\delta-b}{P^*} & -s \end{pmatrix}, \quad C = \begin{pmatrix} -k & k-s \\ \frac{b'-\delta-b}{P^*} & -\frac{(b'-\delta-b)I}{PP^*} - s \end{pmatrix}.$$

We need to determine when $C$ satisfies Beretta and Capasso's condition (b) which is described in Section 2.16.5. By Lemma 2.9, we need $-k \leq 0$, which is always true; $(b' - \delta - b)I/PP^* + s > 0$, which holds if $b' - \delta - b \geq -P^*s$; and

$$\frac{(b' - \delta - b)kI}{P} + skP^* > (k-s)(b' - \delta - b). \tag{2.40}$$

The above equation is clearly true if $b' - \delta - b = 0$, thus the endemic equilibrium is globally asymptotically stable in this case whenever it exists. Otherwise, we note that the condition (2.40) is a linear inequality in $I/P$ on $[0, 1]$, consequently, its minimum value is assumed at one of the two endpoints of this interval. If $b' - \delta - b > 0$, this minimum occurs at $I/P = 0$, while if $b' - \delta - b < 0$, it occurs at $I/P = 1$. Thus, for condition (2.40) to hold we need to have

$$skP^* \geq (b' - \delta - b)(k-s), \quad \text{if} \quad b' - \delta - b > 0,$$
$$-kP^* \leq b' - \delta - b, \quad \text{if} \quad b' - \delta - b < 0.$$

Hence, in the most common case, when $b' - \delta - b < 0$, that is, when the disease reduces the net reproductive capacity of the host, the endemic equilibrium is globally asymptotically stable when

$$b' - \delta - b \geq \min\{-kP^*, -sP^*\}.$$

In the unusual case when the disease increases the net reproductive capacity of the host, that is, if $b' - \delta - b > 0$, the endemic equilibrium is globally asymptotically stable when

$$skP^* \geq (b' - \delta - b)(k-s).$$

These threshold inequalities provide a set of conditions which guarantee the asymptotic stability of the endemic equilibrium.

## 2.12 Parameter Estimation

The models previously discussed afford insight into the possible mechanisms by which pathogens may be sustained within a population, the way in which various parameters enter into the determination of threshold conditions and equilibrium levels, and so forth. In applying these models to real data, one must know good estimates of the actual numerical values of these parameters in the case at hand. Sometimes one can use values that have been already determined by experiment.

On the other hand, the required parameter values for a particular study may not be available and, furthermore, values obtained from laboratory studies may not be correct for the same organisms in the natural environment. In this section, we shall describe the work of Nakasuji et al. [1985] on the rice

dwarf virus that is carried by green rice leafhoppers. In this work, a model
was formulated and parameter values were determined by an experiment carried out in field cages. We include this study in the book as an example of
parameter estimation, and also because it illustrates the fact that vertical
transmission plays a role in plant diseases, not just animal diseases.

Rice dwarf virus (RDV) is a virus that infects rice plants. It is carried by
the green rice leafhopper, *Nephotettix cincticeps Uhler* and two other species
of green leafhoppers. The leafhoppers act as vectors, picking up virus from
plants that are already infected, and transferring the virus to plants on which
they feed. A vector that has acquired RDV orally becomes infectious after a
latent period and remains infectious throughout its life. There is transovarial
vertical transmission of the virus to leafhopper progeny. The infected vector
has a shorter longevity and lower fecundity than a healthy vector.

The Nakasuji model includes equations for the population dynamics of the
rice plants and equations for the dynamics of the vectors. Denote the number
of susceptible (non-infected), latent infected, and infectious rice hills ("clumps
of tillering stalks from planted seedlings") by $S$, $E$, and $I$, respectively, and the
total number by $P$. The number of susceptible, latent infected, and infectious
leafhoppers per rice hill are denoted by $\tilde{S}$, $\tilde{E}$, and $\tilde{I}$, respectively, and the
total number by $\tilde{P}$. The equations for $S$, $E$, $I$ are standard $SEI$ equations
that assume a mass-action type law $\alpha S \tilde{I}$ for infections by infectious vectors
and have the form

$$dS/dt = -\alpha S \tilde{I},$$
$$dE/dt = \alpha S \tilde{I} - \sigma E, \qquad (2.41)$$
$$dI/dt = \sigma E - \omega I.$$

The only change in the number of susceptible rice hills is due to infection by
vectors. The parameter $\alpha$ is the coefficient of transmission, $\sigma$ is the rate at
which latently infected hills become infectious, and $\omega$ is the death rate of rice
hills caused by infection. As usual in such models, $1/\sigma$ may be interpreted
as the average latent period. In the present case, $\omega = 0$, since no rice hills
actually die of RDV infection.

The equations proposed for the dynamics of the leafhoppers are as follows:

$$d\tilde{S}/dt = (\tilde{S} + \tilde{E})a(1 - b\tilde{P}) + (1 - q)\tilde{I}a'(1 - b\tilde{P}) - c\tilde{S} - \beta I \tilde{S},$$
$$d\tilde{E}/dt = \beta I \tilde{S} - (c + \lambda)\tilde{E}, \qquad (2.42)$$
$$d\tilde{I}/dt = q\tilde{I}a'(1 - b\tilde{P}) + \lambda \tilde{E} - c\tilde{I}.$$

These equations may be explained in the following way. The term $\beta I \tilde{S}$ represents the rate at which susceptible leafhoppers are infected by infectious rice
hills. The natural birth rate of susceptible and latent vectors is $a$ and that for
infectious vectors is $a'$ ($a' < a$). The factor $1 - b\tilde{P}$ is introduced because births
are assumed to be regulated by density-dependent processes. All newborn of
susceptible and latent parents go immediately into the $\tilde{S}$ class, but progeny of
infected parents are partly susceptible and partly vertically infected; $q$ denotes
the rate of transovarial transmission. Finally, $c$ is the natural death rate and

$\lambda$ is the rate at which latent vectors become infectious (or $1/\lambda$ is the mean length of latency).

The parameter $\alpha$ was estimated from experimental results of Ishii, Yasuo and Yamaguchi [1970]. In this experiment, rice seedlings were planted in each of five cages, two to seven infectious insects were introduced into each cage and all living insects were removed after 9 to 20 days. After removal, the rice hills were kept free of insects until disease symptoms appeared and the number of infected hills could be counted. Since the number of infectious insects ($\tilde{I}$) was fixed throughout the experiment, it follows from the first equation in (2.41) that

$$S(t) = S_0 e^{-\alpha \tilde{I} t},$$

where $S_0$ is the initial number of healthy rice hills. Thus,

$$\ln[S(t)/S_0] = -\alpha \tilde{I} t.$$

By using a linear regression of $\ln[S(t)/S_0]$ against $\tilde{I}t$ for the data, the estimate $\alpha = 0.15$ hills per infectious vector per day was obtained. The fit was not very good, but the authors attribute this to experimental error "because replications were not done for each experimental plot". Another experiment was performed to estimate $\beta$. In this experiment, different numbers of infectious rice hills were planted at random among healthy hills. Eggs from healthy leafhopper parents were then placed in each cage and allowed to mature into adults. Adults were collected on the 47th day and infection by RDV was determined by a serological test. Since no recruitment of newborn occurred in this experiment, the first equation in (2.42) reduces to

$$\frac{d\tilde{S}}{dt} = -c\tilde{S} - \beta I \tilde{S},$$

and for the total number $\tilde{P}$ of insects one has $d\tilde{P}/dt = -c\tilde{P}$. Therefore

$$\tilde{S}(t) = \tilde{S}_0 e^{-(c+\beta I)t}, \quad \tilde{P}(t) = \tilde{P}_0 e^{-ct}.$$

The proportion of healthy vectors at time $t$ is

$$\tilde{S}(t)/\tilde{P}(t) = (\tilde{S}_0/\tilde{P}_0)e^{-\beta I t} = e^{-\beta I t}.$$

The parameter $\beta$ was then established from the data to be $3.1 \times 10^{-8}$ individuals per infectious hill per day. Again, the fit was not very good. The authors suggest that this was due either to experimental error or to inappropriateness of the term $\beta I \tilde{S}$. In fact, $\beta \tilde{S} \sqrt{I}$ appears to yield a better fit, and it is suggested that more experiments be done to elucidate the relationship.

The other parameters in the model were estimated from various sources of data, and then simulations were run by solving the differential equations. In these simulations, the relative number (prevalence) of infectious vectors decreased for about 50 days, then increased to an equilibrium level of about 8% after about 150 days. The prevalence of infectious rice hills steadily increased and after about 100 days reached an equilibrium level of 83%. The authors of the article conclude that the structure of the model is adequate to describe the important qualitative features of RDV epidemiology. For additional details and comments, the reader should consult Ishii, Yasuo and Yamaguchi [1970].

## 2.13 Models of Chagas' Disease

Chagas' disease is recognized as one of the major public health problems in Latin America with estimates of up to 20 million presently infected people (Scharfstein *et al.* [1985].) The fact that this disease is vertically transmitted in humans was recognized by Chagas [1909] himself, but the extent of the occurrence of this mode of transmission has not yet been determined. The infective agent is *Trypanosoma cruzi* which is horizontally transmitted to humans via blood transfusions or, more commonly, by the bite of various triatomite bugs (*Triatoma dimidiata, T. nitida* and also possibly the North American *T. protracta protracta,* Ponce and Zeledon [1973], Theis *et al.* [1987].) In fact, Theis *et al.* report indications that this infection is starting to make inroads in both the United States and Canada. After an initial acute flare-up, the disease has two forms, a long term low level chronic form and a clinically detectable one. In its clinical form, the disease is fatal, usually because of serious cardiac, lung and digestive tract autonomic degeneration (Coura [1988], Bittencourt [1984].) In endemic areas, a considerable portion of the human population is infected with the disease and Scharfstein *et al.* [1985] report that of 50 donors who were tested at the blood bank of the General Hospital of Tegucigalpa, the capital of Honduras, 28% were found to be serologically positive to the disease. The overall prevalence rates in Central America have been estimated to be between 2% and 8% (see, for example, Salazar *et al.* [1988].) There is currently no therapy to specifically treat chronic Chagas' disease, and it is not usually detected except via serological tests or by typical abnormalities in electrocardiogram patterns. Consequently, there is a definite risk of geographic spread due to vertical and horizontal transmission by immigrants from endemic areas to currently unaffected areas (Theis *et al.* [1987].) Appropriate mathematical models can provide a qualitative assessment of the risk of this serious infection. Such models have only recently been developed by Busenberg and Vargas [1991], and Velasco-Hernandez [1991a,b,c]. We describe some of the work of Busenberg and Vargas here, including one case that has already been completely analyzed.

### 2.13.1 Proportional Mixing and Vector Transmission

We start with a model of this disease of the form

$$\begin{array}{ccccc} \downarrow & & \downarrow & & \\ S & \rightarrow & I & \rightarrow & S \\ \downarrow & & \downarrow & & \end{array}$$

This model takes both the vertical transmission and the horizontal transmission due to blood transfusions and vectors into account but it does not distinguish between the clinical and chronic forms of the infection. More detailed models will be presented later in this section.

For the vector transmission, we assume that there is a constant rate $v$ of infection of the susceptible human population due to the presence of infective vectors. In endemic regions, the horizontal transmission rate due to contaminated blood transfusions would typically be lower than that due to the vectors. However, it may be a more important mode of transmission in unaffected areas which have received immigrants from endemic zones. The form of the term describing the rate of this type of horizontal transmission that we adopt is

$$k\frac{SI}{S+I},$$

where $k$ is a contact rate of susceptibles and $I/(I+S)$ is the proportion of total contacts (through blood transfusions in this case) of each susceptible which occur with infective individuals. As before, $b, b', r, r', c$ and $q$, respectively, denote the birth rates of susceptible and infective individuals, their death rates, the cure rate (complete recovery is, however, very unlikely, Molyneux and Ashford [1983]) and the probability of vertical transmission. The equations of the model are

$$\frac{dS}{dt} = (b - r - v)S + (b'p + c)I - k\frac{SI}{S+I},$$
$$\frac{dI}{dt} = (b'q - r' - c)I + vS + k\frac{SI}{S+I}. \tag{2.43}$$

Letting $P = S + I$, we get

$$\frac{dP}{dt} = (b - r)P + (b' - b + r - r')I$$
$$= (b - r)S + (b' - r')I, \tag{2.44}$$

from which it is seen that the total population $P$ could be either increasing or decreasing. We note that one would typically expect $\alpha = b - b' + r' - r$ to be positive, since the birth rate of the infectives is lower than that of the susceptibles, while their death rate is higher.

We first look at the special case where the total population $P$ is constant. This occurs only if $dP/dt = 0$, hence,

$$S = \frac{r' - b'}{b - r}I, \tag{2.45}$$

which leads to a feasible endemic level only if $(r' - b')/(b - r) > 0$. From (2.43) and (2.45) we obtain the single equation for $I$

$$\frac{dI}{dt} = \left[ b'q - r' - c + v\frac{r' - b'}{b - r} + \frac{k(r' - b')}{b - r + r' - b'} \right] I. \tag{2.46}$$

From (2.45) and (2.46) it is seen that $P$ can remain constant only if the following unusual condition, which implies that $dI/dt = 0$, holds:

$$b'q - r' - c + v\frac{r' - b'}{b - r} + \frac{k(r' - b')}{b - r + r' - b'} = 0. \qquad (2.47)$$

In this case, the population settles to the endemic proportion

$$\frac{I}{P} = \frac{b - r}{b - r + r' - b'} . \qquad (2.48)$$

Note that this form of the endemic proportion does not show the explicit dependence on $v, k, c$, and $q$, which come in because of the condition (2.47). When the condition $(r' - b')/(b - r) > 0$ does not hold, the only possible solution with $P$ constant is the trivial one $I = S = P = 0$.

In order to study the case with $dP/dt \neq 0$, we introduce the notation

$$x = \frac{S}{P}, \quad y = \frac{I}{P}, \quad \alpha = b - r - (b' - r')$$

and, from a direct computation using (2.43), (2.44), and the fact that $x + y = 1$, we obtain the equations

$$\begin{aligned}
x' &= \frac{dx}{dt} = -vx + (c + b'p)y - (k - \alpha)xy, \\
y' &= \frac{dy}{dt} = -(c + b'p)y + vx + (k - \alpha)xy.
\end{aligned} \qquad (2.49)$$

Noting that $x + y = 1$, we obtain the single equation for $y$,

$$y' = v - (v + c + b'p - k + \alpha)y - (k - \alpha)y^2. \qquad (2.50)$$

Because of the simplicity of this equation we have the following complete description of the dynamic behavior of this model.

**Theorem 2.2.** *The model (2.43) has the following behavior if $v \neq 0$.*

*If $P = $ constant, then the population is at the endemic level $\frac{I}{P}$ given by (2.48). When $dP/dt \neq 0$, the system (2.43) has the following behavior.*

**Case 1:** $k = \alpha$. *The only steady state is the endemic level*

$$\frac{I}{P} = y^* = \frac{v}{v + c + b'p}, \qquad (2.51)$$

*and it attracts all solutions with positive initial data.*

**Case 2:** $k > \alpha$. *There is a unique positive equilibrium endemic level $I/P = y^*$ given by*

$$y^* = \frac{-(v + b'p + c - k + \alpha) + \sqrt{(v + b'p + c - k + \alpha)^2 + 4v(k - \alpha)}}{2(k - \alpha)} \qquad (2.52)$$

*which is asymptotically stable and which attracts all solutions with positive initial data.*

**Case 3:** $k < \alpha$. *There is a unique positive endemic level $\frac{I}{P} = y^*$ which lies in the feasible interval $[0, 1]$, and*

$$y^* = \frac{v + b'p + c - k + \alpha - \sqrt{(v + b'p + c - k + \alpha)^2 + 4v(k - \alpha)}}{2(\alpha - k)}. \qquad (2.53)$$

*$y^*$ is asymptotically stable and attracts all solutions with feasible positive initial data.*

*Moreover, in all three cases, the total population $P(t)$ increases without bound if $\beta = b - r - \alpha y^* > 0$, where $y^*$ is given by (2.51), (2.52) or (2.53); and tends to zero if $\beta < 0$.*

The proof of this result is straightforward and we only outline it here. It relies on the easily established fact that equation (2.50) leaves the interval $[0, 1]$ invariant. Since (2.50) is a one dimensional differential equation, its asymptotic behavior in that interval is completely determined by the roots of the quadratic equation obtained by setting its right hand side equal to zero. This yields the expressions for $y^*$ in the theorem. The fact that there is only one root of this quadratic in the interval $(0, 1)$ follows most easily by noting that the value of the quadratic at $y = 0$ is $v > 0$, and at $y = 1$ it is $-c - b'p < 0$, while it tends to either plus or minus infinity when $|y| \to \infty$ depending on the sign of $k - \alpha$. The intermediate value theorem for continuous functions implies that one of the two roots of this quadratic is in the interval $(0, 1)$.

Even though this is a mathematically very simple result, it has some interesting epidemiological implications. First, in all cases, it is easy to see that the endemic proportion $y^* \to 1$ as $v \to \infty$, that is, as the vector transmission increases, so does the proportion of infectives in the total population. Moreover, when $k \leq \alpha + v + b'p + c$, or equivalently, when the threshold

$$R_0 = \frac{k}{\alpha + v + b'p + c} \leq 1,$$

then an endemic level occurs only if $v > 0$, that is, when vector transmission is present. This is so since, in this case, (2.52) and (2.53) imply that $y^* = 0$ when $v = 0$. However, when $R_0 > 1$, the endemic level $y^*$ given by (2.52) remains feasible even when $v = 0$. Thus, in the presence of a strong enough horizontal transmission process within the human population alone, the disease can be sustained by the coupling of vertical and horizontal transmission, even when vector transmission is not present. This implies that this disease could be imported by immigrants from endemic areas into disease free areas where the vectors that transmit it are not present, or else, are not of consequence because of differences in climate or hygienic standards. Note that, as expected, $R_0$ increases as the probability of vertical transmission $q$ increases, and decreases as the cure rate $c$ increases.

Next, it is easily seen that $y^* \to 1$ as $k \to \infty$ and $y^* \to 0$ as $c \to \infty$, two results with obvious epidemiological implications. We can also explicitly compute the change of the endemic level $y^*$ with respect to the cure rate $c$

and note that $\partial y^*/\partial c < 0$. Thus, increases in the cure rate cause decreases in the level of the endemic proportion. From the form of the threshold $\beta$, it is hence seen that $\beta$ increases as $c$ increases, that is, increasing the cure rate increases the population's net reproductive coefficient.

An interesting parameter is $\alpha$, which can be viewed as the *net fitness change* caused by the infection. When $\alpha = k$, then changes in $\alpha$ have no effect on $y^*$. However, when $k < \alpha$, it is easily seen that $y^* \to 0$ as $\alpha \to \infty$, provided all the other parameters in (2.53) of the model are kept fixed. Hence, if the net reproductive coefficient of the disease free population, $b - r$, is large, the population can effectively "flush" the disease by increasing rapidly enough. The disease is always endemic in this situation, however, the endemic proportion $y^*$ becomes small. Given the other common effects of such large population increases, this is not a disease control stategy that can be widely recommended.

In the next section we shall examine in more detail the special case of this model with $v = 0$, paying particular attention to the epidemiological interpretation of the various thresholds which appear in the results. In the more general case with $v \neq 0$ which we have treated here, the threshold conditions and the expressions for the endemic equilibria are sufficiently more complicated that their epidemiological interpretations cannot be expressed in simple terms.

We will now describe a more detailed model of Chagas' disease, again due to Busenberg and Vargas [1991], for which we currently have only partial analytical results. This model takes into consideration the fact that the infection has both a chronic low level form and a clinical form, hence, it separates the infectives into two distinct epidemiological classes $I_1$ and $I_2$, representing the chronically and the clinically ill individuals, respectively. The form of this model is

$$
\begin{array}{ccc}
\downarrow & \downarrow & \\
S & \to \quad I & \to \quad S \\
\downarrow & \downarrow &
\end{array}
$$

$$
\begin{array}{cccc}
& \downarrow & & \downarrow \\
\underline{I}: & \to \quad I_1 & \to & I_2 \quad \to \\
& \downarrow & & \downarrow
\end{array}
$$

and the dynamic equations are

$$
\begin{aligned}
\frac{dS}{dt} &= (b - r - v)S + (b_1'p_1 + c_1)I_1 + (b_2'p_2 + c_2)I_2 - S\frac{k_1 I_1 + k_2 I_2}{S + I_1 + I_2}, \\
\frac{dI_1}{dt} &= (b_1'q_1 - r_1' - c_1)I_1 + vS + S\frac{k_1 I_1 + k_2 I_2}{S + I_1 + I_2} - gI_1, \\
\frac{dI_2}{dt} &= (b_2'q_2 - r_2' - c_2)I_2 + gI_1.
\end{aligned} \tag{2.54}
$$

The parameters in this model have the same meaning as their counterparts that we have already seen in equations (2.43), with the subscripted ones pertaining to the corresponding epidemic classes. The one new parameter, $g$, is the rate at which the chronically ill move into the clinically ill class. For Chagas' disease, $g$ would be very small since $1/g$ is the mean period of stay in the chronic class which is estimated to be of the order of ten to fifteen years. Also, in the case of Chagas' disease, the chronically ill are normally not detected, and even if detected, their probability of being cured is very low. Thus their cure rate $c_1 = 0$, for all practical purposes. The mathematical analysis of the full model (2.54) is complicated, hence, we shall concentrate on some special cases which have particular epidemiological interest.

The significant additional information that this more complicated model can yield concerns the effects of the presence of the more "silent" form of the infection. In particular, one can address the question of what inroads an infection can have, in an initially healthy population, due to the introduction of some chronically infected individuals, even when the vector transmission is not present ($v = 0$), or is very small. This is the question that we shall now address. We, hence, consider the case where the initial population consists of only susceptible individuals and some chronically infected ones, thus $I_2(0) = 0$. Since $g$ is very small, we look at the case when it is zero. This yields a considerable mathematical simplification which will allow us to give a rapid analysis of the question we have raised. We set $P = S + I_1 + I_2$ and define the variables

$$x = \frac{S}{P}, \quad y_1 = \frac{I_1}{P}, \quad y_2 = \frac{I_2}{P}.$$

Noting that $x + y_1 + y_2 = 1$, and setting $\alpha_i = b_i - r_i - (b_i' - r_i')$, $i = 1, 2$, we use (2.54) to obtain the following system for $y_1$ and $y_2$.

$$\frac{dy_1}{dt} = v - (v - k_1 + \alpha_1 + b_1'p_1 + c_1)y_1 + (k_2 - v)y_2$$
$$+ (\alpha_2 - k_1 - k_2)y_1y_2 + (\alpha_1 - k_1)y_1^2 - k_2y_2^2, \qquad (2.55)$$

$$\frac{dy_2}{dt} = -(\alpha_2 + b_2'p_2 + c_2)y_2 + \alpha_1 y_1 y_2 + \alpha_2 y_2^2.$$

The region of interest is $Q = \{y_1, y_2 \in [0,1] \text{ and } y_1 + y_2 \leq 1\}$. A direct computation shows that

$$\left.\frac{dy_1}{dt}\right|_{y_1=0} = (v + k_2 y_2)(1 - y_2) > 0, \quad \left.\frac{dy_2}{dt}\right|_{y_2=0} = 0,$$

and

$$\left.\frac{d(y_1 + y_2)}{dt}\right|_{y_1+y_2=1} = -(b_1'p_1y_1 + b_2'p_2y_2 + c_1y_1 + c_2y_2) < 0.$$

Thus, solutions of (2.55) with initial data in this region remain there for all time. We are interested in solutions with initial data $I_2 = 0$, which implies $y_2 = 0$, hence, from (2.55) we see that $y_2(t) = 0$ for all $t \geq 0$. In this case, the equation for $y_1$ becomes

$$\frac{dy_1}{dt} = v - (v - k_1 + \alpha_1 + b_1'p_1 + c_1)y_1 + (\alpha_1 - k_1)y_1^2.$$

This equation has a unique steady state $y_1^*$ in the interval $(0, 1)$, and

$$y_1^* = \frac{v - k_1 + \alpha_1 + b_1' p_1 + c_1 \pm \sqrt{(v - k_1 + \alpha_1 + b_1' p_1 + c_1)^2 - 4v(\alpha_1 - k_1)}}{2(\alpha_1 - k_1)},$$

with the $+$ sign if $\alpha_1 - k_1 < 0$, and the $-$ sign otherwise. Thus, if the vector population is present, there always is an endemic state.

If $v = 0$, there are two possible steady states

$$y_1^* = \begin{cases} 0, & \text{if } \alpha_1 - k_1 > 0; \\ 1 + \frac{b_1' p_1 + c_1}{\alpha_1 - k_1}, & \text{if } \alpha_1 - k_1 < 0. \end{cases} \tag{2.56}$$

the second being feasible if, and only if,

$$R_0 = \frac{k_1}{\alpha_1 + c_1 + b_1' p_1} > 1. \tag{2.57}$$

Thus, if the horizontal transmission is strong enough, even when the vector transmission is absent, the disease would reach an endemic level if silent infectives are introduced into an otherwise healthy population. Note that vertical transmission by itself cannot sustain an endemic level, since the threshold condition $R_0 > 1$ requires that $k_1 > 0$. Clearly, $R_0$ decreases as $\alpha_1, c$, or $p_1$ increase. This conclusion may have practical implications for certain regions in the United States where there are large concentrations of immigrants from endemic areas. Since the chronic, or silent, form of this disease is not detected, and since there is a tendency of recent immigrants to concentrate in regions with strong ethnic identities, the horizontal transmission, coupled with vertical transmission, may become high enough in such regions to sustain a geographically localized endemic level. The situation would be yet more serious if the disease could establish itself in a local vector population. The experiments of Theis *et al.* [1987] show that this is indeed possible. However, one should not discount the effects of differences in living conditions when considering vector transmission. This is nicely illustrated by a totally different disease, sylviatic plague, whose vector is a flea and which is endemic in the rodent and coyote populations of the San Gabriel mountains in the Los Angeles area. Yet cases of its human counterpart, bubonic plague, which was once justifiably termed the "black death", are an extemely rare occurrence. The horizontal transmission via blood transfusions is more serious and needs to be studied carefully. Since detailed serological data on the incidence of the silent form of Chagas' disease are not currently available, we can only give rough estimates based on our model.

Using the threshold $R_0$ in (2.57) with $c_1 = 0$, $p_1 = 0.4$, $\alpha_1 = 0$, and $b_1' = 0.02/\text{year}$, we see that an endemic condition will occur if $k_1 > 0.008/\text{year}$. Such a horizontal rate of transmission due to blood transfusions would be possible only if 30% of the blood supply in an affected area were contaminated and on the average three persons per one hundred needed a blood transfusion per year. If $p_1 = 0.97$, and the other parameters were kept at the same values as before, then an endemic threshold will occur if $k_1 > 0.019/\text{year}$, essentially doubling the degree of horizontal transmission necessary for endemicity to occur. Since the vertical transmission rates for Chagas' disease are very small, the above calculations suggest that it would be unlikely for the disease to be established in a population which is not subject to vector transmission.

A systematic effort to model Chagas' disease has been undertaken by Velasco-Hernandez [1991,a,b,c] who has analyzed a variety of models of this disease and has compared his results to data from several Latin American countries. This work is promising to shed light on the complicated dynamics of this serious disease.

### 2.13.2 An SIS Model with Proportional Mixing

There are several intricate interactions between the various parameters in the first model of Chagas' disease that we studied in the previous section. These lead to a number of threshold criteria which are quite involved and difficult to understand on an intuitive level. Consequently, it is worthwhile to examine in some detail a special case of that model in order to obtain in this simpler setting a clear understanding of these thresholds, and hopefully help us grasp what is occurring in the more complicated setting. The results we present here can be obtained by letting $v \to 0$ in Theorem 2.2 of the previous section. However, the clearer interpretation that we can give here of the threshold criteria makes it worthwhile to study this simpler case in detail.

We consider the $S \to I \to S$ model with force of infection term $kSI/P$, $P = I+S$, which is obtained by setting $v = 0$ in (2.43). The resulting equations are

$$\frac{dS}{dt} = (b-r)S + (b'p+c)I - k\frac{SI}{S+I} ,$$
$$\frac{dI}{dt} = (b'q - r' - c)I + k\frac{SI}{S+I} . \tag{2.58}$$

Then $P$ satisfies (2.44), and (2.50) for $y = I/P$ becomes

$$\frac{dy}{dt} = (k - \alpha - c - b'p)y + (\alpha - k)y^2. \tag{2.59}$$

We shall make the following additional simplifying assumptions,

$$\alpha = b - r - (b' - r') > 0, \text{ and } k > \alpha.$$

Note that $\alpha$ is the reproductive advantage of the susceptible individuals over the infectives, hence, the condition $\alpha > 0$ is biologically reasonable for the situation that we are modeling.

Since $v = 0$, the equilibrium given by (2.52) reduces to

$$y^* = \frac{k - \alpha - pb' - c}{k - \alpha} = 1 - \frac{pb' + c}{k - \alpha}. \tag{2.60}$$

There are two possible equilibrium values for $y$, namely, $y = 0$ and $y = y^*$. The following threshold parameters will play a role in the dynamics of this model.

$$R = \frac{b}{r}, \quad R_0 = \frac{k}{\alpha + pb' + c}, \quad R_1 = \frac{b}{r + \alpha y*}, \quad R_2 = \frac{k + qb'}{c + r'}.$$

We collect our results for this model in the following theorem.

**Theorem 2.3** *The model equations (2.58) have the following behavior. If $P = $ constant, then the infective proportion $y = I/P$, is given by*

$$y^* = \frac{b - r}{\alpha},$$

*if $R > 1$ and $R_1 = 1$; while if $R \leq 1$, then $P = I = 0$, and $y$ is not defined.*
   *If $P \neq$ constant, we have the following possibilities.*
   *(a) The infective proportion $y(t)$ obeys*

$$\lim_{t \to \infty} y(t) = \begin{cases} y^*, & \text{if } R_0 > 1, \\ 0, & \text{if } R_0 \leq 1, \end{cases}$$

*where $y^*$ is given by (2.60). Moreover, we have the following finer structure in the asymptotic behavior of the population.*
   *(b) If $R_0 \leq 1$, and $R \leq 1$, then $P(t)$, $I(t)$ and $y(t) \to 0$, as $t \to \infty$. However, if $R_0 \leq 1$ and $R > 1$, then as $t \to \infty$,*

$$P(t) \to \infty, \quad y(t) \to 0,$$

*and*

$$I(t) \to \begin{cases} 0, & \text{if } R_2 < 1, \\ \infty, & \text{if } R_2 > 1. \end{cases}$$

   *(c) If $R_0 > 1$, then $y(t) \to y^*$, and*

$$P(t) \to \begin{cases} 0, & \text{if } R_1 < 1, \\ \infty, & \text{if } R_1 > 1, \end{cases}$$

*and*

$$I(t) \to \begin{cases} 0, & \text{if } R_1 < 1, \\ \infty, & \text{if } R_1 > 1. \end{cases}$$

*Remark.* It is important to note that, even though the infective ratio $y(t)$ may tend to zero, the total number of infectives may still be increasing when the total population is increasing. This can happen in case (b) of the theorem. On the other hand, the infective ratio, $y(t)$, may be tending to a positive endemic ratio $y^*$, and yet the total number of infectives will still go to zero if the total population is decreasing. Hence, there are two distinct notions of what it means to eradicate the disease in a population which is not constant. The first notion, which is less strict when the total population is increasing, requires that the proportion $y(t) \to 0$, and the threshold which controls this is $R_0$. The second notion of control requires that the total number of infectives tend to zero, and the thresholds here are $R_1$ and $R_2$. In a decreasing population, this second notion of control is less strict, since the proportion of infectives may go to an endemic level $y^*$, even though the total number of infectives may be decreasing along with the total population. This fine structure of the threshold parameters and its relevance to the different notions of disease transmission has been introduced in the work of Busenberg and van den Driessche [1990], Busenberg, Cooke and Thieme [1991] and Busenberg and Vargas [1991]. Such thresholds were also studied, for the case where the force of infection is of the mass-action type, in the earlier work of Busenberg, Cooke and Pozio [1983] which was described in Section 2.4.

**Discussion of the Threshold Parameters.** There are four different threshold parameters which play a role in this model, while in typical population models one encounters only two. The additional parameters are due to the fact that we are allowing the possibility that the population change size, that is, we are allowing for demographic changes. These parameters can be given an epidemiological interpretation as follows.

$R = b/r$ can be viewed as the *disease-free reproduction coefficient* of the population. In fact, if $I(t) \equiv 0$, we have

$$\frac{dS}{dt} = \frac{dP}{dt} = (b - r)S = r(R - 1)S = r(R - 1)P.$$

$R_0 = k/(\alpha + pb' + c)$ can be regarded as the *net infective value* which measures the relative strength of horizontal transmission and the change in the number of infectives due to the cure rate and the demographic effects.

$R_1 = b/(r + \alpha y^*)$ is the *net reproductive coefficient of the population when the disease is endemic*. In fact, when $I/P$ reaches the endemic level $y^*$, the total population satisfies the equation

$$\frac{dP}{dt} = (b - r - \alpha y^*)P = (r + \alpha y^*)(R_1 - 1)P,$$

hence, $P$ will grow or decay according as $R_1 > 1$ or $R_1 < 1$.

$R_2 = (k + qb')/(r' + c)$ is the *net reproductive coefficient of the diseased population when the total population is increasing and the endemic proportion $I/P$ decreases to zero*. The limiting equation for $I$ when $I(t)/P(t) \to 0$, hence, $S(t)/P(t) \to 1$, can be written in the form

$$\frac{dI}{dt} = (r' + c)\left(\frac{k + qb'}{r' + c} - 1\right)I = (r' + c)(R_2 - 1)I,$$

hence, $I(t)$ will tend to zero or to infinity according as $R_2$ is less than or greater than one.

We now turn to the rather simple proof of Theorem 2.3 which is given by Grabiner [1988].

*Proof.* First, note that $P = $ constant if, and only if, either $P = 0$ or $b - r - \alpha y = 0$. The latter condition implies $y = y^* = (b - r)/(\alpha)$, which is feasible if, and only if, $R > 1$ and $R_1 = 1$. If $R < 1$, then $P = I = 0$ is the only feasible steady state, and hence $y = I/P$ is not defined.

When $P \neq$ constant, then part (a) of the theorem is obtained by noting that (2.59) leaves the interval $0 \leq y \leq 1$, invariant, and hence, $y(t)$ must tend to one of the two steady states of this equation. Now, the derivative of the right hand side of (2.59) with respect to $y$ at $y = 0$, is $k - \alpha - pb' - c$, which is positive if $R_0 > 1$, hence, $y(t) \rightarrow y^* > 0$, and negative if $R_0 < 1$, hence, $y(t) \rightarrow 0$. When $R_0 = 1$, $y = 0$ is the only steady state in $[0, 1]$, hence, $y(t) \rightarrow 0$ in this case also.

The finer structure in the asymptotic behavior is shown as follows. If $R_0 \leq 1$, and $R \leq 1$, then $P'(t) = (b - r)P - \alpha I < 0$, when $R \neq 1$, or $I_0 \neq 0$. If both $R = 1$ and $I_0 = 0$, then $P(t) =$ constant, which is not possible in this case. Thus, $P(t)$, $I(t)$, and $y(t) \rightarrow 0$ as $t \rightarrow \infty$. Next, if $R_0 \leq 1$, but $R > 1$, the limiting form of the equation for $P$: $P'(t) = (b - r - \alpha y)P$, becomes $P'(t) = (b - r)P$, since $y(t) \rightarrow 0$ as $t \rightarrow \infty$. Here, $b - r > 0$, since $R > 1$, and thus, $P(t) \rightarrow \infty$ as $t \rightarrow \infty$. The equation for $I$ can be written as

$$\frac{dI}{dt} = (k + qb' - r' - c - ky)I \rightarrow (k + qb' - r' - c)I$$
$$= (r' + c)(R_2 - 1)I,$$

hence, $I(t) \rightarrow 0$, if $R_2 < 1$, and $I(t) \rightarrow \infty$, if $R_2 > 1$.

Finally, if $R_0 > 1$, $y(t) \rightarrow y^*$, and the limiting form of the equation for $P$ is $P'(t) = (b - r - \alpha y^*)P = (r + \alpha y^*)(R_1 - 1)P$, yielding the conclusion that $P(t) \rightarrow 0$ for $R_1 < 1$ and $P(t) \rightarrow \infty$ for $R_1 > 1$. Since $I(t) = P(t)y^*$, and $y^* > 0$, we see that the behavior of $I(t)$ is the same as that of $P(t)$ in this case. This completes the proof of this result.

### 2.13.3 Logistic Control

The model equations (2.58) lead to exponentially increasing or decreasing populations, a situation which can be expected to occur only for a finite time interval. If this time interval is large in comparison to the time-scale of the dynamics of the disease, as is often the case with diseases in human populations, then the thresholds that are obtained on the basis of such a model could be useful in understanding the dynamics of disease transmission. In animal populations, however, it is often the case that competition for resources exerts a control on the growth of the population. In this section we will describe a model studied by Grabiner [1988] which includes a classical logistic control, and we consider the effect that it has on the disease dynamics. In particular, assume that the population crowding affects the net reproduction terms in (2.59) in proportion to the size of the total population to obtain the following model

$$\frac{dS}{dt} = (b - r)S + (b'p + c)I - k\frac{SI}{S+I} - dPS,$$
$$\frac{dI}{dt} = (b'q - r' - c)I + k\frac{SI}{S+I} - dPI.$$

Then $P$ satisfies

$$\frac{dP}{dt} = (b - r - dP)P - \alpha I,  \tag{2.61}$$

and $y = I/P$ again satisfies (2.59), that is, the special case of (2.50) with $v = 0$. We shall make the following additional assumptions,

$$\alpha = b - r - (b' - r') > 0, \quad b > r, \quad \text{and } k > \alpha.$$

The first of these conditions, $\alpha > 0$, implies that the disease decreases the net reproductive capacity of the host. The second condition implies that the host population would not go extinct in the absence of the disease, and the third condition, as we shall see below, is needed in order to guarantee the existence of an endemic proportion of infected host individuals. These assumptions are not needed in the mathematical analysis and are made in order to focus attention on a biologically interesting situation. We get the same equilibrium $y^*$ given in (2.60) and we have the two cases $R_0 > 1$ where $y(t) \to y^*$, and $R_0 < 1$ where $y(t) \to 0$. In the first case, the limiting form of (2.61) is

$$\frac{dP}{dt} = (b - r - \alpha y^* - dP)P$$

which is the standard logistic equation with carrying capacity $(b - r - \alpha y^*)/d$. Thus, if $b/(r + \alpha y^*) = R_1 \leq 1$ the population will tend to zero; while if $R_1 > 1$ the population will tend to the carrying capacity. Similarly, in the case where $R_0 < 1$, the limiting form of (2.61) is

$$\frac{dP}{dt} = (b - r - dP)P,$$

a logistic equation with carrying capacity $(b - r)/d$. Thus, the population approaches either the carrying capacity or zero according as $b/r = R > 1$ or $R \leq 1$.

Note that the thresholds are identical to those of the model (2.59) without the logistic control. This is due to the fact that these thresholds are determined by the appropriate linear forms of the equations which are the same for both models. An interesting effect that is worth noting is that, in the case where $R_1 > 1$, the carrying capacity of the total population is decreased because of the presence of the disease by an amount

$$\frac{\alpha y^*}{d} = \frac{\alpha(k - \alpha - pb' - c)}{d(k - \alpha)}.$$

Thus, an increase in the vertical transmission probability $q$, hence a decrease in $p$, results in a decrease in the carrying capacity of the population. The vertical transmission mechanism can hence act as a means for controlling the population size. For the study of other couplings of disease induced mortality and logistic population size controls see Brauer [1990].

## 2.14  An SIRS Model with Proportional Mixing

In this section we will describe some recent results which give the complete global analysis of the $S \to I \to R \to S$ model with proportional mixing and vertical transmission when the total population is not assumed to be of constant size. These results are due to Busenberg and van den Driessche [1990] and have been extended to the case with vertical transmission by Busenberg and Hadeler [1990]. These papers describe the various thresholds that occur in this situation, and they develop methods of analysis that are being found to be useful in studying other epidemic models. They illustrate two general methods for handling epidemic models which have a certain natural homogeneity property. In particular, we describe a criterion for ruling out periodic solutions, due to Busenberg and van den Driessche [1990], which provides a basic step in the study of the global behavior of solutions.

In Sections 2.3-2.7 we considered models of vertically transmitted diseases with mass-action contact terms in populations of varying size, and gave a complete global analysis of the model equations. In Section 2.13 we considered $S \to I \to S$ models of Chagas' disease with a proportional mixing contact term in populations of varying size. Here we treat the $S \to I \to R \to S$ model with a proportional mixing contact term. The main result gives a complete global stability analysis, and once again shows the close coupling between the demographics of the population and the dynamics of the disease.

In deriving our model equations, we divide the population into three classes, the susceptible, the infective and the recovered (removed) individuals with total numbers respectively denoted by $S$, $I$ and $R$. We set $P = S + I + R$, and use the following notation:

$b_1 =$ per capita birth rate of the susceptible population.

$b_2 =$ per capita birth rate of the infected population.

$b_3 =$ per capita birth rate of the recovered population.

$q =$ probability of vertical transmission, $0 \le q \le 1$, and $p = 1 - q$.

$d =$ per capita disease free death rate.

$\epsilon =$ excess per capita death rate of infected individuals.

$\delta =$ excess per capita death rate of recovered individuals.

$c =$ per capita recovery rate of infected individuals, assumed to be positive.

$e =$ per capita loss of immunity rate of recovered individuals.

$\lambda =$ effective per capita contact rate of infective individuals.

We assume a proportional mixing contact rate, hence, the rate at which susceptible individuals become infected is given by

$$\lambda \frac{IS}{P}.$$

The above hypotheses lead to the following model equations.

$$S' = b_1 S + p b_2 I + b_3 R - dS - \lambda \frac{SI}{P} + eR,$$

$$I' = q b_2 I - (d + \epsilon + c)I + \lambda \frac{SI}{P}, \tag{2.62}$$

$$R' = -(d + \delta + e)R + cI.$$

The equation for the total population P is obtained by adding Eqs. (2.62),

$$P' = (b_1 - d)P - (\epsilon + b_1 - b_2)I - (\delta + b_1 - b_3)R. \tag{2.63}$$

All the parameters in this model are non-negative, and we are interested in solutions which are also non-negative. It is a simple matter to show that the model equations (2.62) are well-posed in the sense that any initial data for $(S, I, R)$ which are non-negative lead to solutions which are defined and remain non-negative for all time $t > 0$. We shall study this model in situations where the population $P(t)$ is not stationary. We note that $P(t)$ can remain constant when $I(t)$ or $R(t)$ are not identically zero only if special restrictions on the model parameters hold.

A special case of this model with the assumption that $P(t) = $ constant and with no vertical transmission has been studied by Mena-Lorca [1988], who considers the case with $\delta = 0$, and shows that a line of equilibria exists which is neutrally stable. Generally, $P'(t) \neq 0$ and $P(t)$ is not constant, which is the case we consider here. To proceed with the analysis, we consider the proportions of individuals in the three epidemiological classes, namely

$$s = S/P, \ i = I/P \text{ and } r = R/P. \tag{2.64}$$

The dynamical system becomes

$$s' = p b_2 i + b_3 r + er + (\epsilon + b_1 - b_2 - \lambda)si + (\delta + b_1 - b_3)sr,$$

$$i' = (q b_2 - b_1 - \epsilon - c)i + \lambda si + (\delta + b_1 - b_3)ir + (\epsilon + b_1 - b_2)i^2, \tag{2.65}$$

$$r' = -(\delta + e + b_1)r + ci + (\epsilon + b_1 - b_2)ir + (\delta + b_1 - b_3)r^2,$$

and the feasibility region is

$$\mathcal{D} = \{(s, i, r) : s \geq 0, i \geq 0, r \geq 0, \ s + i + r = 1\}. \tag{2.66}$$

We define $\mathcal{D}_0 = \mathcal{D} - \{(1, 0, 0)\}$.

There are two distinct ways of considering a disease as being brought under control in a population of increasing or decreasing total size. The stricter way requires that the total number of infectives $I(t) \to 0$, while a weaker requirement is that the proportion $i(t) \to 0$. This distinction is discussed in some detail in Busenberg and van den Driessche [1990], and Busenberg, Cooke and Thieme [1991] and in the remarks following Theorem 2.3. Here we will only describe the single threshold $R_0$ governing the existence and stability of a proportional endemic state. We refer to the paper of Busenberg and van den Driessche [1990] for a complete discussion of the other thresholds that occur in this type of model. The following result is proved in Busenberg and Hadeler [1990].

**Theorem 2.4** *Consider the epidemiological model* (2.65) *with* $b_1 \geq b_3 \geq b_2 > 0$, $c > 0$, *and all other parameters non-negative. Then*
*(a) The disease free equilibrium proportion* $(s, i, r) = (1, 0, 0)$ *always exists, and is globally asymptotically stable in* $\mathcal{D}$ *whenever* $R_0 < 1$, *and it attracts all solutions with initial data in* $\mathcal{D}$ *when* $R_0 \leq 1$, *where*

$$R_0 = \frac{\lambda}{b_1 - qb_2 + \epsilon + c}. \tag{2.67}$$

*This solution is unstable when* $R_0 > 1$.
*(b) When* $R_0 > 1$, *there exists a unique endemic proportion equilibrium* $(s, i, r) = (s^*, i^*, r^*)$ *with* $i^* > 0, r^* > 0$ *which is globally asymptotically stable in* $\mathcal{D}_0$.

Before we outline the proof of this result, we turn to a discussion of its epidemiological implications. The threshold $R_0$ measures the relative strength of the transmission of the disease via horizontal contacts versus the dilution effect of the infective proportion either through recovery, or through excess death, or else through the increase of the disease-free population via births of uninfected individuals. The effect of vertical transmission is through the term $-qb_2$ which decreases the denominator, and hence increases the value of $R_0$. Thus, the demographics of the population interact with the epidemiology in two different ways. In the presence of vertical transmission, an increase in the birth rate $b_2$ of the infective part of the population (or else an increase in the probability of vertical transmission $q$) leads to an increase in $R_0$. However, an increase in the birth rate $b_1$ of the susceptible part of the population leads to a decrease of $R_0$. The birth rate $b_3$ of the removed or immune part of the population does not affect this threshold. As can be expected, an increase in either the recovery rate or the excess death rate of the infectives leads to a decrease in $R_0$. Thus, the demography can outrun the disease if, keeping all other parameters constant, the birth rate of the susceptible population $b_1$ is increased sufficiently to reduce $R_0$ to a value less than one. However, we note again that even if $i \to 0$, it is still possible in the case of an increasing population to have $I$ increase. That is, the condition $R_0 < 1$ only guarantees that the proportion of infectives and not their total number tends to zero.

We now outline the proof of the Theorem 2.4.

*Proof.* Since $s + i + r = 1$, the solutions of the system (2.65) are located on the two-dimensional region $\mathcal{D}$. In fact, it is easy to see that $(s + i + r)' = 0$ on this region, and that the direction of the vector field defined by the right hand sides of Eqs. (2.65), when evaluated on the boundary of $\mathcal{D}$, points towards its interior. Now, by using some detailed and rather long analysis which we do not present here, it is shown that the condition $R_0 > 1$ is necessary and sufficient for instability of the disease free equilibrium $(1, 0, 0)$ and the existence of a unique locally stable endemic equilibrium $(s^*, i^*, r^*)$ in $\mathcal{D}_0$. The global stability of this second equilibrium follows by first showing that there are no periodic solutions in $\mathcal{D}$ through the use of a result of Busenberg and van den Driessche [1990] which we describe in Theorem 2.5 in Section 2.16.3. In fact, letting $f_i$ for $i = 1, 2, 3$, denote the right hand sides of the three equations (2.65), and using the restriction $s + i + r = 1$, one can obtain a vector valued function $\mathbf{g}(s, i, r)$ which has the properties

$$\mathbf{g} \cdot (f_1, f_2, f_3) = 0, \ \nabla \times \mathbf{g}(s, i, r) \cdot (1, 1, 1) < 0$$

on $\mathcal{D}_0$. These are the hypotheses needed to rule out the existence of periodic solutions that lie in $\mathcal{D}_0$. The global stability of the endemic equilibrium then follows from an application of the Poincaré-Bendixson theorem on $\mathcal{D}$. The local stability analysis can be performed by either doing the standard linearization procedure on the manifold $\mathcal{D}$, or else by noting that the system (2.62) is homogeneous of degree one and using the theory of such systems that is discussed in the book of Hahn [1967]. The first approach is taken in Busenberg and van den Driessche and the second in Busenberg and Hadeler [1990].

## 2.15 Evolution of Viruses

When a viral genome enters a host cell, it frequently happens that new virus particles are produced, the cell is destroyed, and the new viruses are released to enter new cells. On the other hand, in some cases the viral genome integrates into the host cell's DNA and this "provirus" remains in a latent state until the cell replicates, thereby also replicating the virus. One may ask, from the evolutionary point of view, whether these two modes may coexist, and if not, which is likely to persist. In this section, we describe a model of Nowak [1991], who explores this question.

Nowak calls the first mode horizontal transmission, because the viruses burst from a cell to infect other cells. He calls the second mode vertical transmission, because the viral genome is passed from mother cell to daughter cells. That is, division of an infected cell to produce two infected cells is regarded as the asexual analogue of transmission from parent to progeny. Intuitively, the first mode provides a rapid way of reproduction, since a large number of virus particles can be produced from only one cell, whereas the second mode is slower because of the period of latency. Nowak argues that the first mode is at a higher risk level than the second since the new free viruses may not all succeed in infecting a new cell. Several models are proposed to pursue these ideas, but for lack of space only one will be described here.

In this model, the population is divided into three subpopulations. We let $x(t)$ be the number (or density) of uninfected cells. Let $y_1(t)$ and $y_2(t)$ denote the number of infected cells of two types, and let $k$ be the rate of immigration of new uninfected cells. Let $r$ be the net reproduction rate of uninfected cells and let $r_1$ and $r_2$ be the respective net reproduction rates of infected cells. Assume a mass-action law for contacts, where $b_1$ and $b_2$ are the contact coefficients. Then one obtains the model equations

$$\dot{x} = k + x(r - b_1 y_1 - b_2 y_2),$$
$$\dot{y}_1 = y_1(r_1 + b_1 x), \qquad\qquad (2.68)$$
$$\dot{y}_2 = y_2(r_2 + b_2 x).$$

Since the model does not contain a growth-limiting term, we see that if $r_1$ or $r_2$ is positive, then the population of infected cells goes to infinity. Nowak therefore concentrates on the case in which $r$, $r_1$, and $r_2$ are negative. There are then three steady state solutions, in which $(x, y_1, y_2)$ is $(-k/r, 0, 0)$, the disease-free equilibrium, or is

(i) $E_1 = \left( -\dfrac{r_1}{b_1}, \dfrac{kb_1 - rr_1}{-r_1 b_1}, 0 \right)$, or

(ii) $E_2 = \left( -\dfrac{r_2}{b_2}, 0, \dfrac{kb_2 - rr_2}{-r_2 b_2} \right)$.

There is no internal equilibrium, indicating that in this model the two types of virus cannot coexist. Clearly, $E_1$ is feasible if and only if $kb_1 - rr_1 > 0$, and $E_2$ is feasible if and only if $kb_2 - rr_2 > 0$. Thus, the basic reproductive coefficients of virus type one, in the absence of type two, and of type two in the absence of type one, are

$$R_0^1 = \frac{a_1 r - b_1 k}{r d_1} \quad \text{and} \quad R_0^2 = \frac{a_2 r - b_2 k}{r d_2},$$

respectively, where $r = a - d$, $r_1 = a_1 - d_1$, $r_2 = a_2 - d_2$ and the a's represent birth rates and the d's represent death rates. Observe that the condition for feasibility of the equilibrium $E_1$ is that $kb_1 - rr_1 > 0$, which is equivalent to the condition $R_0^1 > 1$, and similarly the condition for feasibility of $E_2$ is $kb_2 - rr_2 > 0$, which is equivalent to $R_0^2 > 1$.

Computing the Jacobian of the system, we find that the eigenvalues of the disease-free equilibrium are $r$, $(rr_1 - b_1 k)/r$, and $(rr_2 - b_2 k)/r$. Consequently this is stable if and only if $rr_1 - b_1 k > 0$ and $rr_2 - b_2 k > 0$, or equivalently $R_0^1 < 1$ and $R_0^2 < 1$. In this case, $E_1$ and $E_2$ do not lie in the feasible region. Now consider the case in which $R_0^1$ and $R_0^2$ are both larger than one, hence $E_1$ and $E_2$ are both feasible. The eigenvalues of $E_1$ are $(r_2 b_1 - b_2 r_1)/b_1$ and the two roots of the equation

$$\lambda^2 - \frac{kb_1}{r_1}\lambda + (kb_1 - rr_1) = 0.$$

Therefore $E_1$ is stable if and only if $R_0^1 > 1$ and $r_2 b_1 - b_2 r_1 < 0$. Similarly, $E_2$ is stable if and only if $R_0^2 > 1$ and $r_1 b_2 - b_1 r_2 < 0$. Hence, if

$$\frac{r_2}{b_2} > \frac{r_1}{b_1}, \qquad\qquad (2.69)$$

then $E_1$ is unstable and $E_2$ is stable, and the situation is reversed if the inequality is reversed. The ratio of the net reproduction rate $r$ to the transmission parameter $b$ therefore determines which virus strain is dominant. In particular, this local stability analysis suggests that persistence of both viruses might not be possible, however, a complete global analysis has not been done.

Nowak now examines the following scenario. Suppose that the cell population is initially infected with virus strain one, with parameters $r_1$ and $b_1$, and $R_0^1 > 1$, and that the system has settled to the equilibrium $E_1$. Assume that a new mutant is generated, with parameters $r_2, b_2$, and $R_0^2 > 1$. If inequality (2.69) holds, then the mutant can invade, spread, and finally displace the original virus strain. This can happen even if $R_0^2 < R_0^1$. Nowak gives a numerical example to illustrate this possibility. Thus, latency can evolve even if the latent strain has a lower basic reproductive coefficient than the original strain. The competition between two viral strains may not necessarily select for increasing the reproductive rate.

The competition between two virus strains, as described above, is analogous to the competition between temperate and virulent bacteriophage. (Bacteriophage are viruses that infect bacteria.) Models of this competition have been developed by Stewart and Levin [1984], whose paper lists a large number of relevant references. Similar questions arise in studying cross-immunity and the competition between highly virulent and less virulent forms in host-parasite interactions. References to this work include Levin and Pimentel [1981], Bremermann and Thieme [1989], and Castillo-Chavez et al. [1989].

## 2.16 The Mathematical Background

This section provides a synoptic discussion of the main mathematical methods that were used in the analysis of the models of Chapter 2. We do not provide a logical development of these topics, since that would require an extensive treatment that is beyond the scope of this monograph. The reader who desires a more detailed treatment of this material will need to make use of the references that we list. We have made no attempt at completeness in either the material we present or the references to the literature. Rather, we have aimed to provide the reader a convenient presentation of material that is not readily available in any one text and which may go beyond the standard mathematical background that can be expected from some of the possible users of this monograph. Throughout this section, it is assumed that the reader has a basic background in calculus, linear algebra and ordinary differential equations on the level that is common in standard undergraduate courses.

There are six subsections dealing with a) Positivity and Invariant Regions, b) Equilibria and Stability Analysis, c) Global Stability in One and Two Dimensions, d) General Global Stability, e) A Special Global Stability Result, and f) Existence and Bifurcation of Periodic Solutions.

## 2.16.1 Positivity and Invariant Regions

The models that we have studied in this chapter are mathematically formulated as systems of differential equations

$$\frac{dx_1}{dt} = f_1(x_1, x_2, \cdots, x_n),$$

$$\frac{dx_2}{dt} = f_2(x_1, x_2, \cdots, x_n),$$

$$\cdots\cdots$$

$$\frac{dx_n}{dt} = f_n(x_1, x_2, \cdots, x_n),$$

(2.70)

which can be written more concisely in vector notation

$$\frac{d\mathbf{x}}{dt} = \mathbf{f}(\mathbf{x}),$$

(2.71)

where $\mathbf{x}$ and $\mathbf{f}$ are vectors with components $x_i$ and $f_i$, respectively. The functions $f_i$ are assumed to be smooth enough so that through each point $\mathbf{x}_0$ there passes a unique solution of (2.70). A simple condition that guarantees this, and which is satisfied by all the equations used in the models we have studied, is that the $f_i$ be differentiable functions of the variables $x_i$. In our models, the dimension of the system, $n$, was usually 2 or 3, and the variables $x_1, x_2, \cdots, x_n$, were S, I, E, R or other quantities of epidemiological interest. The functions $f_i$ were explicit expressions in terms of one or more of the variables S, E, I, R which were determined by the situations that were being modeled.

In the models, the dependent variables $S(t)$, $I(t)$, $R(t)$ represent numbers of individuals, or fractions of the whole population. Therefore, they should be positive or zero for all times $t \geq 0$, and if this fails to hold then the model should probably be discarded since it violates a basic aspect of the biological reality. This suggests that we should formulate the following question.

Let $\mathbf{R}^n$ be n-dimensional space ($n \geq 1$,) and let $\Omega$ be a subset of $\mathbf{R}^n$. We say that $\Omega$ is *positively invariant* for (2.70) if, when $(x_1(0), x_2(0), \cdots, x_n(0))$ is in $\Omega$, the solution starting with these initial values has the property that the trajectory $(x_1(t), x_2(t), \cdots, x_n(t))$ is in $\Omega$ for all $t \geq 0$. A case of particular interest is when $\Omega$ is the so-called nonnegative orthant or cone

$$\mathbf{R}^n_+ = \{(x_1, x_2, \cdots, x_n) : x_1 \geq 0, x_2 \geq 0, \cdots, x_n \geq 0\}.$$

A set $\Omega$ may similarly be called negatively invariant if the trajectory remains in $\Omega$ for $t \leq 0$.

Positive invariance of the nonnegative orthant $\mathbf{R}^n_+$ for a given system (2.70) will be assured if no trajectory can leave $\mathbf{R}^n_+$ by crossing through one of its faces. Consider the face $x_1 = 0$. On it, the *direction field* has components $(f_1(0, x_2, \cdots, x_n), f_2(0, x_2, \cdots, x_n), \cdots, f_n(0, x_2, \cdots, x_n))$ and this defines a vector at each point $(0, x_2, \cdots, x_n)$ on this face. A solution trajectory must have this direction, and if the vector points into $\mathbf{R}^n_+$, the trajectory cannot leave $\mathbf{R}^n_+$. Thus, to show that $\mathbf{R}^n_+$ is positively invariant it suffices to show that the direction field points inward on the boundary of $\mathbf{R}^n_+$. For example, consider (2.1). On the face $S = 0$, we have $\dot{S} = (b + g)R + pb'I$, which is positive except when $R = I = 0$, so that the vector field points inward. On $R = 0$, $\dot{R} = cI > 0$. On the face $I = 0$, we have $\dot{I} = 0$ and the situation is not as clear. However, it can be seen from the equations (2.1) with $I = 0$ that there is a trajectory through each point in the $R, S$ plane face, which remains in that face for $t \geq 0$. Since two trajectories cannot intersect, by the uniqueness theorem for solutions, we see that a trajectory starting from $\mathbf{R}^3_+$ with $I > 0$ cannot touch the $R, S$ plane. Thus, the nonnegative orthant is positively invariant.

In general, the following holds. Suppose that $\Omega$ is a region in $\mathbf{R}^n$, and suppose that at each point $\mathbf{x}$ on the boundary of $\Omega$, the direction field vector $\mathbf{v} = \mathbf{f}(\mathbf{x})$ and the inward normal vector $\mathbf{n}$ have nonnegative inner product, $\mathbf{v} \cdot \mathbf{n} \geq 0$. Then $\Omega$ is invariant for (2.70).

### 2.16.2 Equilibria and Stability Analysis

In analyzing a system of the form (2.70), often the first step is to determine whether there are *steady states*, or *equilibria*. An equilibrium is a constant vector $\overline{\mathbf{x}}$ (i.e., $x_i = \overline{x}_i$, $i = 1, \cdots, n$ are constant) that satisfies the equations. Since this solution is constant, it may be found by solving the equations

$$0 = f_1(\overline{x}_1, \cdots, \overline{x}_n),$$
$$\cdots \tag{2.72}$$
$$0 = f_n(\overline{x}_1, \cdots, \overline{x}_n).$$

A set of values $(\overline{x}_1, \cdots, \overline{x}_n)$ that satisfy (2.72) represents a system state such that if the system is in that state at some time $t_1$, it will remain in that state for all $t \geq t_1$, in the absence of external disturbance.

The effects that disturbances have on an equilibrium are important since they determine whether or not the steady state will persist under the inevitable perturbations that occur in any real situation that is being modelled. Hence, it is necessary to distinguish between stable and unstable equilibria in order to describe the behavior of a solution trajectory that starts, at some time $t = t_0$, near an equilibrium point. This may be accomplished by using linearized analysis, which we now describe restricting ourselves to the case $n = 2$, in order to keep the notation simple. The extension to higher dimensions is direct and will be discussed later. For $n = 2$, equations (2.70) are

$$\frac{dx_1}{dt} = f_1(x_1, x_2),$$
$$\frac{dx_2}{dt} = f_2(x_1, x_2). \tag{2.73}$$

If $(x_1(t), x_2(t))$ is a solution of this system for $t \geq 0$ such that $(x_1(0), x_2(0))$ is near an equilibrium $(\overline{x}_1, \overline{x}_2)$, we may define

$$y_1(t) = x_1(t) - \bar{x}_1, \quad y_2(t) = x_2(t) - \bar{x}_2.$$

Then

$$\frac{dy_1}{dt} = f_1(\bar{x}_1 + y_1(t), \bar{x}_2 + y_2(t)),$$

$$\frac{dy_2}{dt} = f_2(\bar{x}_1 + y_1(t), \bar{x}_2 + y_2(t)).$$

Assuming that the functions $f_1$ and $f_2$ are sufficiently differentiable, these expressions can be expanded in Taylor series:

$$f_1(\bar{x}_1 + y_1, \bar{x}_2 + y_2) = f_1(\bar{x}_1, \bar{x}_2) + a_{11}y_1 + a_{12}y_2$$
$$+ \frac{1}{2}(b_{11}y_1^2 + 2b_{12}y_1y_2 + b_{13}y_2^2) + \cdots,$$

$$f_2(\bar{x}_1 + y_1, \bar{x}_2 + y_2) = f_2(\bar{x}_1, \bar{x}_2) + a_{21}y_1 + a_{22}y_2$$
$$+ \frac{1}{2}(b_{21}y_1^2 + 2b_{22}y_1y_2 + b_{23}y_2^2) + \cdots$$

and since $y_1(t)$ and $y_2(t)$ are assumed to be small displacements from the equilibrium, we drop the terms of degree two or higher and consider the linear parts of these equations. Since $(\bar{x}_1, \bar{x}_2)$ is an equilibrium, $f_1(\bar{x}_1, \bar{x}_2) = f_2(\bar{x}_1, \bar{x}_2) = 0$, and since $a_{11}, a_{12}$, etc., are given by partial derivatives of the $f_i$ evaluated at $(\bar{x}_1, \bar{x}_2)$, we obtain the approximate linear equations

$$\frac{dy_1}{dt} = a_{11}y_1 + a_{12}y_2,$$
$$\frac{dy_2}{dt} = a_{21}y_1 + a_{22}y_2, \tag{2.74}$$

where

$$J = \begin{pmatrix} a_{11} & a_{12} \\ a_{21} & a_{22} \end{pmatrix} = \begin{pmatrix} \frac{\partial f_1}{\partial x_1}(\bar{x}_1, \bar{x}_2) & \frac{\partial f_1}{\partial x_2}(\bar{x}_1, \bar{x}_2) \\ \frac{\partial f_2}{\partial x_1}(\bar{x}_1, \bar{x}_2) & \frac{\partial f_2}{\partial x_2}(\bar{x}_1, \bar{x}_2) \end{pmatrix}$$

is the *Jacobian matrix* of system (2.73), evaluated at $(\bar{x}_1, \bar{x}_2)$. System (2.74) is called the *linearization* of (2.73) near $(\bar{x}_1, \bar{x}_2)$.

The behavior of solutions of (2.74) is determined by the eigenvalues of $J$, which are the roots $\lambda$ of the algebraic (quadratic) equation

$$\det(J - \lambda I) = 0. \tag{2.75}$$

If both roots of (2.75) are negative or are complex with negative real parts, then every solution of (2.74) has the property that $y_1(t) \to 0$ and $y_2(t) \to 0$ as $t \to +\infty$. In that case it can be rigorously proved that any solution of (2.73) with initial value sufficiently close to $(\bar{x}_1, \bar{x}_2)$ will tend to $(\bar{x}_1, \bar{x}_2)$ as $t \to +\infty$, at an exponential rate. Then $(\bar{x}_1, \bar{x}_2)$ is said to be a (locally) *asymptotically stable* equilibrium of (2.73). If one or both eigenvalues are positive or have positive real parts, then most solutions of (2.74) become unboundedly large as $t \to +\infty$ and consequently most solutions of (2.73) do not remain near $(\bar{x}_1, \bar{x}_2)$, even if they start very close. In this case, $(\bar{x}_1, \bar{x}_2)$ is said to be *unstable*. Finally, if both eigenvalues have zero real parts (that is, are zero or pure imaginary) this does not provide sufficient information to decide whether $(\bar{x}_1, \bar{x}_2)$ will be stable or unstable for the nonlinear system (2.73).

If $n$ is greater than 2, the same method applies but the Jacobian will be an $n \times n$ matrix in which $a_{ij}$ is the derivative of $f_i$ with respect to $x_j$, evaluated at the equilibrium $\bar{x}$, and equation (2.75) will be a polynomial equation of degree $n$. The condition for local asymptotic stability is that all eigenvalues of $J$ have negative real parts.

It should be pointed out that local asymptotic stabilty of an equilibrium does not mean that all solutions tend to it as $t \to +\infty$, only that solutions which at some time are near-by to the equilibrium do so. A given system may have several equilibria, some stable and some unstable, and in addition there can be other important types of solutions such as periodic solutions or unbounded solutions. Some of the possibilities are explored in the sections that follow. Hence, knowledge of the local stability of all of the equilibria does not provide a complete picture of the dynamic behavior of the system. In fact, if the regions of attraction of the stable equilibria are small, then this local information may be of very little import in explaining the typical behavior of the situation that the equations are modeling. We stress this fact because the majority of the stability analyses that have been made in biomathematical models are restricted to local stability. Care should be taken in interpreting such results, as was illustrated in one of the cases of the model we treated in Sections 2.3 and 2.4.

It is at times necessary to examine the properties of other subsets of the space which have invariance and stability properties. The individual solution orbits on these sets may be unstable, however, the set as a whole may still attract all nearby solutions, or even all possible solutions. We illustrate this notion with the following simple linear example.

$$\frac{dx_1}{dt} = -x_1, \quad \frac{dx_2}{dt} = 0, \quad \frac{dx_3}{dt} = x_2,$$

whose solution with initial data $(x_{01}, x_{02}, x_{03})$ is

$$x_1(t) = x_{01}e^{-t}, \quad x_2(t) = x_{02}, \quad x_3(t) = x_{03} + x_{02}t.$$

The set $S = \{(0, y_2, y_3) : y_2, y_3 \in \mathbf{R}\} \subset \mathbf{R}^3$, is stable in the sense that any solution tends to $S$ as $t \to \infty$. However, individual solutions whose orbits make up this invariant set may tend to infinity as $t$ increases. This type of behavior occurs with nonlinear systems of the form (2.71) as well, and we define an *integral set* for such a system to be a subset of $\mathbf{R}^n$ consisting of solution orbits. Such a set is a *stable integral set* if for every open set $U$ containing $S$ (we call such an open set *a neighborhood of S*) there exists a neighborhood $V \subset U$ of $S$ with the property that any solution of (2.71) which satisfies $\mathbf{x}(t_0) \in V$ for some $t_0$, remains in $U$ for all $t \in \mathbf{R}$, that is, $\mathbf{x}(t) \in U$. The set is *asymptotically stable* if it is stable and it has a neighborhood $U$ such that $\mathbf{x}(t) \to S$ as $t \to \infty$ for solutions with $\mathbf{x}(t_0) \in U$ for some $t_0$. It is globally asymptotically stable if it is asymptotically stable and the set $U$ which it attracts is the whole space

$\mathbf{R}^n$. An *unstable set* is an integral set which is not stable. In the above simple example, S is an integral set which is globally asymptotically stable, and it is two dimensional. Such integral sets of dimension lower than that of the whole space play an important role in the study of the global behavior of solutions.

In the special case of $\mathbf{R}^2$, an integral set which has dimension one can separate the space into two regions which have the useful property that the points of one of these regions cannot be joined to the points of the other region by a solution of the system (2.73). The term *separatrix* is sometimes used to describe such a set. We have exploited this property in Sections 2.3 and 2.4 when studying the global behavior of the solutions of the model we considered there. This separation property has appropriate generalizations to systems in $\mathbf{R}^n$ for $n > 2$, which we shall not consider here.

### 2.16.3 Global Stability in One and Two Dimensions

The method of linearized stability analysis cannot by itself provide an overview or "global" picture of the behavior of all solutions. In fact, not all trajectories tend to an equilibrium point. For example, a system of differential equations can have a periodic solution, that is a solution such that $x_i(t + p) = x_i(t)$ for all $t$ and $i = 1, 2, \cdots, n$, where $p$ is a fixed non-zero constant called the *period* of the solution. Such a solution is represented in the space $\mathbf{R}^n$ by a closed curve, because the trajectory starting at $x_i(0)$ returns to this point after time $p$. The closed curve is often called a *limit cycle* if it attracts a trajectory that contains some point which does not lie on the limit cycle.

When $n = 2$, so that the trajectories lie in a plane, a knowledge of all equilibria and all limit cycles provides the basis for a complete description of the trajectories. When $n = 1$, the situation is yet simpler since knowledge of the equilibria and their local stability also gives the global stability of the system. We first explain the one dimensional case where we are dealing with a single equation. Since the function $f$ in (2.71) is assumed to be continuous, it can change sign only by going through one of its zeros, that is, through one of the equilibria of the differential equation. Hence, when $f$ has only isolated zeros (which is the only case we need to consider here), $f$ is either uniformly positive or uniformly negative between any two successive equilibria. Since $f(x)$ is equal to the derivative of $x$, the solution of (2.71) is either monotone increasing or monotone decreasing in any such interval. Thus the condition $f'(x_0) < 0$, for local asymptotic stability of an equilibrium $x_0$, is seen to also guarantee global stability of the equilibrium in the largest open interval that contains it and that contains no other equilibrium. We have exploited this simple fact in the global stability analysis of one of the models of Section 2.13.1 and in the models of Sections 2.13.2 and 2.13.3.

To explain the situation for $n = 2$, we introduce a few terms. Let $x_1(t), x_2(t)$ be a solution, let $t_n$ be a sequence of real numbers such that $t_n \to +\infty$ as $n \to \infty$, and let $P_n$ be the point $(x_1(t_n), x_2(t_n))$. If $P_n$ converges to a point $P$ in the plane, then $P$ is said to be an $\omega$ *limit point* of the trajectory $(x_1(t), x_2(t))$. The set of all such points $P$ is called the $\omega$ *limit set* of

$(x_1(t), x_2(t))$. Similarly, if $P_n$ converges to $P$ as $t_n \to -\infty$, then $P$ is called an $\alpha$ *limit point* of the trajectory; the set of all $\alpha$ limit points is the $\alpha$ *limit set*. If a trajectory $(x_1(t), x_2(t))$ lies in a bounded set for $t \geq 0$, its $\omega$ limit set is nonempty, closed, bounded, and connected. The following well-known theorem is fundamental.

**Poincaré-Bendixson Theorem.** *Suppose that $S$ is a bounded invariant set for a two-dimensional system* (2.73), *with $f_1$ and $f_2$ continuously differentiable, and suppose that $S$ contains a finite number of equilibrium points. Let $\Lambda$ be a trajectory that begins in $S$ at $t = 0$. Then one of the following must hold:* (i) *$\Lambda$ is a periodic orbit;* (ii) *the $\omega$ limit set $\Lambda^+$ of $\Lambda$ is a periodic orbit, or* (iii) *$\Lambda^+$ contains equilibria of the system.*

Another useful result, which is part of the background of the above theorem, is the following.

(iv) *Every periodic trajectory of a two-dimensional system contains an equilibrium point in its interior.*

Because of the above result, if periodic orbits can be ruled out in an invariant set $S$, then the global behavior of the solutions in $S$ can be determined by studying the stability of the equilibria of (2.73). Fortunately, for $n = 2$, there is a simple method, described in the following result, which can sometimes be used to show that there are no periodic orbits in a region.

**Bendixson-Dulac Criterion.** *Suppose that there is a continuously differentiable function $g(x_1, x_2)$ defined on a simply connected region $S$ and suppose that*

$$\frac{\partial}{\partial x_1}[g(x_1, x_2) f_1(x_1, x_2)] + \frac{\partial}{\partial x_2}[g(x_1, x_2) f_2(x_1, x_2)]$$

*does not change sign in $S$. Then there are no periodic solutions in $S$.*

A useful generalization of the above result is the following special case of the criterion of Busenberg and van den Driessche [1990].

**Theorem 2.5** *Let $\mathbf{f} : \mathbf{R}^3 \to \mathbf{R}^3$ be continuously differentiable and let $\gamma(t)$ be a closed, piecewise smooth curve which is the boundary of an orientable smooth surface $S \in \mathbf{R}^3$. Suppose that $\mathbf{g} : \mathbf{R}^3 \to \mathbf{R}^3$ is defined and smooth in a neighborhood of $S$, and that it satisfies*

$$\mathbf{g}(\gamma(t)) \cdot \mathbf{f}(\gamma(t)) = 0 \text{ for all } t,$$

*and*

$$(\text{curl } \mathbf{g}) \cdot \mathbf{n} > 0 \text{ (or else } < 0) \text{ on } S,$$

*where $\mathbf{n}$ is the unit normal to $S$. Then $\gamma(t)$ is not a periodic solution, nor the finite union of solution trajectories traversed in one sense relative to $\mathbf{n}$, of the differential equation system $d\mathbf{x}/dt = \mathbf{f}(\mathbf{x})$.*

These theorems were employed in Sections 2.5, 2.10 and 2.14 in the following way, which is fairly typical of the method for establishing the global results described in those sections. We found an invariant set in the $(I, P)$ plane (or on a planar set, in Section 2.14) containing the feasible equilibrium $(I^*, P^*)$ and no other equilibrium point. Also, by using the Bendixson-Dulac Criterion or the generalization of Busenberg and van den Driessche, we showed that there were no periodic solutions in this region. Then (i) and (ii) in the Poincaré-Bendixson Theorem were ruled out, so (iii) had to hold. Since we had shown that there was only one equilibrium point in the invariant set, it followed that every trajectory starting in the set approached $(I^*, P^*)$ as $t \to +\infty$.

### 2.16.4 General Global Stability

For higher dimensional nonlinear systems, that is, systems with more than two differential equations, the Poincaré-Bendixson Theorem is not valid, and in fact, much more complicated dynamical behavior is possible than occurs in two dimensions. Consequently, it is much harder to obtain a global analysis of the system. One method that can sometimes be profitably applied, and which we used in Sections 2.8, 2.9 and 2.11, is called Liapunov's second method and will be described here. It depends on constructing or inventing a function, called a Liapunov or energy function, which is a measure of how "far" a solution is from an equilibrium point. If this measure decreases as we follow a trajectory, then under certain hypotheses we can conclude that the trajectory must be attracted to the equilibrium point. We now give a more precise description of this idea.

Consider a system (2.71) where $\mathbf{x} = (x_1, \cdots, x_n)$ is a vector and $\mathbf{f}(\mathbf{x}) = (f_1(\mathbf{x}), \cdots, f_n(\mathbf{x}))$ is a vector of functions that are defined and continuously differentiable in an open set $G^*$ in $\mathbf{R}^n$ and $G \subset G^*$. Let $V : G \to \mathbf{R}$ be a real-valued function that is continuously differentiable on $G$. The function $V$ is called a Liapunov function for (2.71) on $G$ if the function $\dot{V}(\mathbf{x})$ defined by $\dot{V}(\mathbf{x}) = (\mathrm{grad} V(\mathbf{x})) \cdot \mathbf{f}(\mathbf{x})$ is nonpositive for $\mathbf{x} \in G$. Here $\mathrm{grad} V(\mathbf{x})$ denotes the vector

$$\mathrm{grad} V(\mathbf{x}) = \left( \frac{\partial V}{\partial x_1}, \cdots, \frac{\partial V}{\partial x_n} \right). \tag{2.76}$$

The reason for introducing the function $\dot{V}$ is that if $\mathbf{x}(t)$ is a solution of the system (2.71) and if we let $v(t) = V(\mathbf{x}(t))$, then by the chain rule $dv/dt = \mathrm{grad} V(\mathbf{x}(t)) \cdot (d\mathbf{x}/dt) = \mathrm{grad} V(\mathbf{x}(t)) \cdot \mathbf{f}(\mathbf{x}(t))$, hence, $\dot{V}(\mathbf{x}) \le 0$ on $G$ implies that $v(t)$ is decreasing. A number of theorems relating stability to the properties of Liapunov functions have been proved by Liapunov and subsequent authors. The following, called the La Salle Invariance Principle, is very useful. In the statement of the theorem we use the notation $\overline{G}$ to denote the closure of the set $G$, that is, $\overline{G}$ is the union of the points in $G$ and those on the boundary of $G$. The symbol $V^{-1}(c)$ means the set consisting of all the points $\mathbf{x}$ such that $V(\mathbf{x}) = c$. Finally, by an *invariant* set $M$ we mean a set of points such that any solution of $\mathbf{x}(t)$ of (2.70) with $\mathbf{x}(t_0)$ belonging to $M$, has the property that $\mathbf{x}(t)$ is also in $M$ for all $t \in (-\infty, \infty)$.

**The La Salle Invariance Principle.** *Let $V$ be a Liapunov function on a region $G$. Let $E = \{\mathbf{x} : \dot{V}(\mathbf{x}) = 0, \mathbf{x} \in \overline{G} \cap G^*\}$ and let $M$ be the largest invariant set in $E$. Then every trajectory that is bounded and remains in $G$ for $t \geq 0$ tends to the set $M \cap V^{-1}(c)$ as $t \to +\infty$, for some constant $c$.*

A useful special case of the above theorem is contained in the following corollary.

**Corollary 2.6** *If $\overline{\mathbf{x}}$ is an isolated equilibrium point lying in $G$, if $\dot{V}(\overline{\mathbf{x}}) = 0$ and $\dot{V}(\mathbf{x}) < 0$ for all $\mathbf{x} \in G$ except $\mathbf{x} = \overline{\mathbf{x}}$, then $\overline{\mathbf{x}}$ is asymptotically stable and attracts every trajectory that is bounded and remains in $G$ for $t \geq 0$.*

If one is able to choose a bounded set $G$ which is positively invariant (trajectories starting in $G$ remain in $G$), then under the conditions of the Corollary, $G$ is a "basin of attraction" for $\overline{\mathbf{x}}$. In biological problems, $G$ is usually a subset of the nonnegative orthant $\mathbf{R}_+^n$. The difficulty in applying Liapunov's method lies in having to find a suitable function $V$ and a region $G$. However, the structure of some of the equations of population dynamics allows the construction of a special Liapunov function $V$ leading to a useful method for establishing global stability results, as explained in the following section.

### 2.16.5 A Special Global Stability Result

For several of the models presented in this chapter, it is possible to prove global stability of an equilibrium within the class of feasible (non-negative) solutions. When such a result is available, it unambiguously defines the asymptotic behavior of the solution and thus the ultimate future of the epidemic.

A general procedure for obtaining such global asymptotic stability results for many epidemic systems can be based on a result established by Beretta and Capasso [1986] which relies on the use of a special Liapunov function constructed by Goh [1977, 1978]. We shall describe this method here, and give the auxiliary results that are needed to apply it to models with vertical transmission. The systems considered by Beretta and Capasso have the form

$$\frac{d\mathbf{z}}{dt} = \text{diag}(\mathbf{z})(\mathbf{e} + A\mathbf{z}) + \mathbf{b}(\mathbf{z}) \qquad (2.77)$$

where $\mathbf{z}(t) \in \mathbf{R}^n$, $\mathbf{e} \in \mathbf{R}^n$ is a constant vector, $A$ is an $n \times n$ constant matrix, and $\text{diag}(\mathbf{z})$ is the diagonal matrix with diagonal entries $z_i$. Also

$$\mathbf{b}(\mathbf{z}) = \mathbf{c} + B\mathbf{z} \qquad (2.78)$$

where $\mathbf{c} \in \mathbf{R}_+^n$ is a constant non-negative vector and $B$ is a real constant matrix such that $b_{ij} \geq 0$ for all $i, j = 1, \cdots, n$ and $b_{ii} = 0$ for $i = 1, \cdots, n$.

Many classical epidemic models, as well as models in this book, have the form (2.77). It is assumed in the general discussion that the set

$$\{z \in \mathbf{R}_+^n \; : \; \sum_{i=1}^{n} z_i \leq 1\}$$

or the set

$$\{z \in \mathbf{R}_+^n \; : \; z_i \leq 1, i = 1, \cdots, n\}$$

is positively invariant. The symbol $\Omega^n$ or $\Omega_+^n$ will denote either of these. The hypothesis of the theorem of Beretta and Capasso involves the following definition.

**Definition.** *Let $C$ be a real $n \times n$ matrix. $C$ is called $W$-skew-symmetrizable if and only if there exists a positive diagonal real matrix $W$ such that $WC$ is a skew-symmetric matrix, that is, the entries $a_{ij}$ of $WC$ satisfy $a_{ij} = -a_{ji}$.*

**Definition.** *Let $C$ be a real $n \times n$ matrix. We say that $C$ is in the class $S_W$ if and only if there exists a positive diagonal real matrix $W$ such that $WC + C^T W$ is negative definite. Here, $C^T$ denotes the transpose of $C$.*

Now suppose that (2.77) has an equilibrium $z^* = (z_1^*, \cdots, z_n^*)$, with $z_i^* > 0$ for $i = 1, \cdots, n$. Introduce the Liapunov function $V : \mathbf{R}_+^n \to \mathbf{R}_+$, defined by

$$V(z) = \sum_{i=1}^{n} W_i \left( z_i - z_i^* - z_i^* \ln \frac{z_i}{z_i^*} \right) \tag{2.79}$$

where the $W_i$ are the positive constant diagonal entries of the matrix $W$. It can then be easily seen that the derivative of $V(z)$ along solutions of (2.77) is

$$\dot{V}(z) = (z - z^*)^T W \, \mathrm{diag}(z)^{-1} \dot{z}$$

and further, using the equation satisfied by $z^*$, that

$$\dot{V}(z) = (z - z^*)^T W C (z - z^*), \tag{2.80}$$

where

$$C = \tilde{A} + \mathrm{diag} \left( -\frac{b_1(z)}{z_1 z_1^*}, \cdots, -\frac{b_n(z)}{z_n z_n^*} \right), \tag{2.81}$$

$$\tilde{A} = A + \mathrm{diag}(z^*)^{-1} B. \tag{2.82}$$

Since $\dot{V}(z)$ is a scalar, it is equal to its transpose, and we also have

$$2\dot{V}(z) = (z - z^*)^T (WC + C^T W)(z - z^*). \tag{2.83}$$

The analysis of stability now uses the La Salle Invariance Principle we stated in the previous section.

Two cases will be considered. In the first, assume

(a) $\tilde{A}$ is $W$-skew-symmetrizable. In this case, associate with $\tilde{A}$ a graph according to the following rules.

(i) Each component $z_i$ of $\mathbf{z}$ is represented by a labeled node,

$$\hat{i} \quad \text{if} \quad b_i(\mathbf{z}) \equiv 0, \quad \text{and} \quad i^{\bowtie} \quad \text{otherwise},$$

(ii) Each pair of elements $\tilde{a}_{ij}$, $\tilde{a}_{ji}$ (the product $\tilde{a}_{ij}\tilde{a}_{ji}$ is negative because $\tilde{A}$ is $W$-skew-symmetrizable) is represented by an arc connecting nodes "$i$" and "$j$".

The following result, which is due to Goh [1977, 1978], is needed.

**Lemma 2.7** *Assume that $\tilde{A}$ is $W$-skew-symmetrizable. If the associated graph is either: a tree and $p - 1$ of the $p$ terminal nodes are $\bowtie$; or a chain and two consecutive internal nodes are $\bowtie$; or a cycle and two consecutive nodes are $\bowtie$, then the largest invariant set $M$ for system (2.77) with $V(\mathbf{z})$ given by (2.79) is $M = \{\mathbf{z}^*\}$.*

In the second case, assume

(b) The matrix $C$ defined by (2.81) is in class $S_W$. Then the following theorem holds.

**Theorem 2.8** *If system (2.77) has a positive equilibrium $\mathbf{z}^*$ in $\Omega^n$, and if (a) along with one of the conditions in Lemma 2.7, or else if (b) holds, then the equilibrium $\mathbf{z}^*$ is globally asymptotically stable within $\Omega_+^n$. The uniqueness of $\mathbf{z}^*$ within $\Omega_+^n$ follows from its global asymptotic stability.*

This theorem has been applied to the models in Sections 2.8, 2.9 and 2.11. The following lemma proved by Grabiner [1988] was useful in applying this theorem.

**Lemma 2.9** *A $2 \times 2$ matrix $C = \begin{pmatrix} a & b \\ c & d \end{pmatrix}$ satisfies Beretta and Capasso's condition (b), that is, $C$ is in class $S_W$, if and only if its diagonal elements are negative and its determinant is positive.*

### 2.16.6 Existence and Bifurcation of Periodic Solutions

Time periodic behavior in population dynamics is often associated with diurnal and seasonal fluctuations of the environment. However, there are many periodic phenomena which are not synchronized with environmental periodicities and which are caused by the nonlinear interactions of subpopulations. Such phenomena can be very complicated and, as we shall see in the next chapter, may even lead to dynamic behavior that can appear to be due to random fluctuations. Here we shall look at one of the simplest ways in which non-linearity can give rise to periodic behavior and describe a general result, called the Hopf bifurcation theorem, which has often been used to show that periodic solutions exist. In applying results of this type one is typically interested in the change of behavior of the system as some pertinent parameter is varied. In particular, one seeks to find thresholds for the parameter below which an equilibrium is asymptotically stable, and above which it becomes unstable and an oscillatory solution emerges. We start by describing this type of phenomenon in the two dimensional case $n = 2$, where it assumes its simplest form.

Consider (2.71) with $n = 2$, and written in the form

$$\frac{d\mathbf{x}}{dt} = \mathbf{f}(\mathbf{x}, \mu), \tag{2.84}$$

where we have explicitly shown one of the parameters, $\mu$, that enter in the equation. For example, $\mu$ could be the contact rate between the susceptible and infective individuals of the population, or else a birth or removal rate. Suppose that $\mathbf{x_0}$ is an equilibrium point of (2.84) for all $\mu$, and write (2.84) in the form

$$\frac{d\mathbf{x}}{dt} = A(\mu)\mathbf{x} + h(\mathbf{x}, \mu), \tag{2.85}$$

where $A(\mu)$ is the Jacobian matrix of $\mathbf{f}$ evaluated at the equilibrium $\mathbf{x_0} = (x_0, y_0)$. Here we are writing $\mathbf{x} = (x, y)$, in the traditional component form. Thus

$$A(\mu) = \begin{pmatrix} \frac{\partial f_1}{\partial x_1}(x_0, y_0, \mu) & \frac{\partial f_1}{\partial x_2}(x_0, y_0, \mu) \\ \frac{\partial f_2}{\partial x_1}(x_0, y_0, \mu) & \frac{\partial f_2}{\partial x_2}(x_0, y_0, \mu) \end{pmatrix} \tag{2.86}$$

Let us also assume that there is an invariant region $\mathcal{R}$ of $\mathbf{R}^2$ containing $\mathbf{x_0}$, and containing no other zeros of $\mathbf{f}(\mathbf{x}, \mu)$ for all values of $\mu$. Now, suppose that both eigenvalues of $A(\mu)$ have negative real parts when $\mu < 0$, are pure imaginary when $\mu = 0$, and have positive real parts when $\mu > 0$. Then, as we have seen before, $\mathbf{x_0}$ is asymptotically stable when $\mu < 0$ and unstable when $\mu > 0$. What is interesting here is what happens to solutions which start near $\mathbf{x_0}$ when $\mu > 0$. Clearly, they cannot tend to $\mathbf{x_0}$, and by the Poincaré-Bendixson theorem, they must then tend to some periodic orbit which lies in $R$. Thus the system has gone from a state where it had an asymptotically stable equilibrium at $\mathbf{x_0}$ to one where solutions starting near $\mathbf{x_0}$ approach an oscillatory state. We shall now give one version of a useful result which shows that this phenomenon of creation of periodic solutions occurs under fairly general conditions.

**Hopf Bifurcation Theorem.** *Suppose that $\mathbf{f} : \mathbf{R}^n \times \mathbf{R} \to \mathbf{R}^n$ is twice continuously differentiable, that $\mathbf{f}(\mathbf{x_0}, \mu) = 0$, for all $\mu$, $\mathbf{x_0}$ is an isolated zero of $\mathbf{f}$, that the Jacobian matrix $A(\mu)$ of $\mathbf{f}$ at $\mathbf{x_0}$ is stable for $\mu < 0$, and $A(0)$ has eigenvalues with negative real parts except for two pure imaginary eigenvalues $\pm i\omega$. Let $\lambda(\mu)$ be an eigenvalue of $A(\mu)$ with $\lambda(0) = i\omega$, and suppose that*

$$\frac{\partial \mathrm{Re}(\lambda(\mu))}{\partial \mu}\Bigg|_{\mu=0} > 0,$$

and that $\mathbf{x}_0$ is a locally asymptotically stable equilibrium of $d\mathbf{x}/dt = \mathbf{f}(\mathbf{x}, 0)$. Then there exists $\delta > 0$ such that for $0 < \mu < \delta$, the differential equation

$$\frac{d\mathbf{x}}{dt} = \mathbf{f}(\mathbf{x}, \mu), \tag{2.87}$$

has a periodic solution $\mathbf{x}(\mu, t)$, with period $p(\mu)$ and amplitude $r(\mu) = ||\mathbf{x}_0 - \mathbf{x}(\mu, t)||$, both continuous functions of $\mu$ and obeying $p(0) = 2\pi/\omega$, $r(0) = 0$.

This result is a special case of various more general theorems that bear the same name some of which are discussed and proved in Marsden and Mac-Cracken [1976], Hassard, Kazarinoff and Wan [1981], and Chow and Hale [1982]. The reader can consult Chapter 8 of the book of Edelstein-Keshet [1988] for a detailed description of this phenomenon in the context of biological models. Here we only note that this is a local result, in that it tells us what happens near the equilibrium, but does not give any information about the global behavior of the system. It is usually extremely difficult to obtain such global information in systems where periodic solutions exist and detailed numerical studies are often used to investigate the behavior of the system.

# 3 Difference Equations Models

## 3.1 Introduction

Difference equation formulations have been widely used for insect populations where generations can essentially be regarded as occurring at discrete time intervals. Insects are carriers of a variety of diseases for which they act as vectors, and some of these diseases are vertically transmitted in these insect populations. Several models using discrete dynamical systems have, consequently, been proposed for such situations. In this chapter we shall describe results that have been obtained using such discrete models.

We begin in the next section by presenting a difference equation model for the transmission of Keystone virus. Under some simplifying assumptions this model is completely analyzed and the effects of vertical transmission are seen quite clearly in the endemic threshold criteria that we derive. In Section 3.3 we present a difference equation model for the transmission of rickettsia in ticks. Here we concentrate on one striking aspect of vertical transmission, which is the cumulative effect of some pathogens as they are vertically transmitted through several generations. The mathematical analysis of this model can be carried to the point where the effects of the vertical transmission mechanism on the dynamics of the spread of the pathogen are explicitly seen. The lengthy proofs illustrate several useful mathematical techniques but can be skipped by readers who are mainly interested in the modeling and the epidemiological conclusions. The results in both of these sections are based on the work of Busenberg and Cooke [1982, 1988], Cooke and Busenberg [1982], and Woodson [1987]. In Section 3.4 we describe a difference equation model, due to Régnière [1984], for vertical transmission of diseases in insects. We present a new local stability analysis and describe some of the extensive numerical results that have been obtained for this model. In Section 3.5 we treat a hybrid model due to Busenberg and Cooke [1982] which combines both discrete and continuous dynamics. In this model there is a logistic control on the birth rates and it leads to a situation where the discrete part of the model has chaotic behavior which also drives the continuous part. We present the results of an extensive numerical study of the dynamics of this model and discuss some of the issues that they raise. We also discuss the phenomena that commonly occur in discrete time models and their implications in making epidemiological predictions. In particular we describe the interpretation of epidemiological data in the light of chaotic behavior as given by Schaffer [1985], Schaffer and Kot

[1985], and Schaffer, Ellner and Kot [1986]. In Section 3.6 we treat a variant of the model in Section 3.5 due to Grabiner [1988] with the logistic control in the death terms. Endemic threshold criteria are derived and a complete stability analysis is given. We conclude with a section describing the mathematical background used in the analysis of discrete time models.

## 3.2 A Model for the Transmission of Keystone Virus

Keystone virus is one of the California group of arboviruses. The word "arbovirus" or "arborvirus" has been introduced to indicate a virus that is borne by arthropods (see Simpson [1972]). This virus is vertically transmitted in the mosquito *Aedes atlanticus* and Fine and LeDuc [1978] formulated a mathematical model for its transmission based on field observations. This model was reformulated as a discrete dynamical system in Cooke and Busenberg [1982] and analyzed in Busenberg and Cooke [1988].

In order to derive the model equation, recall that female mosquitoes seek a blood meal as a source of protein before oviposition (laying eggs). The gonotrophic periods (periods between blood meals) are of the order of four to six days for these mosquitoes. In our model we keep track of only the female portion of the population. We introduce the following notation:

$B_k =$ prevalence rate of the virus among all ovipositing females emerging in the $k^{th}$ year, $0 \leq B_k \leq 1$. Thus $B_k$ is the fraction of eggs laid in the $k^{th}$ year that carry the virus.

$q =$ maternal vertical transmission rate, $0 \leq q \leq 1$. Consequently, $B_{k-1}q$ is the prevalence rate of infections among females emerging in the $k^{th}$ year.

$i =$ proportion of hereditarily infected mosquitoes that are infectious to vertebrates, $0 \leq i \leq 1$.

$n_k =$ average number of female mosquitoes per vertebrate host (ground squirrels or rabbits) at the time of the first blood meal in the $k^{th}$ year, $n_k \geq 1$.

$u =$ proportion of female mosquitoes surviving through one gonotrophic cycle, $0 \leq u \leq 1$.

$r =$ number of gonotrophic cycles in one year, $r \geq 1$.

$f =$ probability that a susceptible mosquito which feeds upon a viremic vertebrate will become infected, $0 \leq f \leq 1$.

$s =$ proportion of host animals, bitten by infectious mosquitoes, that become viremic, $0 \leq s \leq 1$.

$g =$ average number of eggs laid per female mosquito, $g \geq 1$.

We note that the term rate as used above does not denote a variable with dimension 1/time, but is commonly used for such proportionality coefficients in discrete models. At the beginning of the $k^{th}$ year, the prevalence rate of emerging females is $B_{k-1}q$, and the number of females is $n_k V$, where $V$ is the number of vertebrate hosts. Here we assume that $V$ is a constant. Hence, $B_{k-1}qi$ is the probability that a mosquito taking its first blood meal is infectious to vertebrates and $(1 - B_{k-1}qi)^{n_k}$ is the probability that none of the $n_k$ mosquitoes feeding on a vertebrate are infectious. We are making the plausible assumption that the feedings of individual mosquitoes on a particular vertebrate are independent random events. Thus,

$$1 - (1 - B_{k-1}qi)^{n_k}$$

is the probability that a susceptible vertebrate host will be fed upon by at least one infectious mosquito, and

$$s[1 - (1 - B_{k-1}qi)^{n_k}]$$

is the proportion of animals that become viremic after the first blood meal of mosquitoes emerging in the $k^{th}$ year. After this first blood meal the females will lay $n_k V g$ eggs, of which $n_k V g B_{k-1} q$ are deposited by infectious females. Assuming that surviving mosquitoes will take a second blood meal, there will be $u n_k V(1 - B_{k-1}q)$ surviving susceptible females each of which engorge on one animal with probability

$$h_k = fs[1 - (1 - B_{k-1}qi)^{n_k}]$$

of acquiring the infection. So, the number of new horizontally acquired infections will be $u n_k V(1 - B_{k-1}q)h_k$. Also, there are $u n_k V B_{k-1} q$ remaining infected mosquitoes, so the prevalence rate among mosquitoes after the second blood meal is

$$B_{k-1}q + (1 - B_{k-1}q)h_k,$$

and this is the prevalence rate among ovipositing females at this time. If there are only two gonotrophic cycles, the overall prevalence rate among females depositing eggs would now be

$$\frac{B_{k-1}q + [B_{k-1}q + (1 - B_{k-1}q)h_k]u}{1 + u}.$$

So, the prevalence rate satisfies the difference equation

$$
\begin{aligned}
B_k &= \frac{1}{1+u}\{B_{k-1}q + uB_{k-1}q \\
&\quad + u(1 - B_{k-1}q)fs[1 - (1 - B_{k-1}qi)^{n_k}]\} \\
&= qB_{k-1} + \frac{ufs}{1+u}(1 - qB_{k-1})[1 - (1 - qiB_{k-1})^{n_k}].
\end{aligned}
\tag{3.1}
$$

Equation (3.1) is the difference equation governing the dynamics of this disease.

Under certain simplifying assumptions a difference equation can be derived when there are more than two gonotrophic cycles. In particular, if, following Fine and LeDuc [1978], we assume that at the second and subsequent blood meals no additional infection is transferred to the vertebrates, and that in the third and subsequent blood meals a negligible amount of new infection is transferred horizontally to the mosquitoes, then if there are $r$ gonotrophic cycles in all, we obtain the following difference equation for $B_k$:

$$B_k = qB_{k-1} + R(1 - qB_{k-1})[1 - (1 - qiB_{k-1})^{n_k}] \qquad (3.2)$$

where

$$R = \frac{u + \cdots + u^{r-1}}{1 + u + \cdots + u^{r-1}} fs = \frac{fsu(1 - u^{r-1})}{(1 - u^r)} \qquad (3.3)$$

can be interpreted as the net horizontal transmission probability. From the first part of (3.3) it is seen that $0 \leq R < 1$. Note that this horizontal transmission of the disease in the mosquito population occurs with the viremic vertebrates acting as vector carriers for the susceptible mosquitoes engorging on them. Clearly, the right hand side of (3.2) is less than $qB_{k-1} + R(1 - qB_{k-1})$ which is less than 1 if $B_{k-1} < 1/q$. In particular, this is so if $B_{k-1} \leq 1$ since $q < 1$. So, the difference equation (3.2) is well-posed in that it maps the interval $[0, 1]$ into itself.

We now discuss the case when $n_k = n$ is constant. Here, the right hand side of (3.2) can be seen to have a negative second derivative with respect to $B$, and consequently, as will be shown later, one can conclude that (3.2) has the steady states

$$B = 0 \quad \text{and,} \quad \text{if} \;\; T = q(inR + 1) > 1, \;\; B = \bar{B} > 0.$$

The trivial steady state is locally asymptotically stable when $T < 1$, and by the convexity of the r.h.s. of (3.2) it is globally asymptotically stable in the set $B \in [0, 1]$ when $T < 1$. When $T > 1$, $B = 0$ loses its stability and the feasible state $B = \bar{B} > 0$ appears. We note that the condition $T < 1$ incorporates the role of vertical transmission in destabilizing the zero steady state and maintaining an endemic level of infection through the maternal vertical transmission parameter $q$, and the proportion $i$ of vertically infected mosquitoes that are infectious to vertebrates. If $q$ is close enough to zero, $q < 1/[1 + infsu\frac{1-u^{r-1}}{1-u^r}]$, the disease dies out in the mosquito population ($B = 0$ is stable). Even though the steady state $\bar{B} > 0$ cannot be explicitly computed when $n > 4$, its stability can be deduced. In order to illustrate this, first, consider the case when $n = 1$ which is, of course, biologically unimportant. Then the equation (3.2) becomes

$$B_k = q(1 + iR)B_{k-1}\left(1 - \frac{Rqi}{1 + iR}B_{k-1}\right). \qquad (3.4)$$

The nontrivial steady state in this case is

$$\bar{B} = \frac{(\alpha - 1)}{Rq^2i}, \quad \alpha = q(1 + iR), \qquad (3.5)$$

and it is seen to be stable whenever $\alpha > 1$, that is, whenever it is feasible. The proof in the general case will be presented below. The dynamic behavior of this model is described in the following result.

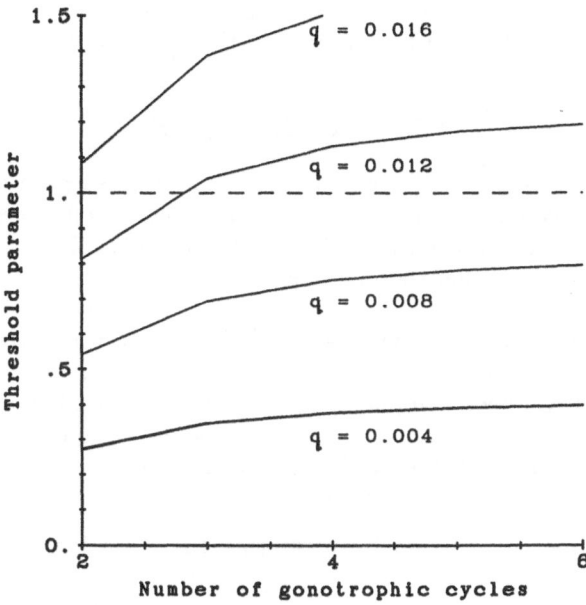

**Fig. 3.1.** Variation of the threshold parameter $T$

**Theorem 3.1** *Assume that $n_k = n$ is independent of $k$. That is, the average number of mosquitoes per vertebrate host at the first blood meal in the $k^{th}$ year is a constant independent of $k$. Then the prevalence rate of the disease in the mosquito population tends to zero as $k$ increases (the disease dies out) if $T < 1$, where*

$$T = q(inR + 1). \tag{3.6}$$

*The trivial steady-state is unstable, and the prevalence rate tends to a constant endemic level $\overline{B} \in (0, 1)$ if $T = q(inR + 1) > 1$.*

Before giving the proof of this result we note that the disease cannot be maintained in the mosquito population without the mechanism of vertical transmission (that is, if $q = 0$), or with weak vertical transmission. The threshold $T$ can be viewed as the *net reproduction factor* of the disease which is also denoted by $R_0$. It represents the total average number of new infectives that a single infective individual causes. In the absence of horizontal transmission ($f = 0$), the net horizontal transmission rate $R$ is equal to zero, and $T = q < 1$, so again the disease dies out. Hence, the maintenance of this infection requires a coupling of the horizontal and vertical transmission mechanisms. Finally, $T$ can be easily shown to be an increasing function of $r$, the number of gonotrophic cycles, and varies from the value $T = q + qinfsu/(1+u)$ when $r = 2$ to $T = q + qinsfu$ as $r \to \infty$. Consequently, the likelihood of the disease reaching an endemic level increases with the number of gonotrophic cycles. This is illustrated in the acompanying graph of $T$ versus $r$ and $q$ where we have taken $f = u = s = 0.5$,   $i = 0.8$ and $n = 1000$.

An interesting limit case occurs when we take $n \to \infty$ (the number of mosquitoes per vertebrate host is large). Here, the equation (3.2) becomes (since $(1 - qiB_{k-1})^n \to 0$),

$$B_k = q(1 - R)B_{k-1} + R, \tag{3.7}$$

a linear difference equation. It is easy to see that, in this case, the only equilibrium is $\overline{B} = R/[1 - q(1 - R)] > 0$ and that it is always globally asymptotically stable since $q$ and $R$ are between zero and one. This conclusion is also supported by the observation that $T \to \infty$ when $n \to \infty$.

*Remark.* The conclusions of Theorem 3.1 are valid for the biologically correct parameter ranges for this model. It is well known, of course, that the difference equation (3.4) can have complicated dynamic behavior when the parameters entering in this equation are not restricted by the assumptions pertinent to the present model. A brief discussion of this situation can be found in Section 3.7.4.

We conclude this section by presenting the main ideas of the proof of Theorem 3.1.

*Proof.* The steady-state solutions of (3.2) when $n_k = n$ is a constant, must satisfy

$$(1 - q)B = R(1 - qB)[1 - (1 - qiB)^n] \tag{3.8}$$

hence, $B = 0$ is one of the steady states. If $B \neq 0$, the right hand side of (3.8) has its first derivative equal to $qinR$ at $B = 0$, its second derivative is negative when $0 \leq B < 1$, and its value at $B = 1$ is less than $1 - q$. So, there is a unique solution of (3.8) in the interval $(0, 1]$, if and only if, $qinR > 1 - q$, and the nontrivial feasible equilibrium exists, if and only if, $T = q(inR + 1) > 1$.

Next, writing (3.2) with $n_k = n$ in the form $B_k = F(B_{k-1})$, we note that, if $0 \leq B \leq 1$, then by the earlier discussion, $0 \leq F(B) \leq 1$, so the dynamical system (3.2) maps the interval $[0, 1]$ onto itself. Computing the derivative of $F$ we conclude that $F'(B) > 0$ and $F''(B) < 0$ for $B \in [0, 1]$. Now, using the observations that $F'(0) = T$, and that $F$ is convex and monotone increasing on the interval $[0, 1]$, it can be shown that, if $T < 1$, then $B_k \to 0$ as $k \to \infty$, while if $T > 1$, then $B_k \to \overline{B}$ as $k \to \infty$. This completes the proof of Theorem 3.1. The details of the arguments supporting these conclusions are in Busenberg and Cooke [1988].

## 3.3 Population Size Control via Vertical Transmission

One of the striking characteristics of vertically transmitted diseases is the possible cumulative effect of the pathogen as it is passed down through several generations. This effect occurs when the pathogen dose that is transmitted by the parent increases as the pathogen load of the parent increases. Thus, vertically infected offspring of a parent with a large pathogen load commence their life with a relatively large load and may reach their reproductive age with a pathogen load that is larger than that of their infective parent. Consequently, the pathogen load may monotonically increase with the generation number of an infective lineage. In some cases, after several generations in an infective lineage, the pathogen load at birth may reach a high enough level to severely impede the reproductive capacity of that generation. As a result of this mechanism, vertical transmission can act as a means for controlling population size.

An example where this type of cumulative mechanism has been observed is *Rickettsia rickettsi* in the tick *Dermacentor andersoni*. This rickettsia causes Rocky Mountain Spotted Fever (RMSF) in humans and other vertebrates, and ticks are the primary vector carriers of the disease. Because of the significant mortality of humans who contract RMSF, there have been careful and extensive laboratory and field studies of this disease (Garvie *et al.* [1978], Burgdorfer [1975]). In this section we present a model due to Busenberg and Cooke [1982, 1988] for the dynamics of one aspect of the transmission of this disease based on the following observations:

(a) The rickettsia are vertically transmitted in the tick population with a transmission rate of about 50%.

(b) The level of the rickettsia load increases with each successive generation of vertically acquired infectivity.

(c) Female ticks of the fifth generation in a lineage of vertically acquired infection carry such a large load of the rickettsia that they cannot undergo successful oviposition and are sterile.

(d) Except for the fifth generation of infected female ticks, the infection does not appreciably affect the behavior of the ticks.

The ticks have discrete generations which depend on seasonal variations. They are active during the summer period (the length of this period varies with geographic latitude) and are dormant, in some stage or other of their development, during the winter months. In Sections 3.3.1 and 3.3.2 we shall discuss a more detailed model of the transmission of this disease, but here we restrict ourselves to modeling the net effects of rickettsia on the tick population size.

There are two basic discrete independent variables in this model. The first is the cohort number $n$ starting at some chosen time origin, and the second is an internal variable or label $\alpha$ that indicates the generation number in an infective lineage. This latter variable takes on the values $\{0, 1, 2, 3, 4, 5\}$, with 0 denoting ticks which have acquired the disease via horizontal transmission, 1 denoting those which have acquired the disease vertically from a parent of infective lineage 0, and so on, with 5 denoting ticks that are vertically infected by a parent of infective lineage 4, and hence, are infertile. We will allow the number of generations in an infected lineage to be an arbitrary variable $m \geq 1$. The basic variables in the model are denoted by:

$m =$ the number of generations in an infected lineage (m=5 in the presei model).

$n =$ the cohort number.

$\alpha =$ the generation number in an infective lineage of vertical transmissic $(\alpha = 0, 1, 2, \cdots, m)$.

$i_n(\alpha) =$ the number of infective ticks in the $n^{th}$ cohort who are of the $\alpha$ infective lineage.

$S_n =$ the number of susceptible ticks in the $n^{th}$ cohort.

$b =$ the birth rate of female ticks adjusted for the proportion of female male ticks in the population. This proportion is assumed to be constai in the model.

$q(\alpha) =$ the probability of a female tick of lineage $\alpha$ to vertically transmit tl infection to its offspring. Here $0 \leq q(\alpha) \leq 1$, and $q(m) = 0$.

$p(\alpha) =$ the probability of a female tick of lineage $\alpha$ to not vertically transm the infection to its offspring. $p(\alpha) = 1 - q(\alpha)$, for $\alpha = 0, 1, \ldots, m -$ and $p(m) = q(m) = 0$.

$d =$ the removal rate of ticks due to death or other causes. $d$ is assumed $t$ be a constant in the present model.

$c =$ the natural survival proportion, $c = 1/(1 + d)$.

$I_n =$ the total number $I_n = \sum_{\alpha=0}^{m} i_n(\alpha)$ of infective ticks in the $n^{th}$ cohor

$P_n = I_n + S_n$, the total number of ticks in the $n^{th}$ cohort.

All the above variables and parameters are non-negative. The rickettsia a transmitted among the ticks both vertically and horizontally. The horizont: transmission occurs when susceptible ticks either engorge on a vertebrate th; is viremic (because it has been infected by an infective tick engorging on it or else via contact with the feces of an infective tick while both the susceptib and infective tick are engorging on the same animal. The viremia induced t rickettsia on small mammals or deer, who are the main vertebrate hosts the ticks, lasts only two or three days. Hence, it is reasonable to assume th; the force of horizontal transmission is a monotone increasing function of tl number of infective and the number of susceptible ticks. This is so becaus the host population is sufficiently plentiful in most circumstances, and henc it does not represent a limiting resource.

In a discrete model, horizontal transmission which occurs over an extende time interval needs to be idealized as occurring at a synchronized specif. instant of time. Since we are following cohort groups which appear at tl beginning of a particular season, we distinguish between those ticks that a born with the infection and those that acquire it via horizontal transmissio We shall assume that the horizontally infective ticks in the $n^{th}$ cohort com from susceptible ticks of the $n^{th}$ cohort who are infected via contact wit infective ticks of the $(n-1)^{th}$ cohort, and not from the new infectives of the own cohort. This assumption allows for the maturation period of newbor infectives before they take their first blood meal, and also takes into accour the lapse of time that is necessary before the vertically acquired pathogen i newborn infectives is large enough to be effectively transmitted via horizont:

contacts. The models we shall present in the next three sections treat this horizontal transmission process more accurately.

The force of horizontal infection is given by $f/S_n$ where $f$ has the form

$$f(S_n, I_{n-1}) = f(S_n, \sum_{\alpha=0}^{m} i_{n-1}(\alpha)), \qquad (3.9)$$

with $f$ a monotone non-decreasing function of $S_n$ and $I_{n-1}$, $f(x,y) = 0$ if either $x = 0$ or $y = 0$, and $f(x,y) > 0$, if $x > 0$ and $y > 0$. If random contact between susceptible and infective ticks is assumed, then a typical form of $f$ would be given by the "mass-action" law

$$f(S_n, I_{n-1}) = kS_n I_{n-1} = kS_n \sum_{\alpha=0}^{m} i_{n-1}(\alpha), \qquad (3.10)$$

where $k$ is a constant transmission factor. Of course, other forms of $f$ may be appropriate in certain circumstances.

Denoting the number of generations of infected vectors by $m$ ($m=5$, in the above case), the dynamic equations of this model are easily derived and are:

$$i_n(0) = cf(S_n, I_{n-1}),$$

$$i_n(\alpha) = cbq(\alpha - 1)i_{n-1}(\alpha - 1), \quad \alpha = 1, 2, \ldots, m, \qquad (3.11)$$

$$S_n = cb \left( \sum_{\alpha=0}^{m-1} p(\alpha)i_{n-1}(\alpha) + S_{n-1} \right) - cf(S_n, I_{n-1}).$$

The above form of the equations does not yield an explicit expression for the vector $\mathbf{x}_n = (i_n(0), i_n(1), \ldots, i_n(m), S_n)$ in terms of $\mathbf{x}_{n-1}$ because the component $S_n$ occurs on the right hand side of the equations. However, since $f(S_n, I_{n-1})$ is monotone non-decreasing in $S_n$, we can rewrite the equation for $S_n$ in the form

$$S_n + cf(S_n, I_{n-1}) = cb \left( \sum_{\alpha=0}^{m-1} p(\alpha)i_{n-1}(\alpha) + S_{n-1} \right),$$

and solve this uniquely for $S_n$:

$$S_n = G \left( c, I_{n-1}, cb \sum_{\alpha=0}^{m-1} p(\alpha)i_{n-1}(\alpha) + cbS_{n-1} \right).$$

Once this expression for $S_n$ is substituted in the first equation in (3.11), we obtain an explicit dynamical system for the vector $\mathbf{x}_n$ in terms of $\mathbf{x}_{n-1}$. We also note that the monotonicity of $f$ implies that whenever $c, b, p(\alpha)$ and $i_{n-1}(\alpha)$ are non-negative, then $S_n = G(c, I_{n-1}, cb \sum_{\alpha=0}^{m-1} p(\alpha)i_{n-1}(\alpha) + cbS_{n-1})$ is also non-negative; and if $c > 0$ and $i_{n-1}(\alpha) > 0$ for some $\alpha$, then $S_n > 0$. This observation immediately implies the well-posedness of the model as given by

(3.11), in the sense that non-negative initial data for $n = 0$ lead to non-negative solutions for $n > 0$. The following result holds (see Section 3.7.1) for the system (3.11) without any further restrictions on the horizontal force of infection $f$.

**Theorem 3.2** *The model equations* (3.11) *preserve positivity in the sense that non-negative initial data yield non-negative solutions. Moreover, if the net reproduction rate cb obeys* $cb < 1$, *zero is the only feasible (non-negative) steady state and all solutions* $(i_n(\alpha), S_n)$ *tend to zero as* $n \to \infty$. *A necessary condition for the existence of a non-trivial feasible solution is that*

$$1 < cb < 1/R_p, \tag{3.12}$$

*where*

$$R_p = \sum_{\alpha=0}^{m-1} p(\alpha)r(\alpha), \tag{3.13}$$

$$r(0) = 1, \quad r(\alpha) = q(0) \cdots q(\alpha - 1)(bc)^\alpha.$$

We shall see below that the exact regions where an endemic equilibrium exists and is stable depend on the forms of the force of infection term, however, in all cases, the restriction implied by (3.12) must hold. Note that, in the absence of vertical transmission $(q = 0, \ p = 1)$, condition (3.12) cannot hold if $cb \neq 1$, and an endemic equilibrium does not exist. In fact, in this case, $i_n(\alpha) = 0$ for $n \geq 1$, $\alpha = 1, 2, \cdots, m$, and

$$S_n + I_n = P_n = cbP_{n-1}.$$

Hence, $P_n \to 0$ as $n \to \infty$ if $cb < 1$, and $P_n \to \infty$ if $cb > 1$. In the absence of horizontal transmission $(f = 0)$, $i_n(\alpha) = 0$ for $\alpha = 0, 1, \cdots, m$, and $P_n = S_n = cbS_{n-1}$, for $n \geq 2$. Again we have $P_n \to 0$ if $cb < 1$ and $P_n \to \infty$ if $cb > 1$. Thus a balanced population can exist only through the effects of the coupling of vertical and horizontal transmission. Of course, this model assumes that there are no environmental constraints to the growth of the tick population.

More detailed conclusions on this model can be obtained once the horizontal transmission force of infection $f$ is specified and we now study the case where $f$ is given by the mass-action law (3.10). We describe these results leaving the proofs to the end of this section. Defining

$$R = \sum_{\alpha=0}^{m} r(\alpha) \tag{3.14}$$

and computing the steady states of (3.11), we find that a feasible steady state exists, if and only if (3.12) holds, and this steady state is given by

$$\overline{S} = 1/ckR, \quad \overline{i}(0) = \overline{S}(cb - 1)/(1 - cbR_p), \quad \overline{i}(\alpha) = r(\alpha)\overline{i}(0), \tag{3.15}$$

where $R$, $R_p$ and $r(\alpha)$ are defined in (3.13) and (3.14 ). The complete stability situation of this steady state has not been determined in general; however, we shall present some numerical simulations which will show that the non-trivial steady-state given by (3.15) can be stable, and, hence, the total population is controlled by the vertical transmission mechanism. In the absence of this mechanism the total population satisfies the equation $P_{n+1} = cbP_n$, and hence, becomes unbounded whenever $cb > 1$.

A horizontal transmission law which exhibits a saturation tendency may be more appropriate in this model, and can take the form

$$f(S_n, I_{n-1}) = \frac{kS_n \sum_{\alpha=0}^{m} i_{n-1}(\alpha)}{k' + \sum_{\alpha=0}^{m} i_{n-1}(\alpha)}. \tag{3.16}$$

We now describe the results of Busenberg and Cooke [1988] on two general forms of $f$ which include those given by (3.10) and (3.16) as special cases. We use the following hypotheses to describe these forms of $f$.

(H$_1$)  $f(x,y)$ is a monotone increasing function of $x$ and $y$ with $f(x,y) = 0$ if either $x = 0$ or $y = 0$. Also, $f$ is continuously differentiable and $f_x(0,0) = f_y(0,0) = 0$.

(H$_2$)  $f$ satisfies (H$_1$) and $f(x,ax)/x$ is a convex function of $x$ for any constant $a > 0$.

(H$_3$)  $f$ satisfies (H$_1$) and $f(x,ax)/x$ is a concave monotone function of $x$ for every constant $a > 0$.

Note that if $f(x,ax)/x = g(x)$ has a second derivative $g''(x)$ then (H$_2$) requires $g''(x) \geq 0$ and (H$_3$) requires $g''(x) \leq 0$. The typical forms of the mass-action and the saturated mass-action forms of the force of infection which the above hypotheses generalize are shown in Fig. 3.2.

The following result from Busenberg and Cooke [1988] describes the behavior of this model when $q(a) = q =$ constant for $\alpha = 0, 1, \cdots, m-1$.

**Theorem 3.3** *Assume that $q(a) = q =$ constant for $\alpha = 0, 1, \cdots, m-1$. If $f$ satisfies hypothesis (H$_2$) then the conclusions of Theorem 3.2 hold and a non-trivial feasible equilibrium exists, if and only if, (3.12) holds (that is, $1 < cb < 1/R_p$). If $f$ satisfies (H$_3$) then the conclusions of Theorem 3.2 hold and:*
*(i) If $f(x, \lambda x)/x \to \infty$ as $x \to \infty$, where*

$$\lambda = \frac{(1 - (cbq)^{m+1})(1 - cb)}{(1 - cbq)(cbR_p - 1)},$$

*then a unique non-trivial equilibrium exists, if and only if, (3.12) holds.*
*(ii) If $f(x, \lambda x)/x \to K < \infty$, then a unique non-trivial equilibrium exists if, and only if, condition (3.12) holds and*

$$K > (1 - cb)/c(cbR_p - 1).$$

The proof of this result can be found in the original paper. Here we note that even though one can readily linearize (3.11) about the positive steady state, the resulting system, in the case $m = 5$, involves a $7 \times 7$ matrix whose stability cannot be easily determined. Numerical and analytical studies of the stability of this steady state have been made for several parameter ranges and for $f$ given by either (3.10) or (3.16). These results have shown that the non-trivial equilibrium is stable whenever it is feasible and $f$ has the form (3.16), while for $f$ given by (3.10), there is a parameter region where this equilibrium is feasible but unstable. When instability occurs, the numerical results show that a stable oscillatory solution exists and the subpopulations undergo bounded periodic variations. Figures 3.3 and 3.4 show the stability regions for these two forms of $f$.

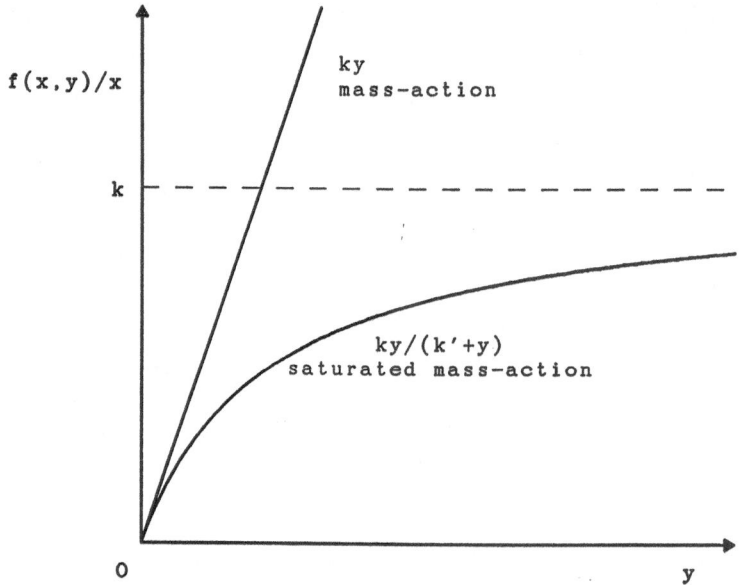

**Fig. 3.2.** The mass-action and saturated mass-action force of infection terms

There are several interesting results concerning the stability regions, the parameter ranges where the populations remain bounded and the nature of the periodic oscillations, which have been obtained in collaboration with James Woodson [1987], and which will be described in the following subsection.

### 3.3.1 Fine Structure of Population Size Control

The presence of sterile ticks in the model we have been considering causes some very interesting dynamic behavior: oscillatory solutions can occur. Moreover, the depressed birth rate due to the presence of sterile ticks may lead to the control of the size of the total population because of the presence of the disease, and it becomes important to determine the parameter regions where the disease can cause the population to remain bounded. We shall present a series

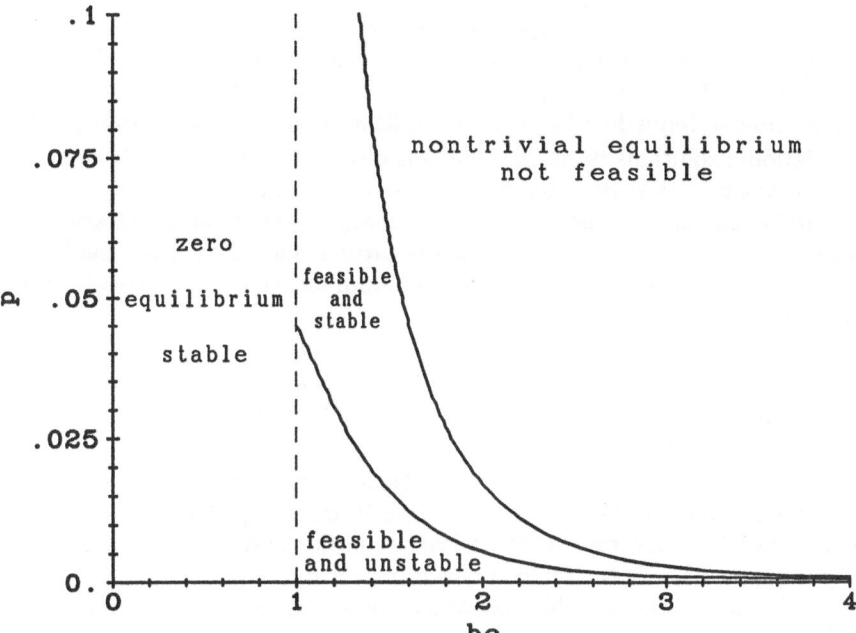

**Fig. 3.3.** Stability regions for $f = kSI$ (regions do not depend on $c$)

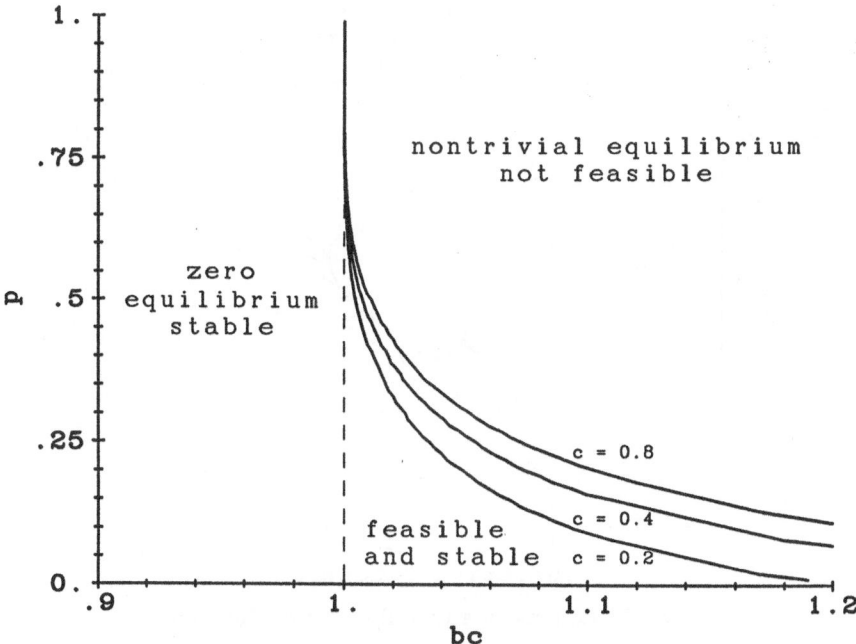

**Fig. 3.4.** Stability regions for $f = kSI/(k' + I)$

of results related to these questions with brief discussions of their significance. Throughout this section, we shall make the simplifying assumption that for $\alpha = 0, 1, \cdots, m-1$, $p(\alpha) = p$ is constant. The proofs of the simpler results are given immediately while the more complicated ones are in Section 3.3.2.

Periodic solutions in discrete models often occur in a specific sequence as the parameters that destabilize the steady state are varied. Particularly, at the first occurrence of such solutions for many widely studied equations, their period is equal to two. However, in the present model we have the following result, where we recall that $m$ is the maximum length of any vertically infected lineage.

**Theorem 3.4** *If $f(S, I) = kSI$ and $m$ is odd, then there are no feasible 2-periodic solutions of the model.*

Figure 3.5 shows an example of a typical periodic orbit which occurs in the case of a mass-action force of infection term. The periods of such solutions which have been observed in numerical simulations are typically large (at least of period seven), and the trajectories, at first sight, can appear to be irregular. We shall discuss the possible role of irregular trajectories in epidemic models in Section 3.5.1.

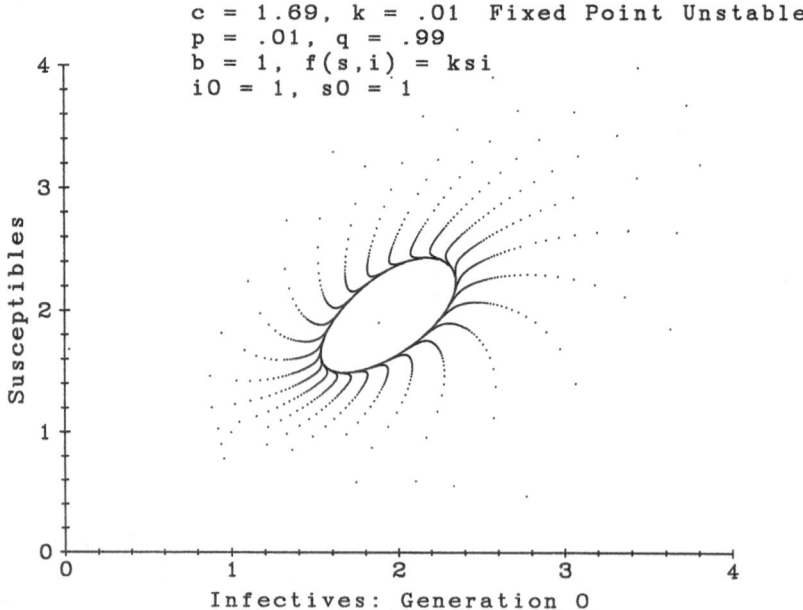

c = 1.69, k = .01   Fixed Point Unstable
p = .01, q = .99
b = 1, f(s,i) = ksi
i0 = 1, s0 = 1

**Fig. 3.5.** An example of a typical periodic solution for $f = kSI$

The next few results discuss the boundedness and growth rate of the population. Note that the specific form of the force of infection term does not play a role in these results. We do assume throughout this section that $f(S, 0) = 0$, that is, the rate of horizontal infection vanishes when there are no infectives present. Since $p$ and $q$ are assumed to be constant, and $\alpha$ ranges from 1 to $m$, the expression for the threshold $R_p$ becomes

$$R_p = p\frac{1 - (cbq)^m}{1 - cbq}.$$

**Theorem 3.5** *If $cbR_p > 1$ the total population is unbounded for all non-negative initial conditions such that $\sum_{\alpha=0}^{m-1} i_0(\alpha) + S_0 > 0$. Moreover, if $cbp > 1$, the total population is unbounded and grows at least as fast as $(cbp)^n$ as $n$ increases.*

*Proof.* Consider the case where $cbp > 1$. We have

$$i_{n+1}(0) + S_{n+1} = cb(p\sum_{\alpha=0}^{m-1} i_n(\alpha) + S_n) \geq cb(pi_n(0) + S_n) \geq cbp(i_n(0) + S_n).$$

Hence $i_n(0) + S_n$ grows at least as fast as $(cbp)^n$. Since $cbp > 1$, the population is unbounded, provided that $i_n(0) + S_n > 0$ for some n. We obtain this easily, however, since

$$i_1(0) + S_1 = cb(p\sum_{\alpha=0}^{m-1} i_0(\alpha) + S_0) > 0.$$

This proves the second part of the theorem. The proof of the first part is longer and is found in Section 3.3.2.

The next result relates the boundedness of the infective part of the population to the growth rate of the susceptible portion.

**Theorem 3.6** *If $cbR_p > 1$, and for some solution $I_n$ is bounded, then there is an integer, $N$, and a positive constant, $K$, (which depends on the initial conditions) such that*

$$S_n > K(cb)^n$$

*for all $n > N$, provided that the initial conditions obey $\sum_{\alpha=0}^{m-1} i_0(\alpha) + S_0 > 0$.*

An immediate corollary of the proof of the above is the following result which applies to bounded force of infection terms.

**Corollary 3.7** *If $f(S, I)$ is bounded and $cbR_p > 1$, then*

$$S_n > K(cb)^n$$

*for all orbits for which the initial conditions obey $\sum_{\alpha=0}^{m-1} i_0(\alpha) + S_0 > 0$.*

The next three results give details on the growth rates of the infected part of the population.

**Theorem 3.8** *If $cbR_p > 1$ and $\sum_{\alpha=0}^{m-1} i_0(\alpha) + S_0 > 0$ then there is an integer $N$, a positive constant $C$, and a constant $r > 1$ such that*

$$i_n(0) + S_n \geq Cr^n$$

*for all $n > N$.*

For specific forms of the force of infection, more detailed information is available, some of which we present in the next three results.

**Theorem 3.9** *If $cbR_p > 1$ and $f = kSI$ then for all initial conditions with $\sum_{\alpha=0}^{m-1} i_0(\alpha) + S_0 > 0$ we have $\lim_{n\to\infty} I_n = \infty$, and there is an integer $N_0$ such that for all $n > N_0$, $S_n < \frac{2b}{k}$. Hence,*

$$\lim_{n\to\infty} \frac{S_n}{P_n} = 0, \quad \text{and} \quad \lim_{n\to\infty} \frac{I_n}{P_n} = 1.$$

Thus, when the endemic threshold is exceeded in an increasing population with a mass-action force of infection, the proportion of the diseased part of the population tends to one. The proportion of susceptibles in the population tends to zero. A different behavior occurs when the force of infection is of the saturated mass-action type, as seen from the following result.

**Theorem 3.10** *If $cbR_p > 1$ and $f = \frac{kSI}{k'+I}$ then*

$$\lim_{n\to\infty} \frac{S_n}{S_n + i_n(0)} = \frac{1}{1 + ck} \quad \text{and} \quad \lim_{n\to\infty} \frac{i_n(0)}{S_n + i_n(0)} = \frac{ck}{1 + ck}.$$

**Theorem 3.11** *If $1 < cb < 1/R_p$, $f = \frac{kSI}{k'+I}$, and $S_n$ is bounded then $I_n$ is bounded.*

The threshold value $cbR_p = 1$ can be computed as a function of $cb$ and $p$, and in Fig. 3.6 we use this fact to illustrate graphically the results on the boundedness of solutions.

The final result concerns the mass-action force of infection terms and relates the stability of the steady state to the various coefficients of the model.

**Theorem 3.12** *The local stability of the steady state for $f = kSI$ and $1 < cb < \frac{1}{R_p}$ does not depend on the value of $k$; further, the stability of the steady state does not depend on $c$ or $b$ independently, but only on their product, $cb$.*

### 3.3.2 Proofs of the Theorems

The proofs in this section, although lengthy, illustrate the use of several methods that are frequently used in analyzing the nonlinear systems of difference

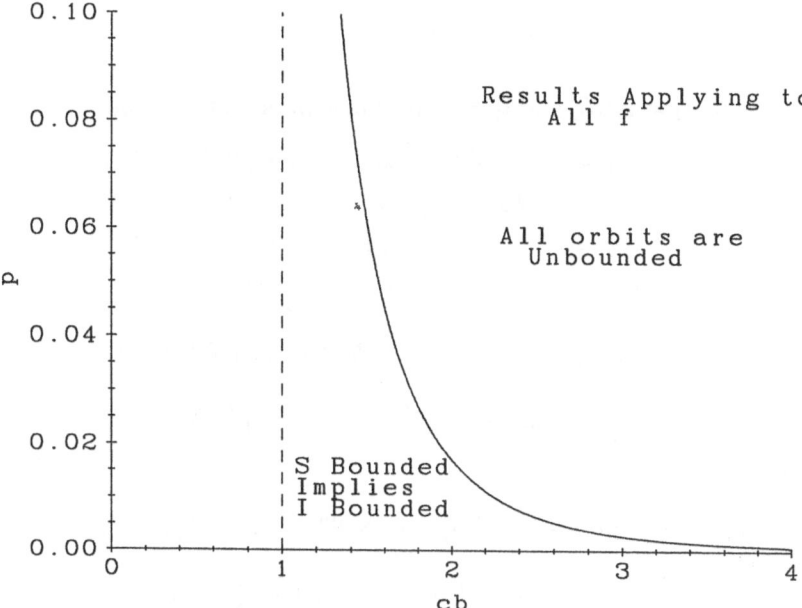

**Fig. 3.6.** Parameter regions where the subpopulations are bounded

equations that arise in epidemic and population models. The proofs also provide insights into the more detailed behavior of the model, but the reader who wishes to concentrate on the study of other models can proceed directly to Section 3.4 without loss of continuity.

*Proof.* (Theorem 3.4) Assume that there is a 2-periodic solution; we will show that it is not feasible. Let the two points in the solution be denoted by subscripts 1 and 2. We have, from (3.11),

$$i_1(0) = ckS_1I_2,$$

$$i_2(0) = ckS_2I_1,$$

$$S_1 = cb\left(p\sum_{\alpha=0}^{m-1} i_2(\alpha) + S_2\right) - ckS_1I_2,$$

and

$$S_2 = cb\left(p\sum_{\alpha=0}^{m-1} i_1(\alpha) + S_1\right) - ckS_2I_1.$$

Thus by adding we obtain

$$S_1 + i_1(0) = cb\left(p\sum_{\alpha=0}^{m-1} i_2(\alpha) + S_2\right),$$

and

$$S_2 + i_2(0) = cb \left( p \sum_{\alpha=0}^{m-1} i_1(\alpha) + S_1 \right).$$

Now, define $i_1 = i_1(0)$, and $i_2 = i_2(0)$. Since $m$ is odd we have

$$
\begin{aligned}
I_1 =& [1 + (cbq)^2 + (cbq)^4 + \ldots + (cbq)^{m-1}]i_1 \\
&+ [cbq + (cbq)^3 + \ldots + (cbq)^m]i_2, \\
I_2 =& [1 + (cbq)^2 + (cbq)^4 + \ldots + (cbq)^{m-1}]i_2 \\
&+ [cbq + (cbq)^3 + \ldots + (cbq)^m]i_1,
\end{aligned}
$$

$$
\begin{aligned}
\sum_{\alpha=0}^{m-1} i_1(\alpha) =& [1 + (cbq)^2 + (cbq)^4 + \ldots + (cbq)^{m-1}]i_1 \\
&+ [cbq + (cbq)^3 + \ldots + (cbq)^{m-2}]i_2,
\end{aligned}
$$

and

$$
\begin{aligned}
\sum_{\alpha=0}^{m-1} i_2(\alpha) =& [1 + (cbq)^2 + (cbq)^4 + \ldots + (cbq)^{m-1}]i_2 \\
&+ [cbq + (cbq)^3 + \ldots + (cbq)^{m-2}]i_1.
\end{aligned}
$$

Thus, by defining

$$
\begin{aligned}
A =& 1 + (cbq)^2 + (cbq)^4 + \ldots + (cbq)^{m-1}, \\
B =& cbq + (cbq)^3 + \ldots + (cbq)^m, \\
D =& cbq + (cbq)^3 + \ldots + (cbq)^{m-2},
\end{aligned}
$$

we have

$$I_1 = Ai_1 + Bi_2, \quad I_2 = Ai_2 + Bi_1,$$

$$\sum_{\alpha=0}^{m-1} i_1(\alpha) = Ai_1 + Di_2, \quad \sum_{\alpha=0}^{m-1} i_2(\alpha) = Ai_2 + Di_1.$$

Hence,

$$i_1 = ckS_1(Ai_2 + Bi_1), \quad i_2 = ckS_2(Ai_1 + Bi_2),$$

$$S_1 + i_1 = cb(p(Ai_2 + Di_1) + S_2), \quad S_2 + i_2 = cb(p(Ai_1 + Di_2) + S_1).$$

Thus,

$$S_1 = (cbpD - 1)i_1 + cbpAi_2 + cbS_2,$$

and

$$S_2 = (cbpD - 1)i_2 + cbpAi_1 + cbS_1.$$

Substituting for $S_1$, we obtain

$$i_1 = ck(Ai_2 + Bi_1)[(cbpD - 1)i_1 + cbpAi_2 + cbS_2],$$

$$i_2 = ck(Ai_1 + Bi_2)S_2,$$

and

$$S_2 = (cbpD - 1)i_2 + cbpAi_1 + cb[(cbpD - 1)i_1 + cbpAi_2 + cbS_2].$$

Thus,

$$S_2 = \frac{(cbpA + c^2b^2pD - cb)i_1 + (cbpD - 1 + c^2b^2pA)i_2}{1 - c^2b^2}.$$

Note that we have $cb > 1$, since for $cb < 1$ the zero steady state is globally stable; if $cb = 1$ and there are no infectives present, then any susceptible population is stable; and if there are infectives present with $cb = 1$, then the population is monotonically decreasing, as is easily seen by using (3.11) to derive the following expression for the total population $P_n = S_n + I_n$,

$$P_n = P_{n-1} - cbi_{n-1}(m) - cf(S_n, I_{n-1}).$$

Substituting for $S_2$ in the equation for $i_1$, we obtain

$$i_1 = ck(Ai_2 + Bi_1) \left[ \left( \frac{cbpD - 1 + c^2b^2pA}{1 - c^2b^2} \right) i_1 + \left( \frac{cbpA + c^2b^2pD - cb}{1 - c^2b^2} \right) i_2 \right],$$

and

$$i_2 = ck(Ai_1 + Bi_2) \left[ \left( \frac{cbpA + c^2b^2pD - cb}{1 - c^2b^2} \right) i_1 + \left( \frac{cbpD - 1 + c^2b^2pA}{1 - c^2b^2} \right) i_2 \right].$$

Now, define two new constants,

$$E = \frac{cbpA + c^2b^2pD - cb}{1 - c^2b^2}, \quad F = \frac{cbpD - 1 + c^2b^2pA}{1 - c^2b^2},$$

and subtract the expression for $i_2$ from that for $i_1$ to get

$$i_1 - i_2 = ck(BF(i_1^2 - i_2^2) + AE(i_2^2 - i_1^2)).$$

We must have $i_1 \neq i_2$, and can divide by $(i_1 - i_2)$ to obtain

$$1 = ck[BF(i_1 + i_2) - AE(i_1 + i_2)] = ck(i_1 + i_2)(BF - AE).$$

Here we see that to have a feasible solution we must have $(BF - AE)$ positive, since all the other terms in the last equation are positive. Thus we need

$$BF - AE = cbqAF - AE > 0$$

to have a feasible solution. Since $A$ is positive we can divide by $A$ to obtain

$$cbqF - E > 0.$$

Substituting for $E$ and $F$, we have

$$cbq \frac{cbpD - 1 + c^2b^2pA}{1 - c^2b^2} - \frac{cbpA + c^2b^2pD - cb}{1 - c^2b^2} > 0.$$

Since $cb > 1$ we need

$$cbq(cbpD - 1 + c^2b^2pA) - cbpA - c^2b^2pD + cb < 0$$

to have a feasible solution. Dividing by $cb$ and using the fact that $A = cbqD + 1$, we obtain

$$cbpqD - q + c^3b^3pq^2D + c^2b^2pq - cbpqD - p - cbpD + 1 < 0.$$

Two of the terms cancel now. Using $1 - p - q = 0$, and dividing by $cbp$ we obtain

$$c^2b^2q^2D + cbq - D = B - D < 0.$$

But $B - D = (cbq)^m > 0$, hence this inequality cannot be true. Thus the condition for having a feasible 2-periodic solution cannot be met, which proves the theorem.

*Proof.* (Theorem 3.5) It only remains to prove the first assertion of this theorem. First we observe that if $cb \leq 1$ then $cbq < 1$ and

$$R_p = p\frac{1 - (cbq)^m}{1 - cbq} < \frac{p}{1 - cbq} < \frac{p}{1 - q} = 1,$$

which is contrary to the hypotheses. Thus, $cb > 1$. Now, if $I_0 = 0$, then we have $S_n = (cb)^n S_0$, with $cb > 1$, and we are done. Thus we need only consider the case where $I_0 > 0$. Hence we have $i_n(\alpha) > 0$ for all $n \geq m + 1$, so if we shift the index, $n$, we can assume that $i_n(\alpha) > 0$ for all $n$. We have

$$i_{n+1}(0) + S_{n+1} = cbp \sum_{\alpha=0}^{m-1} i_n(\alpha) + cbS_n.$$

Now we write the equations as a forced linear system, $X_{n+1} = AX_n + C_n$, where $X_n$ represents the infective population in the $n^{th}$ cohort. Thus

$$X_n = \begin{pmatrix} i_n(0) \\ i_n(1) \\ \vdots \\ i_n(m) \end{pmatrix}, \quad C_n = \begin{pmatrix} cbS_n - S_{n+1} \\ 0 \\ \vdots \\ 0 \end{pmatrix},$$

and the $(m + 1) \times (m + 1)$ matrix $A$ is

$$\begin{pmatrix} cbp & cbp & \cdots & cbp & 0 \\ cbq & 0 & \cdots & 0 & 0 \\ 0 & cbq & 0 & \cdots & 0 \\ \vdots & & \ddots & & \vdots \\ 0 & \cdots & 0 & cbq & 0 \end{pmatrix}.$$

By iterating the equation $X_{n+1} = AX_n + C_n$, we obtain

$$X_{n+2} = A^2 X_n + AC_n + C_{n+1}.$$

Collecting terms, using the fact that $q = 1 - p$, and applying an induction argument, we obtain

$$X_{n+k} = A^k X_n + Y_{n+k} + \begin{pmatrix} 0 \\ 0 \\ \vdots \\ 0 \\ (cbq)^m S_{n+k-m} \\ -(cbq)^m S_{n+k-m} \end{pmatrix}$$

$$+ \begin{pmatrix} 0 \\ 0 \\ 0 \\ (cbq)^{m-1} S_{n+k-4} \\ -(cbq)^{m-1} S_{n+k-4} \\ 0 \end{pmatrix} + \ldots + \begin{pmatrix} cbqS_{n+k-1} \\ -cbqS_{n+k-1} \\ 0 \\ 0 \\ \vdots \\ 0 \end{pmatrix} + \begin{pmatrix} -S_{n+k} \\ 0 \\ 0 \\ 0 \\ \vdots \\ 0 \end{pmatrix}$$

where $Y_{n+k}$ is a positive column vector and the above relation holds for $k \ge m + 1$.

We use this equation to get an expression for $i_n(0) + S_n$. All that is necessary is to extract the top row of the equation which, upon renaming the index $n + k$ to $n$, is an expression for $i_n(0)$, and add $S_n$. Thus we obtain

$$i_n(0) + S_n = [A^n X_0]_1 + [Y_n]_1 + cbqS_{n-1},$$

where $[B]_1$ indicates the first element of the column vector $B$. We know that $[Y_n]_1 + cbqS_{n-1}$ is positive, hence, if $A$ has an eigenvalue greater than 1, the $i_n(0) + S_n$ must be unbounded. To show that this is the case, we compute the characteristic polynomial of $A$

$$P(\lambda) = \lambda(\lambda^m - cbp[\lambda^{m-1} + (cbq)\lambda^{m-2} + \ldots + (cbq)^{m-2}\lambda + (cbq)^{m-1}]),$$

and note that

$$P(1) = 1 - cbp(1 + cbq + (cbq)^2 + \ldots + (cbq)^{m-1})$$
$$= 1 - cb\frac{p(1 - (cbq)^m)}{1 - cbq} = 1 - cbR_p < 0,$$

and since $\lim_{\lambda \to \infty} P(\lambda) = \infty$, there must be a positive real root of $P(\lambda)$ greater than 1. This completes the proof.

*Proof.* (Theorem 3.6) If $(S_n, I_n)$ is a bounded solution, then $F = \{f(S_n, I_{n-1})$ (the set of the values of $f$ on the bounded orbit) must be bounded. Say $cf <$ for all $f \in F$. Then we have

$$S_{n+1} = cbp \sum_{\alpha=0}^{m-1} i_n(\alpha) + cbS_n - cf(S_{n+1}, I_n).$$

Hence $S_{n+1} \geq cbS_n - \kappa$. We have $cbR_p > 1$, implying $cb > 1$, which suggests that if $S_n$ is large enough, then $S_{n+1} > S_n$. In fact, if $S_n > \kappa/(cb-1)$, then $cbS_n - \kappa > S_n$, and hence $S_{n+1} > S_n$.

Thus, if $S_n > \kappa/(cb-1)$, then $S$ grows monotonically after that point. But we know by Theorem 3.5 that the population is unbounded. Thus, since $I_n$ is bounded, $S_n$ must take on arbitrarily large values and we can assume that $S_N > 2\kappa/(cb-1) > \kappa/(cb-1)$ for some $N$. From the above, we know that $S_{n+1} > S_n$ for all $n > N$. In fact, $S_n \geq L_n$, where $L_n$ obeys

$$L_{n+1} = cbL_n - \kappa.$$

The solution to this equation is

$$L_{N+j} = (cb)^j L_N - \kappa \frac{(cb)^j - 1}{cb - 1}.$$

Since we are assuming $S_N > 2\kappa/(cb-1)$, we can take $L_N = 2\kappa/(cb-1)$. Hence

$$L_{N+j} = \frac{2\kappa(cb)^j - \kappa(cb)^j + k}{cb - 1} = \frac{\kappa(cb)^j + k}{cb - 1},$$

and $S_n > L_n > K(cb)^n$ for all $n > N$, where $K = \kappa/((cb)^N(cb - 1))$. This completes the proof.

*Proof.* (Theorem 3.8) If $I_0 = 0$, we have $S_n = (cb)^n S_0$, and we are done since $cb > 1$. Thus we need only consider the case where $I_0 > 0$. From Theorem 3.6, we have

$$i_n(0) + S_n > [A^n X_0]_1,$$

thus it is sufficient to show for some $C$, $r$, and $N$ that $[A^n X_0]_1 \geq Cr^n$ for all $n > N$. To do this, the first step is to show that the matrix $A$ from Theorem 3.6 has a positive, real eigenvalue $\lambda_0 > 1$, such that for any other eigenvalue $\mathrm{Re}(\lambda) < \lambda_0$.

Recall that $A$ is a $(m+1) \times (m+1)$ matrix, and define $A'$ to be the $m \times m$ matrix that results from deleting the last row and last column of $A$. Now, observe that $P(\lambda)$ and $P'(\lambda)$, the characteristic polynomials of $A$ and $A'$, respectively, obey

$$P(\lambda) = (-\lambda)P'(\lambda).$$

This relationship comes from the cofactor expansion on the last column of $A - \lambda I$. Hence, any eigenvalue of $A'$ is also an eigenvalue of $A$. In order to use the Perron-Frobenius Theorem (see Section 3.7.2) we need to note that $A'$ is irreducible, or perhaps more simply, to show that $(A')^n$ is a strictly positive matrix for some n. In fact, it is shown below that $(A')^m$ is strictly positive. For simplicity, positive array entries have been marked with '+'. Then

$$A' = \begin{pmatrix} + & + & \cdots & + & + \\ + & 0 & \cdots & 0 & 0 \\ 0 & + & 0 & \cdots & 0 \\ \vdots & & \ddots & & \vdots \\ 0 & \cdots & 0 & + & 0 \end{pmatrix} \quad (A')^2 = \begin{pmatrix} + & + & \cdots & + & + & + \\ + & + & \cdots & + & + & + \\ + & 0 & 0 & \cdots & 0 & 0 \\ 0 & + & 0 & \cdots & 0 & 0 \\ \vdots & & \ddots & & & \vdots \\ 0 & \cdots & 0 & + & 0 & 0 \end{pmatrix},$$

and each successively higher power of $A'$ adds another positive row. Thus the Perron-Frobenius Theorem applies to $A'$; hence, not only $A'$, but also $A$, has a simple, positive real eigenvalue $\lambda_0$ such that for all the other eigenvalues $|\lambda| < \lambda_0$. Note that $A$ has one more eigenvalue $\lambda = 0 < \lambda_0$ than $A'$.

Associated with $\lambda_0$ are $X'$ and $X^*$, its eigenvectors in $A'$ and $A$ respectively. It is a simple matter to construct $X^*$ from $X'$. If $X'$ has components $x_1, x_2, \cdots, x_m$, then by inspection of $A$, we see that $X^*$ has components

$$x_1, x_2, \cdots, x_m, \frac{cbqx_m}{\lambda_0}.$$

By the Perron-Frobenius Theorem, $X'$ is strictly positive, hence, so is $X^*$.

Now, $\lambda_0$ is the largest eigenvalue of $A$, and by the proof of Theorem 3.5, $A$ has an eigenvalue greater than 1, hence, $\lambda_0 > 1$. Write $X_0$ as follows: $X_0 = aX^* + dX^\perp$, where $X^\perp$ is orthogonal to $X^*$. Recall that we are considering the case where $I_0 > 0$, hence the inner product of $X^*$ with $X_0$ must be positive, which implies that $a$ is positive. However, $X^\perp$ may have negative components. We have

$$A^n X_0 = aA^n X^* + dA^n X^\perp = a(\lambda_0)^n X^* + dA^n X^\perp = (\lambda_0)^n \left( aX^* + \frac{dA^n X^\perp}{(\lambda_0)^n} \right).$$

Now, $\lambda_0$ is a simple eigenvalue, and $A$ leaves the subspace $S^\perp$ of vectors orthogonal to $X^*$ invariant, hence, the spectral radius $\rho$ of the matrix $A$ restricted to $S^\perp$ satisfies $\rho < \lambda_0$. Thus, for any natural matrix norm $\| \; \|$, we have

$$\frac{\|A^n X^\perp\|}{\lambda_0^n} \leq \frac{\|A\|^n \|X^\perp\|}{\lambda_0^n} \leq \left( \frac{\rho}{\lambda_0} \right)^n \|X^\perp\|.$$

For the results from linear algebra which justify the above steps we refer the reader to basic texts in that area, for example, Varga [1962]. Thus, since $(\rho/\lambda_0)^n \to 0$ as $n \to \infty$, there is an $N$ such that for all $n > N$,

$$\left| \frac{dA^n X^\perp}{(\lambda_0)^n} \right| < \beta aX^*,$$

for any $d$, any $a > 0$, and any $0 < \beta < 1$, where $|Y|$ denotes the vector with components equal to the absolute values of the corresponding components of $Y$, and the comparison $(Y < Z)$ is made component by component. Hence, choosing $\beta = \frac{1}{2}$, we have

$$A^n X_0 > (\lambda_0)^n \left( aX^* - \frac{aX^*}{2} \right) = (\lambda_0)^n \left( \frac{aX^*}{2} \right)$$

for $n > N$. Thus, since $X_n = i_n(0) + S_n > [A^n X_0]_1$, we have $X_n > Cr^n$, where $C = a[X^*]_1/2$, and $r = \lambda_0 > 1$. This completes the proof.

*Proof.* (Theorem 3.9) Pick an integer $M$, and assume that $S_n > 2b/k$ for all $n > M$, to get

$$I_{n+1} \geq i_{n+1}(0) = ck I_n S_{n+1} > 2cb I_n$$

for all $n > M$. But, a direct computation shows that

$$P_{n+1} = I_{n+1} + S_{n+1} \leq cb(I_n + S_n) = cb P_n.$$

Hence, $S_{n+1} < cb S_n$ for all $n > M$. Thus we have

$$S_{M+n} < (cb)^n S_M, \text{ and } I_{M+n} > (2cb)^n I_M.$$

Hence

$$S_{M+n+1} = \frac{cb(p \sum_{\alpha=0}^{m-1} i_{M+n}(\alpha) + S_{M+n})}{1 + ck I_{M+n}} \leq \frac{cbp I_{M+n}}{ck I_{M+n}} + \frac{cb S_{M+n}}{ck I_{M+n}}$$

$$\leq \frac{bp}{k} + \frac{(cb)^{n+1} S_M}{ck(2cb)^n I_M} = \frac{bp}{k} + \frac{b S_M}{k 2^n I_M}.$$

This is a contradiction of our assumption that $S_n > 2b/k$ for all $n > M$, since

$$\lim_{n \to \infty} \frac{b S_M}{k 2^n I_M} = 0.$$

Hence, we may assume that $S_n \leq 2b/k$ for some $n > M$.

Since we made no restrictions on the integer $M$, we can assume that we have $S_n \leq 2b/k$ for some arbitrarily large $n$. By Theorem 3.8, though, we have $i_n(0) + S_n > Kr^n$ for some positive constant $K$, some real $r > 1$, and all $n > N$, $N$ a positive integer. Let us pick $M > N$ large enough so that

$$i_n(0) + S_n > \frac{2b}{kq} + \frac{2b}{k}$$

for all $n > M$. Then for some $n > M$ we have $S_n \leq 2b/k$, and hence

$$i_n(0) > \frac{2b}{kq} + \frac{2b}{k} - S_n \geq \frac{2b}{kq}.$$

Let $N_0 > M$ denote a value of $n$ for which these two conditions hold. We will show that they are true for all $n \geq N_0$.

By assumption, we know that the conditions are true for $n = N_0$, so assume that they hold for some $n$ and consider $n + 1$. We have

$$S_{n+1} = \frac{cbp \sum_{\alpha=0}^{m-1} i_n(\alpha) + cb S_n}{1 + ck I_n} < \frac{cbp I_n + cb S_n}{1 + ck I_n} < \frac{cbp I_n}{ck I_n} + \frac{cb S_n}{ck i_n(0)}$$

$$< \frac{bp}{k} + \frac{(2cb)(b/k)}{2cb/q} = \frac{bp}{k} + \frac{bq}{k} = \frac{b}{k} < \frac{2b}{k}.$$

Hence, the conditions still hold for $S_{n+1}$. To see that they still hold for $i_{n+1}(0)$, recall that we have $N_0 > M$, and hence

$$i_{n+1}(0) + S_{n+1} > \frac{2b}{kq} + \frac{2b}{k}.$$

Proceeding as before,

$$i_{n+1}(0) > \frac{2b}{kq} + \frac{2b}{k} - S_{n+1} \geq \frac{2b}{kq}.$$

Thus, by induction, the conditions hold for all $n > N_0$.

In order to see that $I_n \to \infty$ as $n \to \infty$, we need only recall that by Theorem 3.8 we have $i_n(0) + S_n > cr^n$ for some $c > 0$, $r > 1$. Thus, since we have shown $S_n < 2b/k$, for all $n > N_0$, we have $\lim_{n \to \infty} i_n(0) = \infty$; hence $\lim_{n \to \infty} I_n = \infty$. This completes the proof.

*Proof.* (Theorem 3.10) From the basic equations of the model we have

$$S_{n+1} = cb(p \sum_{\alpha=0}^{m-1} i_n(\alpha) + S_n) - \frac{ckS_{n+1}I_n}{k' + I_n}.$$

Hence

$$S_{n+1} = \frac{k' + I_n}{k' + I_n + ckI_n} \left( cbp \sum_{\alpha=0}^{m-1} i_n(\alpha) + cbS_n \right)$$

$$= \frac{k' + I_n}{k' + I_n + ckI_n} (S_{n+1} + i_{n+1}(0)) \quad \text{and}$$

$$i_{n+1}(0) = \frac{ckI_n}{k' + I_n + ckI_n} \left( cbp \sum_{\alpha=0}^{m-1} i_n(\alpha) + cbS_n \right)$$

$$= \frac{ckI_n}{k' + I_n + ckI_n} (S_{n+1} + i_{n+1}(0)).$$

Thus

$$\frac{S_{n+1}}{S_{n+1} + i_{n+1}(0)} = \frac{k' + I_n}{k' + I_n + ckI_n}, \quad \text{and}$$

$$\frac{i_{n+1}(0)}{S_{n+1} + i_{n+1}(0)} = \frac{ckI_n}{k' + I_n + ckI_n}.$$

Hence, if we show that $\lim_{n \to \infty} I_n = \infty$, then we are done. To do this we first show that $I_n$ is unbounded.

Assume that $I_n$ is bounded; i.e. $I_n < I^*$. Then by Theorem 3.6 we have $S_n > K(cb)^n$ for all $n > N$ for some positive $K$ which depends on the initial conditions. Thus we can pick an $M$ such that for all $n > M$ we have

$$S_{n+1} > \frac{2(k' + I^* + ckI^*)}{ck} > \frac{2(k' + I_n + ckI_n)}{ck},$$

and we have

$$I_{n+1} \geq i_{n+1}(0) \geq \frac{ckI_n S_{n+1}}{k' + I_n + ckI_n} > 2I_n$$

for all $n > M$. Thus $I_n$ is unbounded, contradicting our assumption.

Since $I_n$ is unbounded, we have $i_n(0)$ unbounded also. So if we pick a value $i^*$ we can assume $i_n(0) > i^*$ for arbitrarily large $n$. Pick a large $N$ for which $i_N(0) > i^*$, and consider $i_{N+1}(0)$. We have

$$i_{N+1}(0) = \frac{ckI_N}{k' + I_N + ckI_N} \left( cbp \sum_{\alpha=0}^{m-1} i_N(\alpha) + cbS_N \right)$$

$$> \frac{cki^*}{k' + i^* + cki^*} (cbp)(i_N(0) + S_N),$$

since $i/(k' + i + cki)$ is monotone increasing in $i$. By Theorem 3.8 we have $i_n(0) + S_n > Kr^n$ for all $n > M$ for some $K > 0$ and some $r > 1$. Thus

$$i_{N+1}(0) > \frac{cki^*}{k' + i^* + cki^*} (cbp)(Kr^N).$$

From our earlier comments, we can assume $N$ is large enough so that the above inequality yields $i_{N+1}(0) > i^*$. Clearly, then, we have $i_n(0) > i^*$ for all $n > N$ by induction, and thus the above equation gives us a lower bound on $i_n(0)$ which is growing as $(cb)^n$. Thus $i_n \to \infty$, as $n \to \infty$, and hence $I_n \to \infty$ as $n \to \infty$. This completes the proof.

*Proof.* (Theorem 3.11) As in Theorem 3.5, write the system as a linear equation

$$X_{n+1} = AX_n + C_n$$

where $X_n$ represents the state of the infective population, and $C_n$ and $A$ are as in the proof of Theorem 3.5.

Let $S^*$ be the upper bound on $S_n$, that is $S_n < S^*$. Then $C_n < C_{max}$, where

$$C_{max} = \begin{pmatrix} cbS^* \\ 0 \\ \vdots \\ 0 \end{pmatrix},$$

and the comparison is made component by component. The solution to the linear system for $X_n$ is

$$X_n = A^n X_0 + A^{n-1}C_0 + A^{n-2}C_1 + \ldots + IC_{n-1},$$

so if all the eigenvalues of $A$ are such that $|\lambda| < 1$, then we can write

$$X_n < A^n X_0 + (I - A)^{-1}(I - A^n)C_{max}.$$

To see that the eigenvalues are in the interior of the unit disk, we examine $P(\lambda)$, the characteristic polynomial of $A$:

$$P(\lambda) = \lambda^{m+1} - \lambda cbp \left( \lambda^{m-1} + (cbq)\lambda^{m-2} + \ldots + (cbq)^{m-2}\lambda + (cbq)^{m-1} \right)$$
$$= \lambda^{m+1} - G(\lambda).$$

Let $g_i$ be the coefficient of $\lambda^i$ in $G(\lambda)$, and apply Rouché's theorem from complex analysis. We have

$$\sum_{i=0}^{m} |g_i| = cbp \sum_{i=1}^{m} (cbq)^{i-1} = cbR_p < 1.$$

Hence, $|G(\lambda)| < 1 = |\lambda^{m+1}|$ when $|\lambda| = 1$. Thus, $P(\lambda) = \lambda^{m+1} - G(\lambda)$ has as many roots in the interior of the unit disk as does $\lambda^{m+1}$; that is, $m + 1$. Hence, the roots of $P(\lambda)$ are inside the unit disk and $\lim_{n\to\infty} A^n = 0$. From the above inequality for $X_n$, $\lim_{n\to\infty} X_n \le (I - A)^{-1} C_{\max}$, thus $X_n$, and hence $I_n$, is bounded.

*Proof.* (Theorem 3.12) In order to study the local stability, we will linearize the model about the steady state, and examine its Jacobian (see Section 3.7.2). We have the equations of the model for $f = kSI$:

$$S_{n+1} = \frac{cb(p\sum_{\alpha=0}^{m-1} i_n(\alpha) + S_n)}{1 + ckI_n},$$

$$i_{n+1}(0) = ckS_{n+1}I_n = ckI_n\frac{cb(p\sum_{\alpha=0}^{m-1} i_n(\alpha) + S_n)}{1 + ckI_n}, \quad \text{and}$$

$$i_{n+1}(\alpha) = cbqi_n(\alpha - 1), \quad \alpha = 1, 2, \ldots, m.$$

Hence the Jacobian is of the form

$$\begin{pmatrix} A & B & B & \cdots & B & C \\ D & E & E & \cdots & E & F \\ 0 & G & 0 & \cdots & 0 & 0 \\ \vdots & & & \ddots & & \vdots \\ 0 & \cdots & 0 & 0 & G & 0 \end{pmatrix},$$

where

$$A = \frac{\partial S_{n+1}}{\partial S_n} = \frac{cb}{1 + ckI_n},$$

$$B = \frac{\partial S_{n+1}}{\partial i_n(\beta)} = \frac{cbp}{1 + ckI_n} - \frac{ckcb(p\sum_{\alpha=0}^{m-1} i_n(\alpha) + S_n)}{(1 + ckI_n)^2}$$

$$= \frac{cbp}{1 + ckI_n} - \frac{ckS_{n+1}}{1 + ckI_n} = \frac{cbp - ckS_{n+1}}{1 + ckI_n}, \quad \beta = 0, 1, \ldots, m - 1,$$

$$C = \frac{\partial S_{n+1}}{\partial i_n(m)} = \frac{-ckcb(p\sum_{\alpha=0}^{m-1} i_n(\alpha) + S_n)}{(1 + ckI_n)^2} = \frac{-ckS_{n+1}}{1 + ckI_n},$$

$$D = \frac{\partial i_{n+1}(0)}{\partial S_n} = ckI_n\frac{\partial S_{n+1}}{\partial S_n} = \frac{ckcbI_n}{1 + ckI_n},$$

$$E = \frac{\partial i_{n+1}(0)}{\partial i_n(\alpha)} = ckS_{n+1}\frac{\partial I_n}{\partial i_n(\alpha)} + ckI_n\frac{\partial S_{n+1}}{\partial i_n(\alpha)}$$

$$= \frac{cbpckI_n + ckS_{n+1}}{1 + ckI_n}, \quad \alpha = 0, 1, \ldots, m - 1,$$

$$F = \frac{\partial i_{n+1}(0)}{\partial i_n(m)} = ckS_{n+1}\frac{\partial I_n}{\partial i_n(m)} + ckI_n\frac{\partial S_{n+1}}{\partial i_n(m)} = \frac{ckS_{n+1}}{1 + ckI_n},$$

$$G = \frac{\partial i_{n+1}(\alpha)}{\partial i_n(\alpha - 1)} = cbq.$$

All the other partial derivatives are zero.

We can solve the equations (3.11) of the model at equilibrium to obtain an explicit formula for the steady state solution. We have

$$\frac{(1 - cb)\bar{S}}{cbR_p - 1} = cf\left(\bar{S}, \left(\frac{1 - (cbq)^{m+1}}{1 - cbq}\right)\left(\frac{1 - cb}{cbR_p - 1}\right)\bar{S}\right),$$

$$\bar{i}(0) = \frac{(1 - cb)\bar{S}}{cbR_p - 1}, \quad \text{and}$$

$$\bar{i}(\alpha) = (cbq)^{\alpha}\,\bar{i}(0), \quad \alpha = 1, 2, \ldots, m.$$

Substituting $f = kSI$, we obtain

$$\frac{(1 - cb)\bar{S}}{cbR_p - 1} = ck\bar{S}\left(\frac{1 - (cbq)^{m+1}}{1 - cbq}\right)\left(\frac{1 - cb}{cbR_p - 1}\right)\bar{S}.$$

Hence

$$\bar{S} = \frac{1 - cbq}{ck(1 - (cbq)^{m+1})}.$$

Thus

$$\bar{I} = \left(\frac{1 - (cbq)^{m+1}}{1 - cbq}\right)\bar{i}(0) = \left(\frac{1 - (cbq)^{m+1}}{1 - cbq}\right)\left(\frac{1 - cb}{cbR_p - 1}\right)\bar{S} = \frac{1 - cb}{ck(cbR_p - 1)}.$$

To complete the proof, we observe that since both $\bar{S}$ and $\bar{I}$ are proportional to $1/ck$, all the $k$'s in the Jacobian cancel out when $\bar{S}$ and $\bar{I}$ are substituted in it. Hence, the stability of the steady state does not depend on $k$. Similarly, after the substitution is made $c$ and $b$ always appear together. Thus the stability of the steady state does not depend on either independently, but only on their product, $cb$.

## 3.4 Vertical Transmission in Insect Populations

J. Régnière [1984] formulated a model for vertical transmission of diseases in insect populations with discrete non-overlapping generations. He had in mind infections by parasitic or pathogenic microorganisms, including viruses and microsporidian protozoa, and made the suggestion that a possible cause of the eruptions of spruce budworm in North American forests could be the effects of vertically transmitted diseases in the absence of stronger regulating agents. We shall commence by explaining this model, and return to a description of the inferences to be drawn from it later in this section.

Régnière's model differs from the ones in the previous sections in several ways. The pathogen is assumed to be directly transmitted, either horizontally from host to host or vertically from parent to offspring, and thus the model does not involve a vector carrier. The model equations are not derived by the sort of hypotheses concerning the underlying population dynamics that were used in Section 3.2, but rather by assuming certain proportionality relations, as will be explained below. Finally, the basic variables in the model, instead of being the prevalence ratio $B_k$, are the following[3]:

$S_n = $ the number of disease-free, susceptible, hosts at the beginning of generation $n$.

$I_n = $ the number of infected hosts at the beginning of generation $n$.

For convenience, only female hosts are considered. It is assumed that a diseased female is capable of reproduction, and transmits infection to a fraction $q$ of her offspring. The model is derived by following the life cycles of hosts in the groups $S_n$ and $I_n$. Set

$q = $ the proportion of the offspring of an infected female that are also infected. We set $p = 1 - q$.

$l_1 = $ the fraction of infected hosts that survive to the end of their generation (or to the end of their reproductive age).

$l_2 = $ the fraction of all susceptible hosts that survive to the end of their generation (or to the end of their reproductive age).

Of the original $I_n$ infected insects, $l_1 I_n$ survive to reproduce, and produce $l_1 m_1 I_n$ offspring, where

$m_1 = $ the fecundity of vertically infected females.

Of these offspring, $q l_1 m_1 I_n$ are infected and $(1 - q) l_1 m_1 I_n$ are not. Now, consider the susceptibles $S_n$. Let

$p_n = $ the proportion of susceptible hosts that become horizontally infected. We set $q_n = 1 - p_n$.

The particular form of $p_n$ as a function of $I_n$ will be discussed below. Assuming that horizontal infection occurs before laying eggs, we see that $l_2 p_n S_n$ is the number of these females that survive to lay eggs. Let

$m_2 = $ the fecundity of horizontally infected females.

Then $l_2 m_2 p_n S_n$ eggs are laid, and $q l_2 m_2 p_n S_n$ offspring are infected, while $p l_2 m_2 p_n S_n$ are not infected at birth. Finally, of the original $S_n$ hosts, $q_n S_n$ do not become horizontally infected. For these $q_n S_n$ hosts, set

$l_3 = $ the fraction of these that survive to the end of their generation,

$m_3 = $ the fecundity of these survivors.

These individuals give rise to $l_3 m_3 q_n S_n$ non-infected offspring. Figure 3.7 may assist in visualizing the relations between the various parts of the population that we have been discussing.

From the above discussion, we obtain

$$S_{n+1} = (1 - q)(l_1 m_1 I_n + l_2 m_2 p_n S_n) + l_3 m_3 (1 - p_n) S_n,$$
$$I_{n+1} = q(l_1 m_1 I_n + l_2 m_2 p_n S_n).$$

---

[3] In Régnière's paper, these variables are called $y_t$ and $x_t$, respectively, instead of $S_n$ and $I_n$. We also use $P_n$ to denote the total population $S_n + I_n$, instead of $z_t$.

Born diseased                          Born disease free

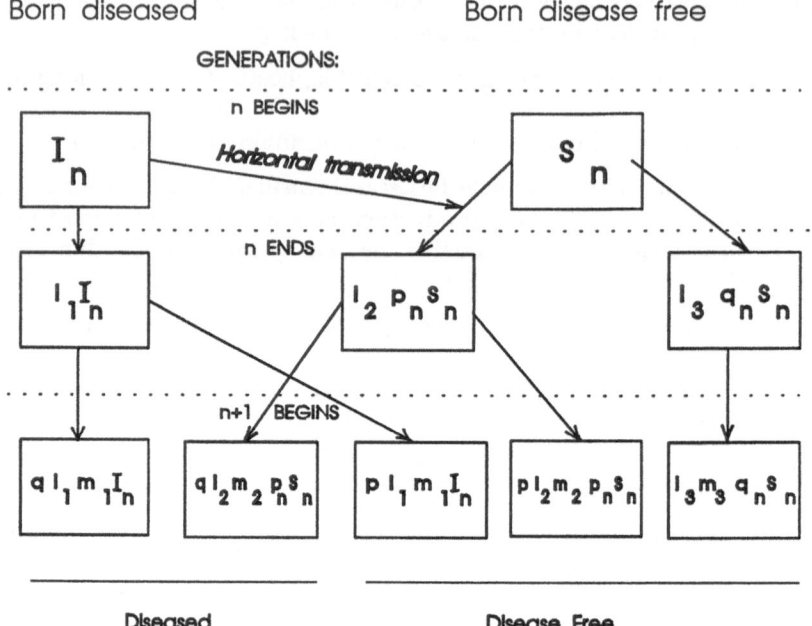

**Fig. 3.7.** The disease transmission dynamics

To simplify the notation, let $a = l_1 m_1$, $b = l_2 m_2$, $c = l_3 m_3$. Then we get

$$
\begin{aligned}
S_{n+1} &= (1-q)(aI_n + bp_n S_n) + c(1-p_n)S_n, \\
I_{n+1} &= q(aI_n + bp_n S_n).
\end{aligned}
\tag{3.17}
$$

It is assumed that $a, b, c, q$ are constants, although Régnière remarks that in actuality the first three are likely to be density dependent.

The two difference equations (3.17) are the basic equations of this model, but if we let

$$
P_n = S_n + I_n,
$$

then we also have

$$
P_{n+1} = aI_n + (bp_n - cp_n + c)S_n.
\tag{3.18}
$$

In order to complete the model, Régnière makes the assumption that $p_n$, the proportion of horizontally infected susceptibles, has the form

$$
p_n = f(I_n),
\tag{3.19}
$$

where $f(I)$ is a function of general saturation type (for example, $f(I) = kI/(\tilde{k} + I)$) satisfying

$$
\lim_{I \to 0} f(I) = 0, \quad \lim_{I \to \infty} f(I) = 1, \quad f'(I) > 0 \text{ for } 0 < I < \infty.
$$

Note that this differs from the mass-action type of assumption, $f(I) = \beta I$, but is included in the more general form of infection terms considered in the previous section (note that in the notation used in Section 3.3 the force of infection term is denoted by $f/S$.)

It is also assumed that

$$0 < a < 1,\ c > 1,\ a \le b \le c,\ 0 < q \le 1. \tag{3.20}$$

The constraint $a \le b \le c$ is most likely biologically, because the survival and fecundity are likely to be greatest for disease-free hosts, and least for hosts that were infected at birth. This assumption can be compared to the model in the previous section where vertically infected lineages of ticks eventually became infertile. The conditions $a < 1,\ c > 1$ are needed because, if both were less than one or both were greater than 1, and $a \le b \le c$, the population $P_n$ would either go to 0 or to $\infty$, unless the population is at an unstable equilibrium level. The condition $c < 1,\ a > 1$, is rejected because it would represent a helpful disease.

We can now find the conditions for equilibrium in this system. Let $S^*, I^*, P^*$, represent equilibrium values, if they exist, and let $p^* = f(I^*)$. Then

$$
\begin{aligned}
S^* &= (1 - q)(aI^* + bp^*S^*) + c(1 - p^*)S^*,\\
I^* &= q(aI^* + bp^*S^*),\\
P^* &= aI^* + (bp^* - cp^* + c)S^*.
\end{aligned}
\tag{3.21}
$$

From these equations we obtain

$$M \begin{bmatrix} S^* \\ I^* \end{bmatrix} = \begin{bmatrix} 0 \\ 0 \end{bmatrix},$$

where

$$M = \begin{bmatrix} (1 - q)bp^* - cp^* + c - 1 & (1 - q)a \\ qbp^* & qa - 1 \end{bmatrix}.$$

A necessary and sufficient condition for the existence of a nontrivial solution $(S^*, I^*)$ is that the determinant of $M$ be zero. This condition leads to the equation

$$p^* = \frac{(1 - aq)(c - 1)}{c - b + q(b - ac)}. \tag{3.22}$$

We require for the model that $0 \le p^* \le 1$. Since $p^* \le 1$, we must have

$$q \ge \frac{b - 1}{b - a} \tag{3.23a}$$

or, equivalently,

$$b \le \frac{1 - aq}{1 - q}. \tag{3.23b}$$

From (3.22), we see that the equilibrium value $p^*$ does not depend on the function $f$, only on the parameters $a, b, c, q$. Also, given $p^*$, the unique value of $I^*$ is the solution of $f(I^*) = p^*$, or $I^* = f^{-1}(p^*)$, and $S^*$ may be computed from (3.21). Moreover, from the second equation in (3.21) and from (3.22), we get

$$\frac{I^*}{S^*} = \frac{qbp^*}{1 - aq} = \frac{bq(c-1)}{c - b + q(b - ac)}, \tag{3.24}$$

thus the prevalence is not dependent on the function $f$, and is positive when (3.20) holds.

Let us now think of $b$ as a parameter that may be varied, and let

$$q_c = \frac{b-1}{b-a}$$

be the critical value of $q$. Thus, $q \geq q_c$ is the condition in order that $p^* \leq 1$. We observe that $q_c$ is a strictly increasing function of $b$ that is zero at $b = 1$ and asymptotically approaches 1 as $b \to \infty$. For $a < b \leq 1$, $q_c$ is negative, and any $q$ in the allowable range $0 < q \leq 1$ will satisfy (3.23a). As $b$ varies with $b \geq a$, $p^*$ increases, with value $(1 - qa)(c - 1)/[c - 1 + q(1 - ac)]$ at $b = 1$, and value $p^* = 1$ at $b = (1 - aq)/(1 - q)$. The prevalence is also strictly increasing with $b$, with prevalence equal to $aq(c - 1)/(c - a)$ at $b = a$, to $q(c - 1)/[c - 1 + qc(1 - a)]$ at $b = 1$, and to $q$ at $b = (1 - aq)/(1 - q)$. We shall extend the discussion of Régnière by investigating the stability of the equilibrium $S^*, I^*$ under small perturbations. That is, the local stability of this constant solution. The functions on the right side of equation (3.17) are

$$g(S, I) = (1 - q)[aI + bSf(I)] + cS[1 - f(I)],$$
$$h(S, I) = q[aI + bSf(I)].$$

The Jacobian matrix of $g, h$ is therefore

$$\begin{bmatrix} (1 - q)bf(I) + c[1 - f(I)] & (1 - q)a + Sf'(I)[(1 - q)b - c] \\ qbf(I) & qa + qbSf'(I) \end{bmatrix},$$

and the characteristic equation is

$$\lambda^2 - \beta\lambda + \gamma = 0,$$

where $\beta$ is the trace of $J$ and $\gamma$ is the determinant of $J$, evaluated at the equilibrium. Using the fact that $f(I^*) = p^*$, and letting $f'$ denote $f'(I^*)$, we find that

$$\beta = \operatorname{tr} J = [(1 - q)b - c]p^* + c + qa + qbS^*f',$$
$$\gamma = \det J = cq[a(1 - p^*) + bS^*f'].$$

Since $p^* < 1$ and $f'(I^*) > 0$, it is clear that $\gamma > 0$. Also,

$$\beta = -[c - b + q(b - ac)]p^* - qacp^* + c + qa + qbS^*f',$$

and using (3.22) we obtain

$$\beta = 1 + qac(1 - p^*) + qbS^*f' > 1.$$

We shall now use the following lemma[4]

**Lemma 3.13** *Both roots $\lambda$ of the quadratic equation $\lambda^2 - \beta\lambda + \gamma = 0$, where $\beta$ and $\gamma$ are real, satisfy $|\lambda| < 1$, if and only if*

$$2 > 1 + \gamma > |\beta|.$$

In our case, $\beta$ is positive, and we only need to check the conditions $\gamma < 1$ and $\beta < 1 + \gamma$. The second of these takes the form

$$-[c - b + qb - qac]p^* + c + qa - 1 - cqa < qb(c - 1)S^* f'.$$

Using the expression for $p^*$ in (3.22), we find that this reduces to $0 < qb(c - 1)S^* f'$, which is satisfied since $c > 1$ and $f'(I^*) > 0$. The condition $\gamma < 1$ is

$$S^* f'(I^*) < \frac{1 - acq(1 - p^*)}{bcq}. \tag{3.25}$$

We have shown that the equilibrium $(S^*, I^*)$, is locally asymptotically stable if and only if (3.25) is satisfied.

We shall consider two special forms of $f(I)$. First, suppose that $f(I) = kI$, where $k$ is a constant, that is, that $f$ is of the mass-action form. Although this does not have the saturating form suggested by Régnière, the previous analysis is valid. In this case, we have $kI^* = p^*$, $S^* = (1 - qa)/(bqk)$, and (3.25) becomes

$$\frac{1 - qa}{bq} < \frac{1 - acq(1 - p^*)}{bcq}$$

or

$$p^* > \frac{c - 1}{acq}.$$

From (3.22), this has the form

$$\frac{1 - qa}{c - b + q(b - ac)} > \frac{1}{acq},$$

which cannot hold when $q = 1$ since $0 < a < 1$, while when $0 < q < 1$ the denominator is positive, and the inequality is equivalent to

$$b > \frac{c(1 - aq)^2}{1 - q}.$$

However, the expression on the right is greater than $c$ since $0 < a < 1$, and this inequality cannot be satisfied because of the assumption that $b \leq c$. Consequently, the equilibrium is never stable if $f(I) = kI$.

The second special form is the one proposed by Régnière,

---

[4] See Hassell and May (1973), page 693. An elementary proof may be found in Edelstein-Keshet (1988), page 57.

$$f(I) = (1 - e^{-\alpha I})^\delta, \qquad (3.26)$$

with $\delta \geq 1, \alpha > 0$. The equilibrium values are then

$$I^* = -\frac{1}{\alpha} \ln(1 - \sqrt[\delta]{p^*}),$$

$$S^* = \frac{(1 - qa)}{qbp^*} I^*,$$

and

$$f'(I^*) = \nu = \alpha\delta(1 - e^{-\alpha I^*})^{\delta-1} e^{-\alpha I^*},$$

$$= \alpha\delta(p^*)^{\frac{\delta-1}{\delta}}(1 - \sqrt[\delta]{p^*}).$$

Now (3.25) can be written as

$$\frac{\nu(1 - aq)}{qbp^*} I^* < \frac{1 - acq(1 - p^*)}{bcq},$$

or

$$p^*[1 - acq + acqp^*] > -\frac{c\nu}{\alpha}(1 - qa)\ln(1 - \sqrt[\delta]{p^*}). \qquad (3.27)$$

The range of values of the parameters for which (3.27) and (3.23) hold could be examined numerically. Régnière's paper includes numerical simulation results which we present graphically in Fig. 3.8, with the regions of stable equilibrium or oscillations delineated.

Now consider the saturating function

$$f(I) = \frac{I}{k + I}, \quad (k > 0), \qquad (3.28)$$

which has the properties $f(0) = 0, f(\infty) = 1, f'(I) = k/(k + I)^2 > 0$. From $f(I^*) = p^*$, we get

$$I^* = \frac{kp^*}{1 - p^*},$$

$$S^* = \frac{(1 - qa)I^*}{qbp^*} = \frac{1 - qa}{qb}\frac{k}{1 - p^*},$$

$$f'(I^*) = \frac{(1 - p^*)^2}{k} > 0.$$

Therefore, (3.27) implies

$$p^* > \frac{c(1 - qa) + qac - 1}{c(1 - qa) + qac} = \frac{c - 1}{c}.$$

Using (3.22), this becomes

$$\frac{1 - qa}{c - b + q(b - ac)} > \frac{1}{c},$$

which reduces to $0 > (q - 1)b$ or $b > 0$. In this case, therefore, the equilibrium is always asymptotically stable when the parameters satisfy (3.20) (for any

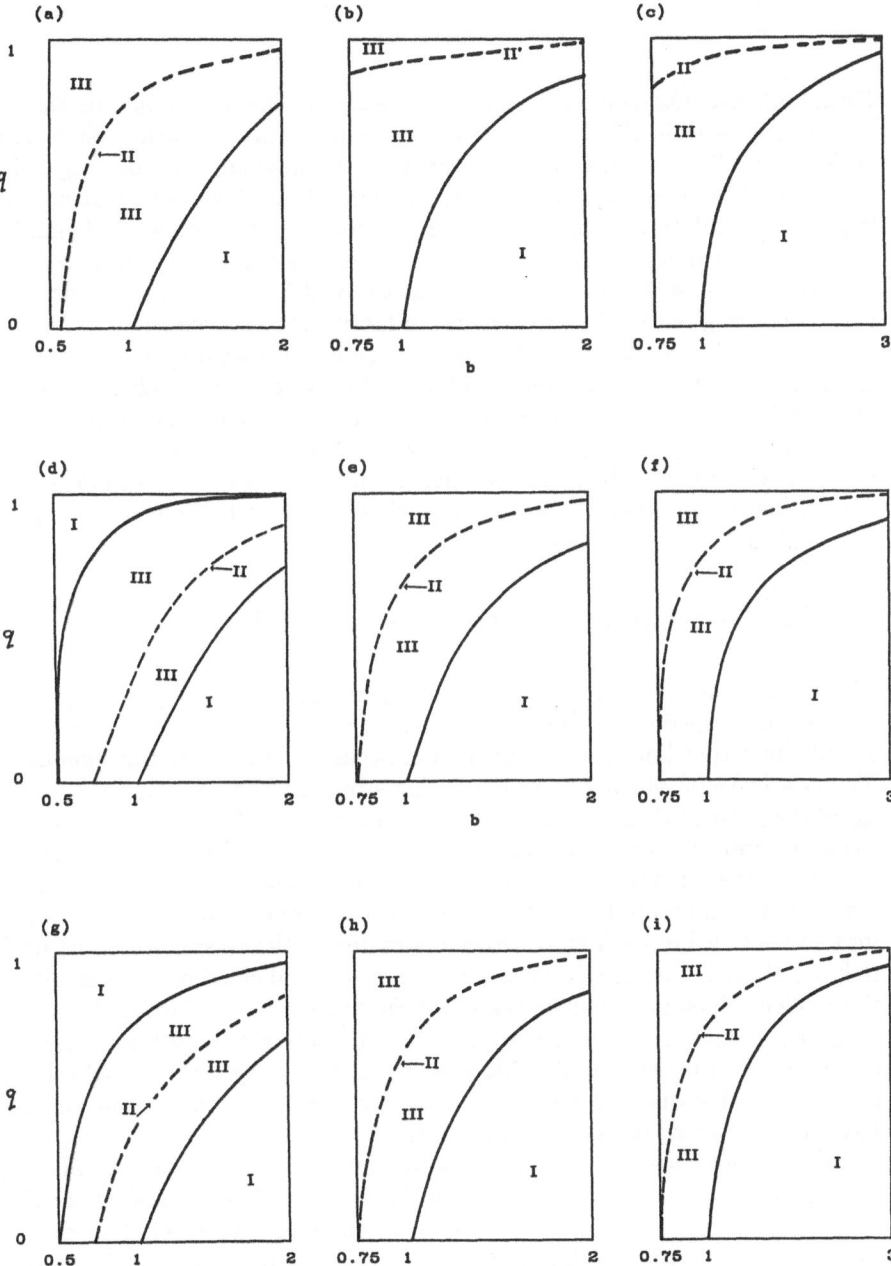

**Fig. 3.8.** Parameter regions with different dynamic behavior. $\delta = 1$ for (a), (b), (c), $\delta = 2$ for (d), (e), (f), and $\delta = 3$ for (g), (h), (i). The lower and upper limits of $b$ are equal to $a$ and $c$, respectively. Region I : Unstable oscillations or absence of equilibrium. Region II : Limit cycles. Region III : Damped oscillations.

$k > 0$). Thus a saturation function $f$ such as that in (3.28) is more stabilizing than the linear mass-action function $f(I) = kI$.

**Conclusions.** Régnière has observed by using numerical simulations that for $f(I)$ of the form in (3.26), there are regions of parameter space where limit cycles (periodic oscillations) occur, but if $q = 1$, these are unstable, regardless of the other model parameters. He concludes that if vertical transmission is perfect, regulation of the population cannot be achieved. A mathematical verification of this assertion is left as an open question which has not been addressed to date. He also observes that the width of the region of unstable oscillations is greater when the net reproductive rate of diseased insects, $a$, is low. "Thus, diseases which are highly pathogenic, and are dispersed widely yet thinly in their host's environment ($\delta >> 1$) must have little effect on newly infected individuals and must be transmitted to a relatively small proportion of the host's progeny in order to achieve regulation. In the limit ($\delta \to \infty$), regulation is not possible." For further discussion of the implications of this model, the reader should refer to the original paper of Régnière.

## 3.5 Logistic Control in the Reproduction Rate

We present here a model due to Busenberg and Cooke [1982] which takes into account both the discrete generations that occur in certain vector populations and the fact that horizontal transmission occurs continuously throughout the life span of these vectors. The particular situation that is being modeled is again the vertical transmission of *Rickettsia rickettsi* in the ticks *Dermacentor variabilis* and *Dermacentor andersoni* . This model is more realistic from the viewpoint that it does not lump all of the dynamics that occur during the season between ovipositions of the rickettsia into one point in time. It allows for more detailed modelling of the dynamics during the season of activity of the tick population. On the other hand, it is not as complicated mathematically as the models which include delays and internal structure that we shall study in Chapters 4 and 5, and consequently, much more detailed analytical conclusions can be derived for this model. Models of this type may well be useful in the analysis of other diseases which are vertically transmitted in populations that have rather narrow reproduction periods.

The model relies on the population dynamics of the tick vectors and Figure 3.9 gives a schematic description of the seasonal dynamics of one of these arthropod vectors, *Dermacentor variabilis* (American dog tick). This description is based on the detailed studies reported in Burgdorfer [1975] and, in particular, on the work of Sonenshine [1971]. These ticks hatch into their larval form from eggs laid by female adults. The larvae and nymphs engorge with a blood meal before moulting and emerging as adults. The larvae and the nymphs feed on small mammals; the adults, however, feed on large mammals, including man, before mating and laying eggs.

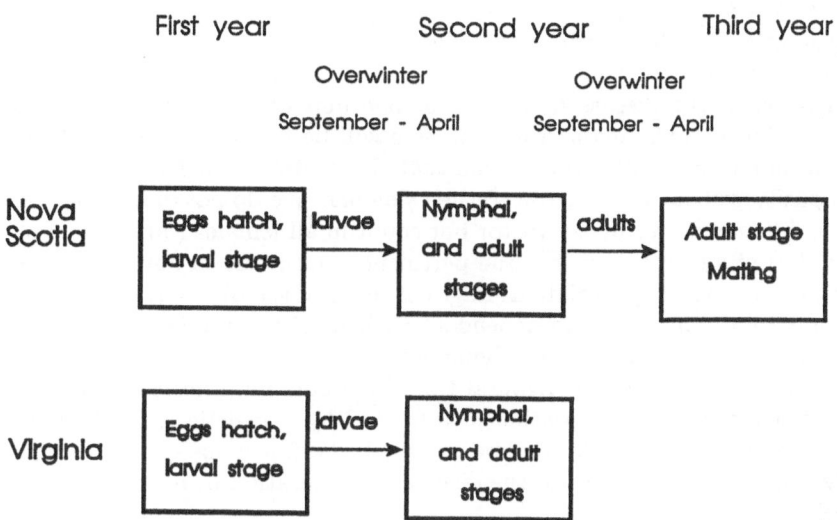

**Fig. 3.9.** Seasonal dynamics of *Dermacentor variabilis* in the Eastern USA

Based on these observations, we propose the model that is described below in order to be able to assess the influence of the two modes of transmission of the disease. This model is not intended to provide a detailed description of the intricate relations between the various stages of the ticks, their environment, the hosts on which they feed, and the temporal progress of the rickettsial infection. Rather, it is designed to collect a few salient parameters that affect the progress of this disease in the ticks and to give qualitative estimates of their relative influence and importance. The model is based on the following assumptions:

(i) The progress of the disease can be described by keeping track of the female portion of the tick population. These females are separated into two classes, those susceptible to the disease and those who are infectious. Once infected a tick remains infected for the balance of its life.

(ii) The infected females pass on the disease to a proportion of their offspring. The generations are discrete and the infection is transmitted from one generation to the next by this vertical path only.

(iii) Individuals within a given generation transmit the disease horizontally via contact (through feeding on common hosts) between infectious and susceptible ticks. The degree of this contact is a function of the number of susceptible and infectious females only. This function includes the contribution of the infected part of the male population.

(iv) Oviposition by mated adult females is preceded by a maturation period during which the ticks go through the changes that transform larvae into adults and also are exposed to horizontal transfer of the disease among members of the same generation.

We let $S_n(t)$ and $I_n(t)$ denote the portion of the female population of generation $n$ which is, respectively, susceptible and infected at time $t$. We will normalize the time variable so that each generation or cohort group is involved in the disease dynamics for one unit of time. For example, for $D.$ $variabilis$ in Nova Scotia a unit of time will be two years while in Virginia it will be one year. We also assume that the environment has a finite carrying capacity which we normalize to the value one. We do not distinguish between the different forms of the vector but count in all females (larvae, nymphs and adults) of generation $n$. So, the pertinent parameters in our model will have values that are appropriate averages of those of the different forms of the tick population, and are time dependent with period one reflecting the seasonal variations in tick population dynamics.

If we assume that horizontal transfer occurs via a mass-action term and that oviposition of generation $n$ is limited by a logistic term dependent on the total female population, we arrive at the following system of equations describing the dynamics of the disease for generation $n$, $n = 1, 2, 3, \ldots$

$$\frac{dI_n}{dt} = -cI_n + kS_nI_n, \quad n < t \leq n+1,$$

$$\frac{dS_n}{dt} = -cS_n - kS_nI_n, \quad n < t \leq n+1,$$

(3.29)

and for $n = 2, 3, \ldots$,

$$I_n(n) = \frac{(1-p)}{m_2 - m_1} \int_{m_1+n-1}^{m_2+n-1} b_I(t)I_{n-1}(t)[1 - I_{n-1}(t) - S_{n-1}(t)]dt,$$

$$S_n(n) = \frac{1}{m_2 - m_1} \int_{m_1+n-1}^{m_2+n-1} [b_S(t)S_{n-1}(t) + pb_I(t)I_{n-1}(t)]$$

(3.30)

$$[1 - I_{n-1}(t) - S_{n-1}(t)]dt,$$

$$0 \leq m_1 \leq m_2 \leq 1,$$

where

$$I_1(1) = I_0, \quad S_1(1) = S_0.$$

(3.31)

Since we normalized the total population so that the carrying capacity of the environment is one, the term $1 - I_{n-1}(t) - S_{n-1}(t)$ represents the logistic control on the oviposition. The death rate, $c$, the birth rates $b_I$ and $b_S$, the horizontal transmission factor $k$, the maturation window limits $m_1$ and $m_2$ and the proportion $0 \leq q = 1 - p \leq 1$ of infected offspring of an infected female, and the initial data $I_0$ and $S_0$ are considered as known. All time dependent parameters are assumed to be continuous, positive and periodic with period one.

The quantities of interest from the viewpoint of epidemiology are the proportion of the carrying capacity consisting of infected and susceptible vectors in the current generation. So, we let

$$S(t) = S_{[t]}(t), \quad I(t) = I_{[t]}(t), \ t \geq 1,$$

(3.32)

where $[t]$ denotes the greatest integer less than or equal to $t$. We call the pair $(S, I)$, the solution of the "sequential differential difference system" (3.29)-(3.31). We note that existence and uniqueness of solutions of the systems (3.29)-(3.31) follow directly from simple applications of standard theorems.

In order to analyze the effects of the various parameters on the dynamics of this model we shall treat two distinct special cases before looking at the general model. As we shall see below, the dynamics of even this simple model can be quite involved.

We first note that if $m_1 = m_2 = 0$, that is, if no maturation period is present, the disease is not transmitted horizontally in the reproducing population, and the only mode of perpetuation of the infection is via vertical transmission. To treat this case we first let $m_1 \to m_2 = m$, and reduce equations (3.30) to

$$
\begin{aligned}
I_n(n) &= (1-p)b_I(n-1+m)I_{n-1}(n-1+m) \\
&\quad [1 - I_{n-1}(n-1+m) - S_{n-1}(n-1+m)], \\
S_n(n) &= [b_S(n-1+m)S_{n-1}(n-1+m) \\
&\quad + pb_I(n-1+m)I_{n-1}(n-1+m)] \\
&\quad [(1 - I_{n-1}(n-1+m) - S_{n-1}(n-1+m)].
\end{aligned}
\tag{3.33}
$$

These equations replace (3.30) when maturation occurs synchronously $m$ units of time after the start of the generation. Now, letting $m \to 0$ in (3.33) we get

$$
\begin{aligned}
I_n(n) &= (1-p)b_I(n-1)I_{n-1}(n-1)] \\
&\quad [1 - I_{n-1}(n-1) - S_{n-1}(n-1)], \\
S_n(n) &= [b_S(n-1)S_{n-1}(n-1) \\
&\quad + pb_I(n-1)I_{n-1}(n-1)] \\
&\quad [1 - I_{n-1}(n-1) - S_{n-1}(n-1)].
\end{aligned}
\tag{3.34}
$$

We will start by looking at the simplest of these systems consisting of (3.29) and (3.34). However, we note that in all cases (3.29) can be explicitly integrated to yield the following expressions for $I_n(t)$ and $S_n(t)$ for $n \le t \le n+1$:

$$
I_n(t) = \frac{I_n(n)P_n(n)e^{-\int_0^{t-n} c(s)ds}}{I_n(n) + S_n(n)e^{-P_n(n)\int_0^{t-n} k(u)e^{-\int_0^u c(s)ds}du}},
\tag{3.35}
$$

$$
S_n(t) = \frac{S_n(n)P_n(n)e^{-\int_0^{t-n} c(s)ds}}{S_n(n) + I_n(n)e^{P_n(n)\int_0^{t-n} k(u)e^{-\int_0^u c(s)ds}du}},
\tag{3.36}
$$

where $P_n(t) = S_n(t) + I_n(t)$ is the total normalized population of generation $n$ at time $t$.

In the case where $m = 0$, (3.34) is independent of the solution (3.35)-(3.36) of (3.29). We also note that $b_I(n-1) = b_I(1), b_S(n-1) = b_S(1)$ do not depend on $n$ because of their periodicity, and for simplicity we write them as $b_I$ and $b_S$ in the next two results.

**Theorem 3.14** *Let $S_n(n)$ and $I_n(n)$ be a solution of* (3.34). *Then the "prevalence rate" $r_n = I_n(n)/P_n(n)$, has the following behavior:*
    *(a) If $(1-p)b_I \leq b_S$, then $r_n \to 0$ as $n \to \infty$.*
    *(b) If $(1-p)b_I > b_S$, then $r_n \to ((1-p)b_I - b_S)/(b_I - b_S)$ as $n \to \infty$.*

This theorem gives a simple threshold condition for the maintenance of the infection through vertical transmission only ($m = 0$). It states that an endemic level will be sustained via vertical transmission in the absence of a maturation period, if and only if, the rate of reproduction of infectious offspring exceeds the rate of reproduction of susceptible offspring from susceptible parents.

The above result concerns the prevalence rate $r_n$ while the next speaks about the dynamics of the total population $P_n(n)$.

**Theorem 3.15** *Let $a = \max\{b_S, (1-p)b_I\} \leq 4$ and consider the quadratic map*

$$x_n = ax_{n-1}(1 - x_{n-1}). \tag{3.37}$$

*Then for each $x_1 \in [0, 1]$ there exists $P_1(1) \in [0, 1]$ such that the total population $P_n(n)$ obeys $|x_n - P_n(n)| \to 0$ as $n \to \infty$, and hence, has the same dynamic behavior as the solutions of* (3.37). *Moreover, if $(1-p)b_I \leq b_S$, then $|x_n - S_n(n)| \to 0$, while if $(1-p)b_I > b_S$, $|S_n(n)(b_I - b_S)/pb_I - x_n| \to 0$ and $|(b_I - b_S)I_n(n)/((1-p)b_I - b_S) - x_n| \to 0$ as $n \to \infty$.*

The above results show that, as is not uncommon with discrete nonlinear difference equations, the population levels may experience very complicated chaotic dynamic behavior. The behavior of the quadratic map (3.37) has been extensively described and we refer the reader to Section 3.7.4 for a brief introduction and to the books by Devaney [1986] and by Lasota and Mackey [1985] for further details. In Fig. 3.10 we illustrate this chaotic behavior by plotting $S(n)$ and $I(n)$ for one special case of (3.34). Numerical plots of this type are very easy to produce using even rudimentary personal computers, and we shall be content with showing only the one case in this figure at this point. We will return to a discussion of the significance of this type of dynamic behavior in the next subsection.

We now move on to the more complicated case where $0 \neq m_1 \neq m_2$, but first assume that $b_I = b_S = b$. This is a reasonable hypothesis for *rickettsia* infestations in *Dermacentor variabilis*. We have the following result which provides expressions which show the effects of the maturation period on the dynamics of the model.

**Theorem 3.16** *Let*

$$a = \frac{1}{m_2 - m_1} \int_{m_1+n-1}^{m_2+n-1} b(t) e^{-\int_0^{t-n+1} c(s)ds} dt, \qquad (3.38)$$

*and*

$$d = \frac{1}{m_2 - m_1} \int_{m_1+n-1}^{m_2+n-1} b(t) e^{-2\int_0^{t-n+1} c(s)ds} dt, \qquad (3.39)$$

*and consider equation (3.37) with a given by (3.38). Then the total population $P_n(n)$ at the start of generation $n$ satisfies equations (3.29)-(3.30) with $b_I = b_S = b$, and obeys the relation $P_n(n) = x_n/d$, where $x_n$ solves (3.37) with $x_1 = dP_1(1)$.*

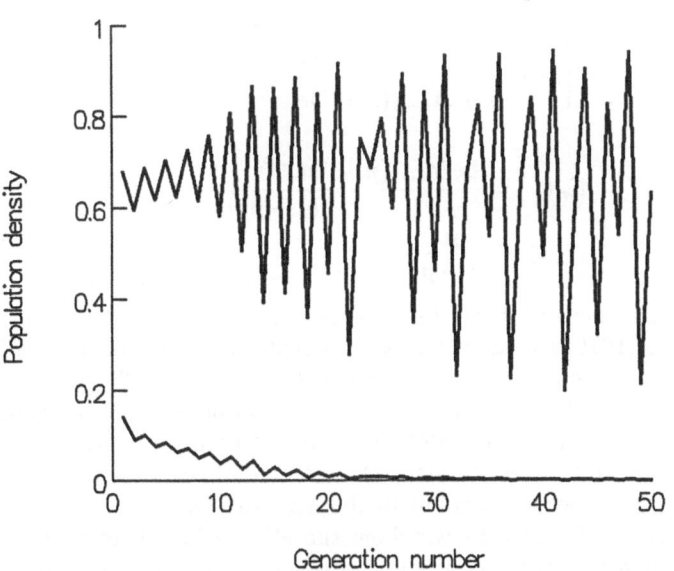

**Fig. 3.10.** Dynamic behavior of the susceptible and infected populations with $p = 0.01$, $b_S = 3.8$, $b_I = 3.6$. The upper graph is $S(n)$ and the lower graph is $I(n)$ in (3.34). The points on the orbits have been connected as a visual aid.

The effect of the maturation period on the total population dynamics comes through the parameters $a$ and $b$. In simplistic terms, the dynamics of (3.37) becomes more complicated as $a$ increases. Here we see that an increase in the birth rate $b(t)$ or a decrease in the death rate $c(t)$ have the effect of increasing $a$. However, a change in the maturation window involves an interaction between birth and death terms that is given by (3.38) and cannot be described in a simple manner. One case where we can give a simple description is when $b$ and $c$ are constant. Here, (3.38) yields $a = b(e^{-cm_1} - e^{-cm_2})/(c(m_2 - m_1))$, which shows that an increase in $m_1$, with $m_2 - m_1$ constant has the effect of reducing the value of $a$, that is, if the maturation window occurs later, then

$a$ is decreased. In the yet more special case where $m_1 = m_2 = m$, we get $a = be^{-cm}$, and it is seen here that as the combination $cm$ (the product of the death rate and the maturation time) increases, $a$ decreases. It is worth noting that the horizontal transmission rate $k$ plays no role in the dynamics of the total population. The role of this parameter is seen by examining equations (3.29), and noting that an increase in $k$ causes a decrease in $S'_n$ and an increase in $I'_n$.

The dynamic behavior of the general case with $b_I \neq b_S$ is fairly complicated. However, if for simplicity we take $m_1 = m_2 = m$, and $c, b_I$ and $b_S$ are made constant, it can be seen that the total population $P_n(n)$ and the ratio $R_n(n) = S_n(n)/I_n(n)$ of susceptible to infected individuals at the start of generation $n$ obey the system of difference equations

$$P_n(n) = e^{-cm} P_{n-1}(n-1)[1 - e^{-cm} P_{n-1}(n-1)]$$
$$\times \left[ b_S + \frac{b_I - b_S}{1 + R_{n-1}(n-1)e^{-P_{n-1}(n-1)(1-e^{-cm})\frac{k}{c}}} \right], \tag{3.40}$$

$$R_n(n) = \frac{b_S R_{n-1}(n-1)e^{-P_{n-1}(n-1)(1-e^{-cm})\frac{k}{c}}}{(1-p)b_I}$$
$$+ \frac{p}{1-p}. \tag{3.41}$$

In this form one can treat $b_I - b_S$ as a parameter and use the techniques of Marotto [1979] to show that when chaotic behavior occurs for $P_n(n)$ with $b_I = b_S = b$, then it also occurs when $b_I - b_S$ is small. Of course, the case where $b_I = b_S = b$ has already been discussed above in a more general setting. We will not pursue a more detailed analysis here, but note that the explicit form of these equations has made them amenable to numerical studies of their dynamics which we will exploit in the next subsection.

In Figs. 3.11 and 3.12 we show the effect of changes in the maturation period, when all other parameters are kept constant. Here we have plotted $I(n)$ versus $S(n)$ for generation number $n$ ranging between 101 and 1,000 and with the parameter values $b_I = 4.0, b_S = 3.6, c = 0.01, k = 4.0, p = 0.01$ and initial data $I(1) = 0.3, S(1) = 0.6$. In the parameter ranges that we have chosen the dynamics of this system is more complicated than these plots would indicate since the population values move in a seemingly random manner from one generation to the next and the points in these graphs are not visited in any type of discernible temporal order. We will examine this behavior in more detail below. We finally note that, in some applications, the quantity of interest may be the total population $T(t)$ at time $t$. This is given by $T(t) = \sum_{n=1}^{[t]} P_n(t)$, and in the case of our model it can be written as

$$T(t) = e^{-\int_{[t]}^{t} c(s)ds} \sum_{n=1}^{[t]} e^{-\int_{[t]}^{n} c(s)ds} P_n(n),$$

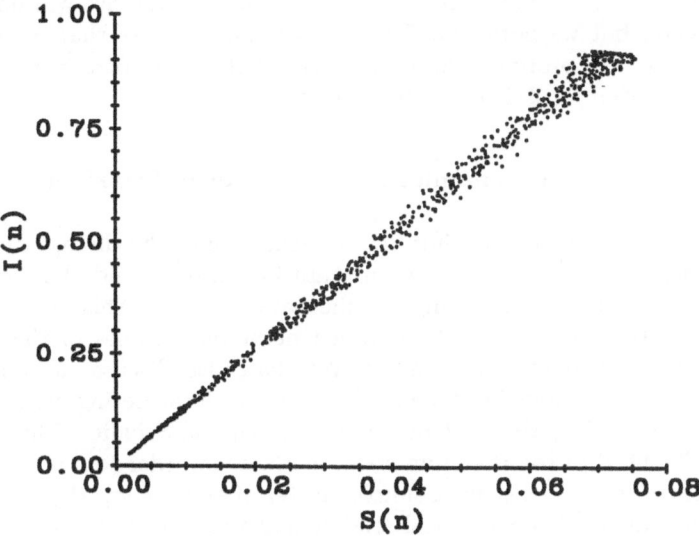

**Fig. 3.11.** Dynamics of the susceptible and infected populations for $m = 0.02$

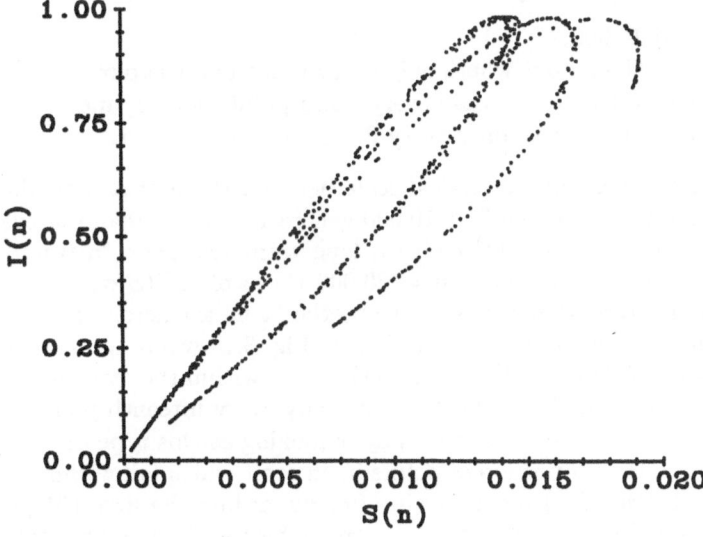

**Fig. 3.12.** Dynamics of the susceptible and infective populations for $m = 0.5$

if we assume that equations (3.40)-(3.41) hold for all $t \geq n$. So, given the dynamic behavior of $P_n(n)$, one is able to compute $T(t)$. We will not give the details here, but we note that for the particular disease that we have been modeling, it is appropriate to assume that $P_n(t) = 0$ for $t > n + 1$, so the above expression for $T$ is not valid in this case.

### 3.5.1 Complicated Dynamics and Long Term Transients

As noted above, there is an intricate dependence of the disease dynamics of this model on the measure of the maturation rate $m$, and chaotic behavior can be expected in a wide range of the parameters. In this section we turn to some of the issues raised by detailed numerical studies of this model as $m$ and other parameters are varied. We shall also discuss the possible use of the modern methods in dynamical systems in interpreting epidemiological data as suggested by the work of Schaffer [1985] and Schaffer, Ellner and Kot [1986]. The need to resort to numerical methods in order to study qualitative properties of the model is not a simple matter of expediency. Rather, there are basic phenomena that numerical studies make strikingly obvious but which cannot be treated with current methods of mathematical analysis. One of these phenomena is the occurrence of the type of very long term transient behavior which we illustrate in figures 3.13–3.15.

In Figs. 3.13(a) and 3.13(b) we plot $I(n)$ versus $S(n)$ with the parameter values $b_S = 4.0$, $b_I = 3.6$, $c = 0.01$, $k = 4.0$, $m = 0.05$, $p = 0.01$, initial data $I(1) = 0.3$, $S(1) = 0.6$, and for generation number $n$ ranging between

(a) 101 and 10,000,
(b) 101 and 50,000 but where only every tenth point is plotted,
(c) 101 and 100,000 with only every tenth point plotted, and
(d) 101 to 200,000 with only every fifteenth point plotted.

Noting the change of vertical scale between the first and the latter three plots, we see that for the first 10,000 generations the dynamics, even though complicated, remains confined to a long term transient "attractor" within which $I(n) < 0.4$. At about $n = 20,000$ the orbit of $(S(n), I(n))$ exits this region and enters what turns out to be the "true attractor" which lies above the original region, and which we show in Fig. 3.14 where we have plotted the orbit with initial data $I(1) = 0.5$, $S(1) = 0.35$ within the "true attractor" and for $n$ ranging from 101 to 200,000 with only every fifteenth point plotted.

In Fig. 3.15 we show another way of looking at this type of data. Here we have plotted the proportion of points in an orbit which fall within a particular area of the $I(n), S(n)$ plane, again after discarding the first 101 points. The parameter and initial values are the same as for Fig. 3.14 and the total number of generations varies as shown on the graphs. The same two types of attractors, the transient and the true, are perhaps more easily seen here, with the first of these being the dominant one for up to $n$ near 10,000 and with the latter becoming increasingly dominant as $n$ reaches and grows beyond 40,000.

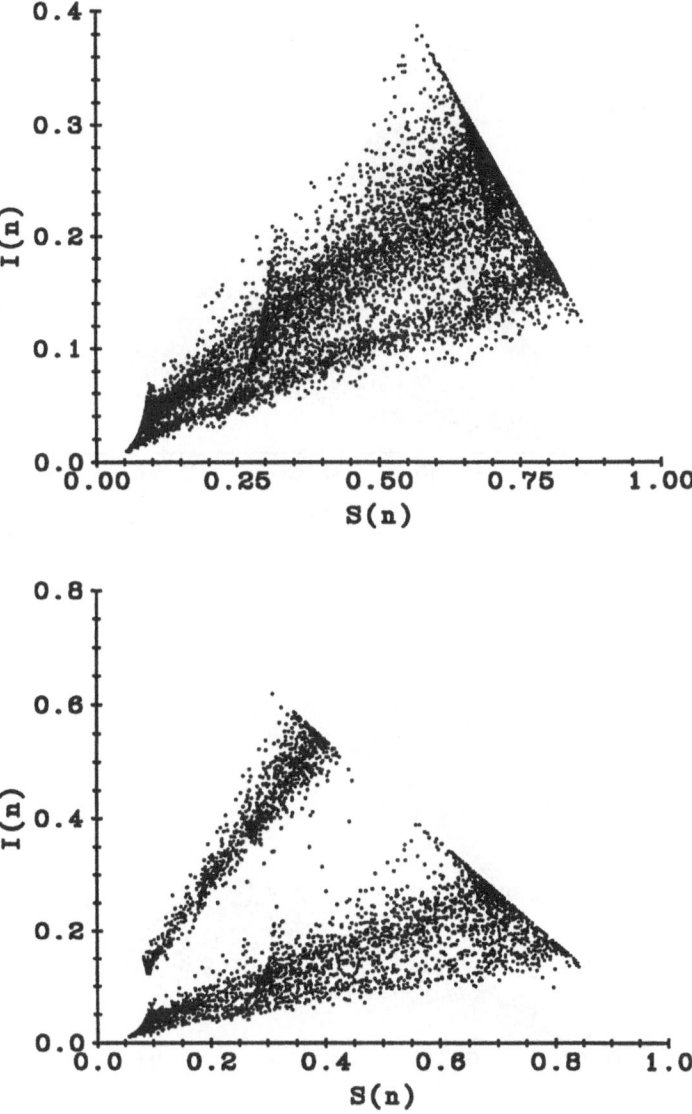

**Fig. 3.13(a).** Dynamics of the susceptible and infective populations for $b_S = 4.0, b_I = 3.6, c = 0.01, k = 4.0, m = 0.05, p = 0.01$, initial data $I(1) = 0.3, S(1) = 0.6$ and for $n$ ranging from 101 to a) 10,000; and b) 50,000 (one of every tenth point on the orbit is plotted).

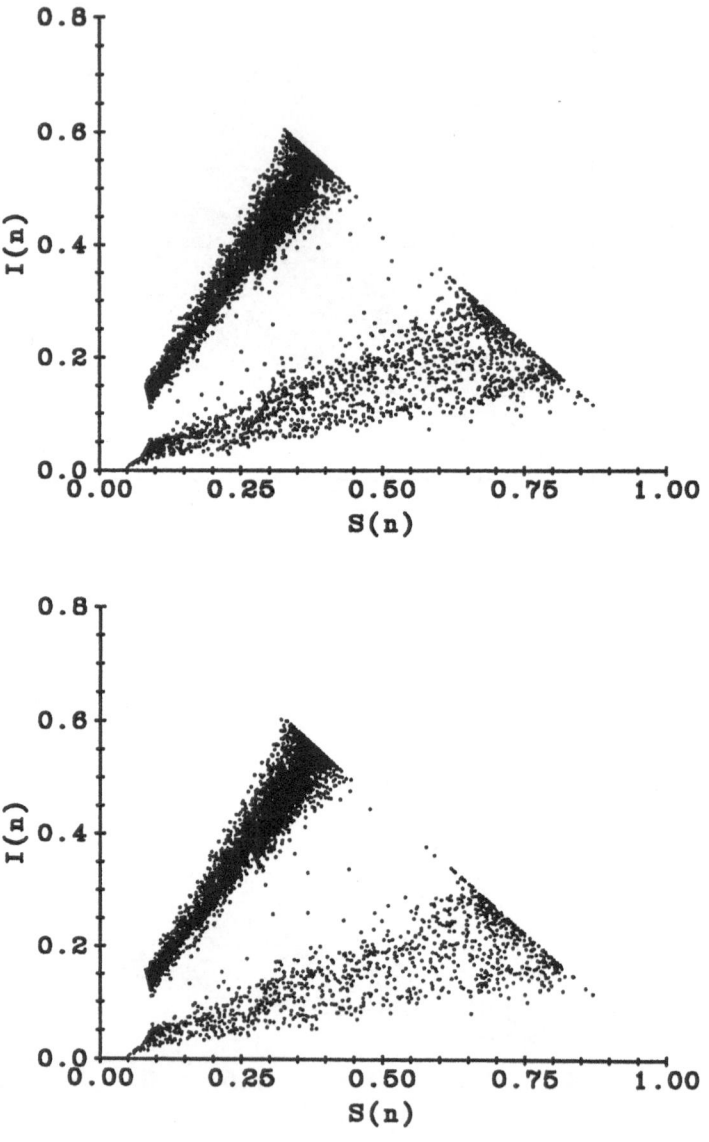

**Fig. 3.13(b).** Dynamics of the susceptible and infective populations for $b_S = 4.0, b_I = 3.6, c = 0.01, k = 4.0, m = 0.05, p = 0.01$, initial data $I(1) = 0.3, S(1) = 0.6$ and for $n$ ranging from 101 to c) 100,000 (one of every tenth point is plotted); and d) 200,000 (one of every fifteenth point is plotted).

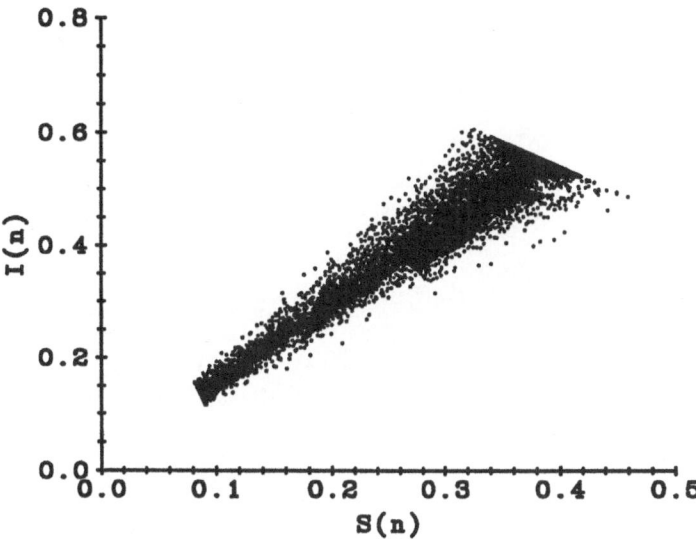

**Fig. 3.14.** Dynamics of the susceptible and infective populations for $b_S = 4.0, b_I = 3.6, c = 0.01, k = 4.0, m = 0.05, p = 0.01$, initial data $I(1) = 0.5, S(1) = 0.35$ and for $n$ ranging from 101 to 200,000. One of every fifteen points on the orbit is plotted.

Current methods of analysis allow us to describe this second region and to also study, via linearization and asymptotic methods, the initial transient behavior essentially contained in the first 101 points of the orbit that we have not plotted. However, mathematics has little to offer that can describe the long term transient. For much of the initial data lying near or below this transient attractor, the population will tend to it and remain there for 10,000 to 20,000 generations. Since in this model each generation amounts to one year, it is clear that this transient is a significant region, and numerical experimentation is the only presently available tool for studying it. This points out the importance of obtaining estimates of the time that is needed before solutions approach an attractor, even when it is known that it is globally asymptotically stable. For, even though the structure of the attractor may be very simple, the dynamical behavior of the system may be such that during the time interval of interest from the biological point of view, the orbit may be in a transient mode that remains far from the eventual attractor. In such a setting the question of the stability of the attractor is not important, rather what is needed is an accurate description of the transient orbit. For this purpose numerical methods seem to provide the best currently available approach.

The "chaotic" aspect of the dynamics that we have been describing raises questions concerning the predictive value of this type of population models. Assuming that the models do indeed give a valid qualitative view of the actual population dynamics, we need to address the fact that small changes in initial

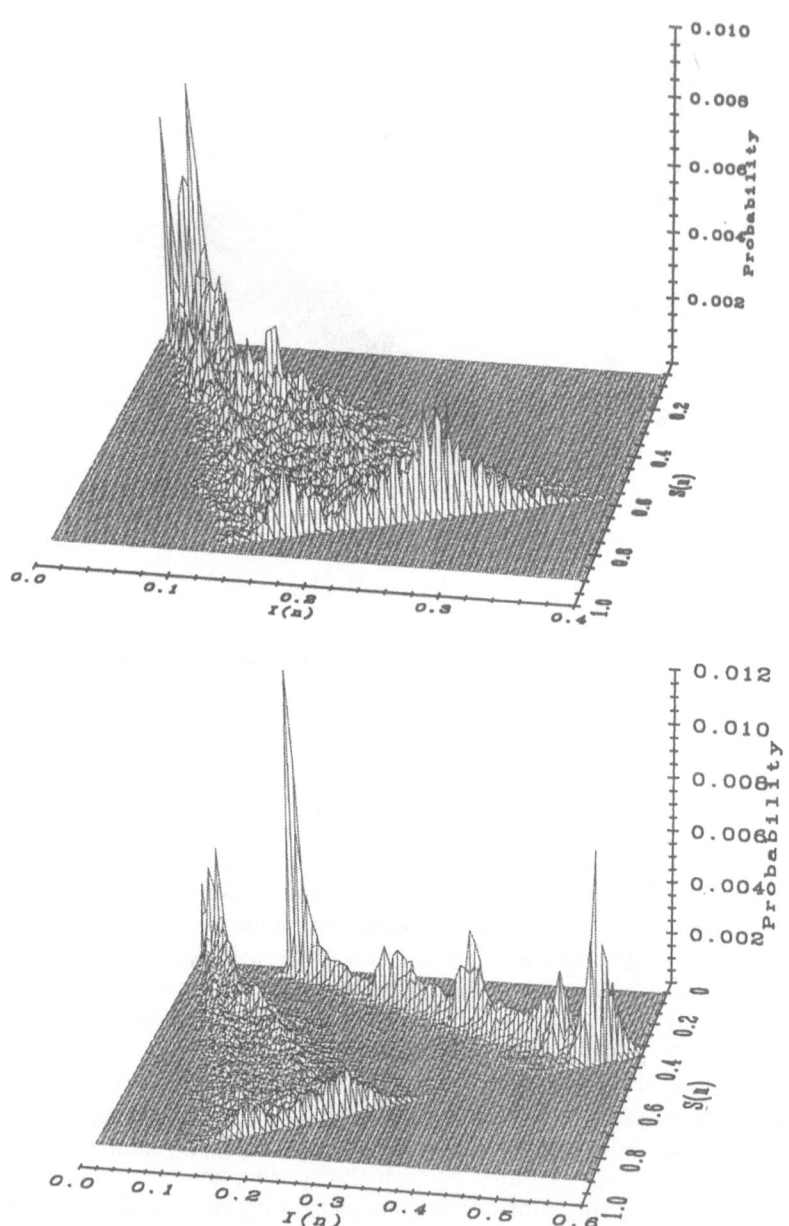

**Fig. 3.15(a).** Proportion of times that a point $(I(n), S(n))$ lies in a given region for $b_S = 4.0, b_I = 3.6, c = 0.01, k = 4.0, m = 0.05, p = 0.01$, initial data $I(1) = 0.3, S(1) = 0.6$ and for $n$ ranging from 101 to a) 10,000, and b) 40,000.

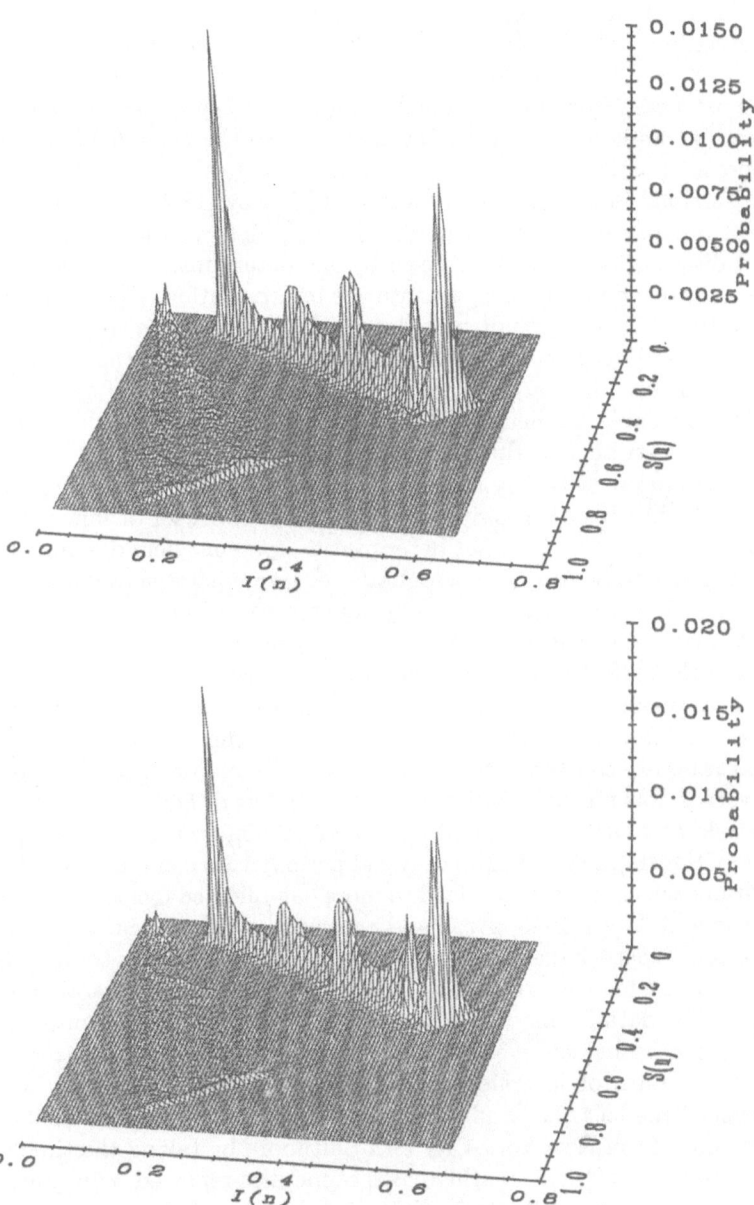

**Fig. 3.15(b).** Proportion of times that a point $(I(n), S(n))$ lies in a given region for $b_S = 4.0, b_I = 3.6, c = 0.01, k = 4.0, m = 0.05, p = 0.01$, initial data $I(1) = 0.3, S(1) = 0.6$ and for $n$ ranging from 101 to c) 100,000, and d) 140,000

data, which often are based on very inaccurate field observations, can cause huge variations of the orbits. This dictates an approach that views the statistical properties of large numbers of such orbits as the only relevant results that can be extracted from such models, or indeed, of any quantitative conclusion that can be made on the basis of even the most exhaustive field observations. This point of view is backed by a solid mathematical foundation which is lucidly described in the book of Lasota and Mackey [1985]. The mathematical models, when analyzed from this viewpoint, point out the nature of the statistical distributions that are caused by the deterministic nonlinearities, and hence, provide additional insights into the interpretation of field data and into the question of what type of such data is most relevant in making statistical predictions and parameter estimations. The uncertainty in the predictions appears as an essential part of these nonlinear models, but is quantifiable via currently available mathematical methods which allow the calculation of the probability distributions that govern the behavior of the model.

The adoption of the dynamical systems viewpoint in treating epidemiological data has been strongly promoted in the work of Schaffer [1985] and his collaborators. The fact that deterministic systems yield dynamic behavior which appears to be caused by stochastic or unpredictable random events has led Schaffer to suggest that the traditional statistical analysis of epidemiological data may not be the most appropriate way of understanding the underlying processes that affect the transmission of the disease.

A convenient parting point in describing this work is the standard $S \to E \to I \to R$ model with seasonal fluctuations in the contact rates. When the contact rates are constant, this model does not exhibit complicated dynamics. However, as was strongly indicated in the studies of Dietz [1976], Grossman, Gumowski and Dietz [1977], and Grossman [1980], and proved in the seminal papers of Smith [1983a, 1983b], seasonal periodicities can induce subharmonic oscillations which, in fact, can lead to more complicated dynamics as shown by Schwartz and Smith [1983], Aron and Schwartz [1984], and Schwartz [1985]. In these latter papers the seasonal periodicities have been shown to cause the type of period doubling cascades that are often connected with chaotic dynamical systems. The data for measles epidemics in large cities in developed countries show both seasonal fluctuations due to the effects of school attendance on the contact rates of juveniles, as well what appear to be purely stochastic variations. Schaffer [1985] and in further work Schaffer and Kot [1985] analyze measles data from New York City and Baltimore by taking the time series of the number, say $x(t)$, of monthly cases of measles reported by physicians and plotting the trajectory in three dimensional space of the vector $(x(t), x(t + 3), x(t + 6))$, where t is measured in month units. The resulting plots show a strong resemblance to the trajectories of three dimensional dynamical systems. The basic idea here, which has been proposed by Takens [1980] and others, is to use the data from the one state variable that is measured and to shift it appropriately in time in order to obtain information that reflects the behavior of other variables which are not available. If a small number of dimensions suffice to produce an orbit that appears similar to one caused by deterministic chaotic systems, then what appear to be stochastic effects may well be best described by a deterministic nonlinear system rather than by purely statistical methods. This is a method that may provide a good link between complicated data and deterministic models that are based on a mathematical formulation of the underlying disease transmission and demographic mechanisms, and the reader is referred to the original papers for the detailed description of the results that have been obtained by these means. We note in closing that there has not yet been a systematic study and development of a formal process by which this type of interpretation of the data can be used as part of a parameter estimation method for chaotic deterministic systems. We believe that this step needs to be taken in order that this method provide a viable alternative to the traditional statistical methods for the quantitative interpretation of data.

## 3.6 Logistic Control through the Death Terms

The previous sequential-continuous model assumes that there is no logistic control of the total population within a generation, but that oviposition is limited by a logistic term, that is, it is the birth rather than the death terms which are being controlled by possible crowding or environmental constraints. If there is competition for a resource, such as a habitat that provides protection from predators, then the death rate has a logistic control while the oviposition remains proportional to the population. In this section we will describe the behavior of such a model and show that it is radically different from the case we have treated above where the logistic control was on the birth terms. In fact, we shall see that the complicated dynamics we encountered there cannot occur in the present case, and the population stabilizes to a constant distribution, as the generation number $n$ becomes large. Theorems 3.17 and 3.19 of this section proving this stabilization are due to Grabiner [1988], but we provide more direct proofs of these results.

   We use a variant of the notation in the previous section, with $\hat{S}_n(t)$, $\hat{I}_n(t)$, and $\hat{P}_n(t) = \hat{S}_n(t) + \hat{I}_n(t)$, respectively denoting the susceptible, the infective and the total population of generation $n$ at time $t$. There are two basic forms of the model, a simple form which assumes that all oviposition takes place at the end of the generation (when $t = n+1$), and a more general form which allows oviposition at any time during the year. We treat each of these in a separate subsection. We shall introduce the variable $\tau$ with $0 \leq \tau \leq 1$ to denote the time in a season, normalized to total length one. Thus, in generation $n$, we have $t = \tau + n \in [n, n+1]$. We use the symbols $I_n(\tau)$, $S_n(\tau)$, $P_n(\tau)$, respectively, to denote the number of susceptible, of infective and the total population of generation $n$ at epoch $\tau$.

### 3.6.1 Synchronous Oviposition

The simple form of the model with oviposition occurring at the end of each gneration is:

$$\frac{dS_n(\tau)}{d\tau} = -\left(r(\tau) + \sigma(\tau)P_n(\tau)\right)S_n(\tau) - k(\tau)S_n(\tau)I_n(\tau),$$

$$\frac{dI_n(\tau)}{d\tau} = -\left(r(\tau) + \sigma(\tau)P_n(\tau)\right)I_n(\tau) + k(\tau)S_n(\tau)I_n(\tau),$$

(3.42)

and

$$S_{n+1}(0) = b\,S_n(1) + pb\,I_n(1),$$
$$I_{n+1}(0) = qb\,I_n(1),$$

(3.43)

where, as usual, $p + q = 1$. The time-dependent parameters $r(\tau)$, $\sigma(\tau)$, and $k(\tau)$ represent, respectively, the death rate, logistic term in the death rate, and horizontal transmission term at a time $\tau$ in the season. They may be constants or non-negative continuous functions. We will assume that $\sigma(\tau)$ and $k(\tau)$ are not identically zero; the cases where one of them is zero are treated later. The following results do hold for $r(\tau)$ negative, a case which is of no biological importance for the model consisting of (3.42) and (3.43), but which will be needed later for an equation which reduces to this form. Note that by taking these parameters to depend on $\tau$ only and not on $n$, we are assuming that there is an annual periodicity which results in the recurrence of the same parameters for each generation.

**Theorem 3.17** *Consider the model consisting of* (3.42) *and* (3.43) *and define the basic reproduction rate $R$ to be*

$$R = be^{-\int_0^1 r(\tau)d\tau}.$$

*Then, if $R \leq 1$ the total population $P_n(\tau) \to 0$ as $n \to \infty$, while if $R > 1$, there exists a unique positive steady state population $\tilde{P}(\tau)$ and non-negative subpopulation levels $\tilde{I}(\tau), \tilde{S}(\tau)$ such that*

$$(S_n(\tau), I_n(\tau), P_n(\tau)) \to (\tilde{S}(\tau), \tilde{I}(\tau), \tilde{P}(\tau)), \quad \text{as } n \to \infty.$$

*The limits as $n \to \infty$ are uniform for $0 \leq \tau \leq 1$.*

*Proof.* From (3.42) and (3.43), we have

$$\frac{dP_n(\tau)}{d\tau} = -\left(r(\tau) + \sigma(\tau)P_n(\tau)\right)P_n(\tau),$$

(3.44)

with initial conditions

$$P_{n+1}(0) = bP_n(1).$$

(3.45)

Equation (3.44) can be integrated via elementary methods (setting $y = 1/P_n$, (3.44) reduces to a linear equation for $y$) to obtain

$$P_n(\tau) = \frac{P_n(0)}{e^{\int_0^\tau r(s)ds} + P_n(0)\int_0^\tau e^{\int_s^\tau r(u)du}\sigma(s)ds}.$$

(3.46)

Now, define the map $\phi : [0, \infty) \to [0, \infty)$, given by

$$\phi(P_n(0)) = P_{n+1}(0) = bP_n(1) = \frac{bP_n(0)}{e^{\int_0^1 r(s)ds} + P_n(0)\int_0^1 e^{\int_s^1 r(u)du}\sigma(s)ds}.$$

From this equation it is clear that $\phi$ is a monotone increasing, concave function on its domain of definition, that $\phi(0) = 0$ and

$$\phi(x) \to \frac{b}{\int_0^1 e^{\int_s^1 r(u)du}\sigma(s)ds} \quad \text{as } x \to \infty.$$

The behavior of $P_n(0)$ as a function of $n$ is given by the orbit of $P_1(0)$ which is determined by the iterates of $\phi$:

$$x_{n+1} = \phi(x_n), \quad x_1 = P_1(0). \tag{3.47}$$

From the above properties of $\phi$ we note that $x = 0$ is a fixed point of (3.47), and a nontrivial fixed point $\tilde{x} > 0$ exists if, and only if, the derivative $d\phi(x)/dx$ at $x = 0$ is larger than one. Moreover, when $x = 0$ is the only fixed point, all solutions of (3.47) tend monotonically to it; and whenever $\tilde{x}$ exist, it attracts all solutions of (3.47) for which $x_1 > 0$. Moreover, for such solutions, $x_n \to \tilde{x}$ monotonically.

From the expression for $\phi(x)$ we get $\phi'(0) = R$. Thus, if $R \le 1$ we have $P_n(0) \to 0$, while if $R > 1$ we have $P_n(0) \to \tilde{x} > 0$.

Suppose that $R > 1$. Denoting by $\tilde{P}(\tau)$ the solution of (3.44) with initial data $P(0) = \tilde{x}$, and using the continuous dependence of solutions of (3.44) on initial data and the fact that $\tau$ lies is a bounded interval, we get

$$P_n(\tau) \to \tilde{P}(\tau), \quad \text{as } n \to \infty,$$

the convergence being uniform in $\tau$. Similarly, when $R \le 1$, the solutions $P_n(\tau) \to 0$ uniformly in $\tau$ as $n \to \infty$, and since it is easy to see that $0 \le I_n \le P_n$ and $0 \le S_n \le P_n$, we also have that $I_n$ and $S_n$ tend to zero in this case.

In order to complete the proof for the case $R > 1$, we rewrite (3.42) and (3.43) as

$$\frac{dS_n(\tau)}{d\tau} = -(r(\tau) + \sigma(\tau)P_n(\tau))S_n(\tau) - k(\tau)S_n(\tau)(P_n(\tau) - S_n(\tau)),$$

$$\frac{dI_n(\tau)}{d\tau} = -(r(\tau) + \sigma(\tau)P_n(\tau))I_n(\tau) + k(\tau)I_n(\tau)(P_n(\tau) - I_n(\tau)),$$

and

$$S_{n+1}(0) = bS_n(1) + pb(P_n(1) - S_n(1)),$$
$$I_{n+1}(0) = qbI_n(1).$$

Each of the above equations is decoupled from the other, and hence we are dealing with two equations in one variable whose solutions in the limit as $n \to \infty$ tend to the solutions of the limiting form of the equations. The limiting equations are

$$\frac{dS_n(\tau)}{d\tau} = -\big(r(\tau) + \sigma(\tau)\tilde{P}(\tau)\big)S_n(\tau) - k(\tau)S_n(\tau)\big(\tilde{P}(\tau) - S_n(\tau)\big),$$

$$\frac{dI_n(\tau)}{d\tau} = -\big(r(\tau) + \sigma(\tau)\tilde{P}(\tau)\big)I_n(\tau) + k(\tau)I_n(\tau)\big(\tilde{P}(\tau) - I_n(\tau)\big),$$

(3.48)

with

$$S_{n+1}(0) = bS_n(1) + pb\big(\tilde{P}(1) - S_n(1)\big),$$

$$I_{n+1}(0) = qbI_n(1).$$

(3.49)

The equation for $dI_n/d\tau$ in (3.48) can be rewritten as

$$\frac{dI_n(\tau)}{d\tau} = -\big(r(\tau) + \sigma(\tau)\tilde{P}(\tau) - k(\tau)\tilde{P}(\tau) + k(\tau)I_n(\tau)\big)I_n(\tau).$$

Now, if we let $\hat{r}(\tau) = r(\tau) + \sigma(\tau)\tilde{P}(\tau) - k(\tau)\tilde{P}(\tau)$, $\hat{\sigma}(\tau) = k(\tau)$, and $\hat{b} = qb$, we have the system

$$\frac{dI_n(\tau)}{d\tau} = -\big(\hat{r}(\tau) + \hat{\sigma}(\tau)I_n(\tau)\big)I_n(\tau),$$

$$I_{n+1}(0) = \hat{b}\,I_n(1).$$

(3.50)

System (3.50) has the same form as system (3.44), (3.45), and we can apply the same reasoning to it to obtain the following threshold result which also completes the proof of Theorem 3.17.

**Theorem 3.18** *Let*

$$R_0 = qbe^{-\int_0^1 \hat{r}(\tau)d\tau},$$

*then if $R_0 \le 1$ $I_n(\tau) \to 0$ as $n \to \infty$ uniformly for $0 \le \tau \le 1$, while if $R_0 > 1$, there exists a unique initial state $\tilde{I} > 0$ and a corresponding endemic solution of (3.50) $\tilde{I}(\tau) > 0$ such that $I_n(\tau) \to \tilde{I}(\tau)$. Moreover, $S_n(\tau) \to \tilde{P}(\tau) - \tilde{I}(\tau) = \tilde{S}(\tau)$ as $n \to \infty$, uniformly in $0 \le \tau \le 1$.*

Note that the problem has two thresholds, the demographic threshold $R$ and the endemic $R_0$. Clearly, when $R \le 1$, we have $\tilde{P} = 0$, and consequently $R_0 = qR \le 1$. However, when $R > 1$ the endemic threshold $R_0$ may be greater or less than one depending on the magnitudes of $k$ and $q$. Clearly, $R_0$ is an increasing function of the vertical and horizontal transmission coefficients $q$ and $k(t)$. The coupling between the demographics and the disease dynamics occurs through $q$ and the dependence of $\hat{r}(\tau)$ on $\tilde{P}(\tau)$. This coupling is similar to other situations that we have seen earlier in this chapter as well as in Chapter 2, and which we will encounter again in some of the age-dependent models studied in Chapter 5.

The two threshold parameters $R$ and $R_0$ have natural interpretations. Since $r(\tau)$ is the natural rate of removal due to mortality, the probability of an individual surviving for the full season is $\exp(-\int_0^1 r(\tau)d\tau)$. The product of this with the birth rate $b$ is $R$ and yields the expected number of offspring for an average individual over a full season. Thus, $R \le 1$ means that each individual in the population gives birth to one or fewer offspring, and in the presence of the excess mortality due to the logistic term, this results in the eventual extinction of the population. When $R > 1$, the average individual produces more than one offspring and the population settles to an equilibrium level $\tilde{P}(\tau)$ which is determined by both the natural birth-death process and the logistic terms.

The endemic threshold $R_0$ has a similar but more complicated interpretation. Here the birth into the infective class is $\hat{b} = qb$, and the contribution of each infective over a season consists of the product of the probability of surviving for the whole season, and the expected number of new infectives that horizontal contacts with this one infective produce, that is $\exp(-\int_0^1 \hat{r}(\tau)d\tau)$. Thus the product of these two terms, which is $R_0$, yields the expected number of new infective offspring that one infective individual will produce over a season. Note that $R_0$ increases with the horizontal contact rate $k$, and decreases with the logistic removal rate $\sigma$. For the time intervals in the season where $k(\tau) > \sigma(\tau)$ $R_0$ increases with the total population $\tilde{P}(\tau)$, while for those intervals where the logistic removal rate exceeds the horizontal contact rate, $R_0$ decreases with $\tilde{P}(\tau)$. Thus the coupling between the demographic process and the disease transmission process can vary from one part of the season to another.

The following special cases are of some interest. If $\sigma(\tau)$ is identically zero (no logistic effects), then the above analysis of (3.44) is not valid. Instead, we have

$$P_n(1) = P_n(0)e^{-\int_0^1 r(\tau)\,d\tau}.$$

The population will only be stable if $R = 1$; otherwise, it will either grow or die out at the rate $R^n$. If the population is stable, then the analysis of (3.50) is still valid, because we have $\hat{\sigma}(\tau) = k(\tau) \geq 0$ and not identically zero.

If $k(\tau)$ is identically equal to zero (no horizontal transmission), then, once the population has stabilized to the equilibrium distribution $\tilde{P}$, we have $I_{n+1}(0) = qI_n(0)$. This is seen by noting that (3.44) can be integrated to yield

$$P_n(1) = P_n(0)e^{-\int_0^1 (r(\tau)+\sigma(\tau)P_n(\tau))d\tau},$$

hence, at equilibrium we have,

$$\tilde{P}(0) = b\tilde{P}(1) = b\tilde{P}(0)e^{-\int_0^1 (r(\tau)+\sigma(\tau)\tilde{P}(\tau))d\tau}.$$

Thus,

$$be^{-\int_0^1 (r(\tau)+\sigma(\tau)\tilde{P}(\tau))d\tau} = 1.$$

Now, when $k$ vanishes, the equation for $I_n$ in (3.48) yields

$$I_{n+1}(0) = qbI_n(1) = qbI_n(0)e^{-\int_0^1 (r(\tau)+\sigma(\tau)\tilde{P}(\tau))d\tau} = qI_n(0).$$

Thus, the disease will die out unless $q = 1$, that is, unless vertical transmission is complete.

## 3.6.2 Distributed Asynchronous Oviposition

A more general model than the one we have just studied allows oviposition at any time during the generation, rather than just at the end of the generation. It consists of (3.42) and

$$
\begin{aligned}
S_{n+1}(0) &= \int_0^1 \big(S_n(\tau) + p(\tau)I_n(\tau)\big)\,db(\tau), \\
I_{n+1}(0) &= \int_0^1 q(\tau)I_n(\tau)\,db(\tau), \qquad p(\tau) + q(\tau) = 1,
\end{aligned}
\tag{3.51}
$$

with $db(\tau)$ a finite measure on $[0,1]$. Often we can take $db(\tau) = b'(\tau)d\tau$ with $b'$ a continuous non-negative function, and readers not familiar with Stieltjes integrals may think of the integral in (3.51) in these terms. However, the form using the measure allows this term to include delta functions, and hence, specific instances of time when oviposition occurs. For example, if the measure of any set not including $\tau = 1$ is zero, and the measure of any set including $\tau = 1$ is a constant $b$, then (3.51) reduces to (3.43), and we have the model that we have studied already.

It is assumed in what follows that the logistic term actually has an effect on the population, which requires that for some $\tau_0$ with $0 \le \tau_0 \le 1$, we have $\int_0^{\tau_0} \sigma(\tau)\,d\tau > 0$ and $\int_{\tau_0}^1 db(\tau) > 0$. As before, we are allowing $r(\tau)$ to be negative even though it is biologically uninteresting in the equation for $P_n$. This is so because it occurs in the equation for $I_n$ in the same way as it did in equation (3.50) above. Using the same reasoning as in the proofs of Theorems 3.17 and 3.18 we obtain the following analogous results.

**Theorem 3.19** *For the model* (3.51), *define the basic demographic reproduction number $R$ by*

$$
R = \int_0^1 e^{-\int_0^\tau r(t')\,dt'}\,db(\tau),
$$

*and make the further hypotheses that for some $\tau_0 > 0$, $\int_{\tau_0}^1 q(\tau)db(\tau) > 0$ and $\int_0^{\tau_0} k(\tau)d\tau > 0$. Then, if $R \le 1$, the total population $P_n(\tau) \to 0$ as $n \to \infty$. If $R > 1$, and if also $\sigma(\tau) > 0$ and $\int_0^\epsilon db(\tau) \to 0$ as $\epsilon \to 0$, then there is a unique nontrivial population distribution $\tilde{I}(\tau), \tilde{S}(\tau), \tilde{P}(\tau)$ to which the subpopulations tend as $n \to \infty$.*

As far as the endemic threshold is concerned, we define

$$
R_0 = \int_0^1 q(\tau)e^{-\int_0^\tau \hat{r}(t')\,dt'}\,db(\tau),
\tag{3.52}
$$

where, as before

$$
\hat{r}(\tau) = r(\tau) + \sigma(\tau)\tilde{P}(\tau) - k(\tau)\tilde{P}(\tau),
$$

and have the following analogue of Theorem 3.18.

**Theorem 3.20** *Under the hypotheses of Theorem* 3.19, *if* $R_0 \leq 1$ *then* $\tilde{I}(\tau) = 0$, *and the disease dies out, while if* $R_0 > 1$, *there is an endemic equilibrium distribution* $\tilde{I}(\tau) > 0$ *to which* $I_n(\tau)$ *converges and the disease persists in the population.*

Again we note that since $0 \leq q(\tau) \leq 1$, when $R \leq 1$ then $R_0 \leq 1$. Moreover, $R_0$ increases with both the vertical transmission coefficient $q(\tau)$ and the horizontal transmission rate $k(\tau)$ and will exceed the threshold value one as $k$ increases.

*Remark.* We can allow a horizontal transmission term of the form $kSI/P$ instead of $kSI$ in the above models, replacing the term $k(\tau)S_n I_n$ in (3.42) by $k(\tau)S_n I_n/P_n$, or even by $k(\tau)S_n I_n f(P_n)$, where f is an arbitrary continuous nonnegative function. This is so because this term does not enter in the equation for $P_n$, hence, once the population has stabilized at $P_n(\tau) = \tilde{P}(\tau)$, we can let $\check{k}(\tau) = k(\tau)f(\tilde{P}(\tau))$, which reduces the modified system to the original limiting system (3.48). The discrete renewal equations (3.43) or else (3.51) remain unchanged. Thus the above results are valid for these alternative forms of the horizontal transmission term.

## 3.7 Mathematical Background

This section provides a brief discussion of the main mathematical methods that were used in the analysis of the models of Chapter 3. We follow the direction we took in the previous chapter and do not attempt to give a complete logical development of the topics we discuss. Rather, we aim to provide the reader with a convenient presentation of material that is not readily available in one place. The material in this section parallels to a large extent that in the corresponding Section 2.16 on differential equations methods. There are four subsections dealing with 1) Positivity and Invariant Regions, 2) Equilibria and Stability Analysis, 3) Global Stability, 4) Periodic Solutions, Bifurcation and Chaos.

### 3.7.1 Positivity and Invariant Regions

The models that we have studied in this chapter have the form

$$
\begin{aligned}
x_n^1 &= f_1(x_{n-1}^1, x_{n-1}^2, \ldots, x_{n-1}^d), \\
x_n^2 &= f_2(x_{n-1}^1, x_{n-1}^2, \ldots, x_{n-1}^d), \\
&\;\;\vdots \\
x_n^d &= f_d(x_{n-1}^1, x_{n-1}^2, \ldots, x_{n-1}^d),
\end{aligned}
\tag{3.53}
$$

where $x^1, x^2, \ldots, x^d$ are the variables, the subscript $n$ takes the successive values $1, 2, 3, \ldots$, and $f_1, \ldots, f_d$ are given functions. For example, in Section 3.3

the variables $x^1, \ldots, x^7$ were $S$ and $i(\alpha)$ for $\alpha = 0, 1, \ldots, 5$. The independent variable $n$ usually represents a time or generation number. These systems may be written more compactly in the form

$$\mathbf{x}_n = \mathbf{f}(\mathbf{x}_{n-1}), \quad n = 1, 2, 3, \ldots \tag{3.54}$$

where $\mathbf{x}$ denotes a vector with components $x^1, x^2, \ldots x^d$, and $\mathbf{f}$ denotes a vector with components $f_1, f_2, \ldots, f_d$. Equation (3.54) is a difference equation system. It is often also described as a mapping, since $\mathbf{f} : \mathbf{R}^d \to \mathbf{R}^d$ is a mapping. It is clear that if the initial value $\mathbf{x}_0$ and the function $\mathbf{f}$ are known, then $\mathbf{x}_n$ is determined from (3.54) by iteration. Thus, the question of existence and uniqueness of a solution is easily handled.

On the other hand, in our epidemic models, the biological interpretation makes it necessary that the variables not take on negative values for any $n$. Consequently, for a "well-posed" model, one desires to show that the nonnegative cone

$$\mathbf{R}_+^d = \{\mathbf{x} : \text{ each component of } \mathbf{x} \text{ is } \geq 0\}$$

is positively invariant with respect to system (3.54). A set $S$ is called positively invariant for (3.54) if $f(S) \subset S$ (compare Section 2.16.1). For the case of ordinary differential equations, this could be done by showing that on each face of the cone, the corresponding derivative was nonnegative. For mappings, this approach is not valid, because the sequence of values $\mathbf{x}_n$ is discrete, not continuous, and so it is possible to "jump over" a face. Instead, we argue as follows. First, for $\mathbf{x}$ and $\mathbf{y}$ in $\mathbf{R}^d$, we define the symbol $\mathbf{x} > \mathbf{y}$ to mean that $x^i > y^i$ for each $i = 1, \ldots d$. Likewise we define $\mathbf{x} \geq \mathbf{y}$ to mean that $x^i \geq y^i$, and similarly when the inequalities are reversed. We let $\mathbf{0} = \{0, \ldots, 0\}$ denote the vector all of whose coordinates are zero. The following result is then obvious.

**Proposition.** *Suppose that* $\mathbf{f}(\mathbf{x}) \geq \mathbf{0}$ *whenever* $\mathbf{x} \geq \mathbf{0}$. *Then the nonnegative cone* $\mathbf{R}_+^d$ *is positively invariant.*

A very special but important class of systems which preserve positivity is the class of linear systems of the form

$$\mathbf{x}_n = A\mathbf{x}_{n-1},$$

where $A$ is a $d \times d$ *non-negative matrix*, that is, its entries are non-negative, $a_{i,j} \geq 0$. Such systems are easily seen to satisfy the conditions of the above proposition, and hence, to preserve positivity. Linear systems with non-negative matrices have other special properties which we used in Section 3.3.2, and which will be discussed in the next section.

### 3.7.2 Equilibria and Stability Analysis

An equilibrium of the difference equation (3.54) is a vector $\mathbf{x}$ in $\mathbf{R}^d$ that does not change under the iteration, that is

$$\mathbf{x} = \mathbf{f}(\mathbf{x}). \tag{3.55}$$

The vector $\mathbf{x} = (x^1, x^2, \ldots, x^d)$ then represents a state of the system that will not change as $n$ increases, unless some external perturbation is applied. Such a vector $\mathbf{x}$ is also called a *fixed point* of the mapping $\mathbf{f}$. One of the first things that one typically does with a difference system is to determine whether such equilibria exist. If $\mathbf{f}$ is a linear or affine function, $\mathbf{f}(\mathbf{x}) = A\mathbf{x} + \mathbf{b}$ where $A$ is a $d \times d$ matrix and $\mathbf{b}$ is a $d \times 1$ vector, this requires solving the equation $\mathbf{x} = A\mathbf{x} + \mathbf{b}$, hence $\mathbf{x} = (I - A)^{-1}\mathbf{b}$, if the matrix inverse exists. In our models, however, $\mathbf{f}$ is almost always nonlinear, and some kind of special argument is needed in order to establish the existence of a steady state (other than the trivial or null steady state $\mathbf{x} = \mathbf{0}$ that exists when $\mathbf{f}(\mathbf{0}) = \mathbf{0}$). When $f$ is a scalar function, as it was for example in the Keystone virus model, methods of calculus may make it possible to show that the graph of $f$ intersects the line $y = x$ in one or several points, and the value of $x$ at each such point is a fixed point of $f$.

Once an equilibrium is found, its stability should be examined. An equilibrium point $\mathbf{x}^*$ of (3.54) is called stable if, given $\epsilon > 0$, there exists $\delta > 0$ such that for every $n = 1, 2, \cdots$, if $||\mathbf{x}_0 - \mathbf{x}^*|| < \delta$ then $||\mathbf{x}_n - \mathbf{x}^*|| < \epsilon$. Here $||\cdot||$ denotes a norm in $\mathbf{R}^d$. We could also extend this definition slightly by saying that if for some $n = n_0$, $\mathbf{x}_{n_0}$ is within $\delta$ of $\mathbf{x}^*$ then $\mathbf{x}_n$ is within $\epsilon$ of $\mathbf{x}^*$ for all $n > n_0$. $\mathbf{x}^*$ is called unstable if it is not stable. It is called asymptotically stable if $\mathbf{x}^*$ is stable and $\mathbf{x}_n$ converges to $\mathbf{x}^*$ as $n \to \infty$. Similarly, we can define a set $S$ to be stable or asymptotically stable if it is positively invariant and satisfies these definitions with $S$ replacing $\mathbf{x}^*$ and $||\mathbf{x} - S|| := \inf_{y \in S}\{||\mathbf{x} - \mathbf{y}||\}$. The stability properties of an equilibrium can often be determined by considering the linearization of (3.54) at $\mathbf{x}^*$. Just as in Chapter 2, the linearization may be found by computing the Jacobian matrix $J$, in which the element in row $i$, column $j$, is the partial derivative of $f_i(\mathbf{x})$ with respect to variable $x_j$, evaluated at $\mathbf{x}^*$. One then considers the system

$$\mathbf{y}_n = J\mathbf{y}_{n-1}, \qquad (3.56)$$

in which the unique equilibrium $\mathbf{y} = \mathbf{0}$ corresponds to the equilibrium $\mathbf{x} = \mathbf{x}*$ of the original system. From (3.56) we obtain $\mathbf{y}_n = J^n\mathbf{y}_0$. It is known from linear algebra that $J^n \to 0$ as $n \to \infty$ if and only if all eigenvalues of $J$ have modulus less than one. The following result follows.

**Proposition.** *If all eigenvalues $\lambda$ of $J$ satisfy $|\lambda| < 1$ then the equilibrium $\mathbf{x}^*$ of* (3.54) *is asymptotically stable.*

If one of the eigenvalues of $J$ has modulus greater than one, then there are solutions of (3.56) that grow unboundedly, and therefore $\mathbf{x}^*$ is unstable. If all eigenvalues of $J$ lie inside or on the circle of radius one in the complex plane, and some eigenvalues are on the circle, then more detailed information is needed in order to determine the stability properties of $\mathbf{x}^*$.

Just as was the case for differential equations, local asymptotic stability of an equilibrium $\mathbf{x}^*$ does not mean that all solutions tend to it as $n \to \infty$, only that a solution that is sufficiently close to $\mathbf{x}^*$ at $n = 0$ will remain close for all larger $n$. Other solutions may approach different equilibria or have other behavior. For information on global stability analysis, see the next section.

Linear systems (3.56) with a matrix $J$ which is essentially non-negative occur very often in epidemic models and other population biology problems, and played a major role in the results we presented in Section 3.3. There is a substantial literature dealing with properties of such matrices, and the reader who wishes a simple introduction is referred to Chapter 6 in Luenberger (1979), while a more detailed discussion is found in the book of Varga (1962). Here we will describe the basic results that were needed in Section 3.3.

We start by giving some necessary definitions. For a given matrix $A$, the index $i$ is said to be connected to the index $j$ if the entry $a_{ij} \neq 0$. The $n \times n$ matrix $A$ is called *irreducible* if for each pair of indices $i$ and $j$, there exists a sequence $i_1, i_2, \cdots, i_k$ of indices, such that $i_1 = i$, $i_k = j$ and $i_l$ is connected to $i_{l+1}$ for $l = 1, 2, \cdots, k - 1$. The following fundamental result, known as the Perron-Frobenius Theorem, holds.

**Theorem Perron-Frobenius** *Let $A$ be an $n \times n$, irreducible, real, non-negative matrix. Then*

*(1) $A$ has a positive eigenvalue $\lambda_0$ which is equal to its spectral radius $\rho(A)$. Thus, $|\lambda| \leq \lambda_0$ for all eigenvalues $\lambda$ of $A$.*

*(2) $\lambda_0$ is a simple eigenvalue of $A$.*

*(3) The eigenvector $\mathbf{x}_0$ corresponding to $\lambda_0$ is positive (that is, all of its components are positive.*

One of the useful corollaries of this result is

**Corollary.** *If $A$ is strictly positive, that is $a_{ij} > 0$ for all $i, j$, then the conclusions of the above theorem hold. In fact, if for some integer $N$, $A^N$ is a strictly positive matrix, then the same conclusions hold.*

These results greatly simplify the stability analysis of a large class of biological models which when linearized about the zero equilibrium naturally lead to positive Jacobian matrices. An example of this can be seen in the proof of Theorem 3.8. Extensions of these theorems to much more complicated systems have been developed and effectively applied, and in fact, form the basis for a number of the results that will be presented in Chapter 5.

### 3.7.3 Global Stability

In beginning this section, we point out that for two-dimensional systems of difference equations, there is no Poincaré-Bendixson type of theory and no Bendixson-Dulac Criterion to simplify matters. The problem is that a solution is geometrically an orbit that is a sequence of points $\mathbf{x}_n$, rather than a continuous curve. Consequently, an orbit may so-to-speak jump over itself. On the other hand, there is a global stability theory of the Liapunov type, which we now describe.

**Definition.** Let $S \subset \mathbf{R}^d$ and let $V : S \to \mathbf{R}$ be a real-valued map. Then $V$ is called a Liapunov function of the difference equation (3.54) if and only if (i) $V$ is continuous on $S$, and (ii) $\dot{V}(\mathbf{x}) := V(\mathbf{f}(\mathbf{x})) - V(\mathbf{x}) < 0$ for all $\mathbf{x}$ in $S$.

We denote by $E$ the set $E := \{\mathbf{x} \in S : V(\mathbf{x}) = 0\}$ and by $M$ the largest invariant set in $E$. That is, $M$ is contained in $E$, $f(M) = M$, and $M$ contains any other set that has these two properties. Also, we define $V^{-1}(c) = \{\mathbf{x} \in \mathbf{R}^d : V(\mathbf{x}) = c\}$. We then have the following result of LaSalle [1976].

**Theorem 3.21** *let $V$ be a Liapunov function of (3.54) on $S$, and let $\mathbf{x}_n$ be a solution which is in a closed, bounded set $G \subset S$ for all $n$. Then, there exists a real number $c$ such that $\mathbf{x}_n$ converges to $M \cap V^{-1}(c)$ as $n \to \infty$.*

For difference equations, as for differential equations, it is difficult to find or construct a Liapunov function appropriate to a given situation. We have not utilized this method in this chapter. However, the book of LaSalle [1986] contains simple illustrations, and LaSalle [1976] contains an application of the method in analyzing a discrete epidemic model for gonorrhea. Applications to ecological models are given in Goh [1980] and in Luenberger [1979].

### 3.7.4 Periodic Solutions, Bifurcation and Chaos

Periodic and other more complicated solutions of nonlinear difference equations played a major role in the models that were discussed in this chapter. In order to describe part of the mathematical theory of such solutions, we start with some basic definitions.

**Definition.** Let $\mathbf{f}(\mathbf{x})$ denote a map from $\mathbf{R}^d$ to $\mathbf{R}^d$, as above. We denote by $\mathbf{f}^0$ the identity map, and by $\mathbf{f}^2$ the composite map of $\mathbf{f}$ with itself, that is, $\mathbf{f}^2 = \mathbf{f}(\mathbf{f})$. In general, we define $\mathbf{f}^k = \mathbf{f}(\mathbf{f}^{k-1})$ for $k = 1, 2, \dots$. By the orbit of a point $\mathbf{x}$ we mean the sequence of points $\mathbf{f}^k(\mathbf{x})$, $k = 0, 1, 2, \dots$.

**Definition.** The point $\mathbf{x}$ is a fixed point of $\mathbf{f}$ if $\mathbf{f}(\mathbf{x}) = \mathbf{x}$. The point $\mathbf{x}$ is a periodic point of period $n$ if $\mathbf{f}^n(\mathbf{x}) = \mathbf{x}$. The least such positive integer $n$ is called the prime period of $\mathbf{x}$, but for abbreviation usually just the period of $\mathbf{x}$. Note that each point on the orbit of $\mathbf{x}$ is also a point of period $n$.

In the context of the model equation (3.54) a point $\mathbf{x}$ of period $n$ represents a state of the system to which the system returns after $n$ time periods. The orbit of $\mathbf{x}$ consists of a sequence of states through which the system moves and returns to $\mathbf{x}$. Such an orbit is also called a periodic solution of the difference equation.

One of the objectives in analyzing a model is to determine whether periodic solutions (orbits) exist. As we have already stated, there is no analogue of the Bendixson-Dulac criterion which can be used to rule out periodic solutions. In Section 3.3.2, a fairly elaborate argument was used to show that no orbit of period 2 could exist. It is also generally difficult to prove the existence of periodic orbits for particular equations, especially when the dimension $d$ is greater than one. The book of Devaney [1986] contains an introduction to this problem and related matters. One method that is very fruitful is the approach via bifurcation from a fixed point. Let us consider a family of difference equations

$$\mathbf{x}_n = \mathbf{f}(\mathbf{x}_{n-1}, \mu), \tag{3.57}$$

where $\mu$ is a parameter. Stated in other terms, consider a family of mappings $\mathbf{f}(\mathbf{x}, \mu)$. Suppose, without loss of generality, that $\mathbf{x} = \mathbf{0}$ is a fixed point of the mapping. As we saw above, $\mathbf{0}$ is asymptotically stable if the eigenvalues of the Jacobian $J$ satisfy $|\lambda| < 1$, but is unstable if there is an eigenvalue with $|\lambda| > 1$. Let us suppose that as $\mu$ varies through a critical value $\mu_0$, an eigenvalue crosses the unit circle. Then $\mathbf{0}$ destabilizes, and one possibility is that another fixed point $\mathbf{x}(\mu)$ bifurcates from $\mathbf{0}$ and assumes its stability. This has been the case in many of our models, where stability of the disease-free steady state was lost when the basic reproductive number exceeded one, and an endemic steady state became stable.

Let us illustrate this for the one-dimensional quadratic map $f_\mu(x) = \mu x(1 - x)$. It is easy to see that $x = 0$ is a fixed point, and there is no positive fixed point if $0 < \mu \le 1$. For $\mu > 1$, there is a positive fixed point $x = 1 - \frac{1}{\mu}$; it is said to bifurcate from $x = 0$ at $\mu = 1$. Note that $f'_\mu(0) = \mu$ has the value 1 at $\mu = 1$ and is greater than 1 for $\mu > 1$. Since $f'_\mu(0)$ is the Jacobian at 0 in this one-dimensional case, we see that this bifurcation occurs as the eigenvalue $\mu$ passes through 1.

It can be shown that the fixed point $1 - \frac{1}{\mu}$ is stable for $1 < \mu < 3$. However, another bifurcation occurs at $\mu = 3$. In this case, $f'(1 - \frac{1}{\mu}) = 2 - \mu$, and this equals -1 at $\mu = 3$. The eigenvalue passes through -1 and is less than -1 for $\mu > 3$. What happens is that the fixed point becomes unstable, and a stable orbit of period 2 arises. This is called a period-doubling bifurcation. It is known that for the quadratic map, additional period doubling bifurcations occur for larger values of $\mu$. There are a number of sources where these are described in detail, for example, see Devaney [1986].

In dimensions $d > 1$, we may also consider families of maps $\mathbf{f}_\mu(\mathbf{x})$, $\mathbf{x} \in \mathbf{R}^d$, and a bifurcation may occur when an eigenvalue of the Jacobian matrix crosses through the unit circle in the complex plane. If the eigenvalue $\lambda$ crosses at $\lambda = 1$, a new fixed point may occur. If it crosses at $\lambda = -1$, a period doubling may occur. But it is also possible that a complex eigenvalue crosses the unit circle at some other point. In that case, since we are dealing with real Jacobian matrices, the conjugate eigenvalue will also cross the circle at the conjugate point. In this case, the so-called Hopf bifurcation for maps may occur. What this means is that an invariant circle may arise from a fixed point. By an invariant circle is meant a closed curve, topologically equivalent to a circle, such that each point on the curve is transformed into another point on the curve by the mapping. Since we have not used this result in this chapter, we omit further explanation and discussion of the complicated story of bifurcations of mappings. These matters, including the Hopf bifurcation, are discussed in the books of Devaney [1986], Chow and Hale [1982], and elsewhere.

Nonlinear difference equations can have very complex dynamic behavior, and a whole theory is being rapidly developed which is providing analytical tools for the study of chaotic behavior of such equations. Chaos is a term coined by Li and Yorke [1975] who gave a formal definition and proved a very striking and useful result which we shall state below. The books of Lasota and Mackey [1985] and of Devaney [1986] provide good introductions to this topic. There are several definitions of chaos that are currently being used, however, we shall restrict ourselves to giving only a modification of the original one of Li and Yorke which is extended to apply to maps in $\mathbf{R}^d$.

**Definition.** The difference equation (3.57) is *chaotic* if there exists an integer $N$ such that
(1) for each integer $p \geq N$, there is a periodic solution of period $p$;
(2) for each integer $p \geq N$, there exists an uncountable set $S_p$ containing no periodic points of $\mathbf{f}$, with:
(a) for every $\mathbf{x}$, $\mathbf{y} \in S_p$ with $\mathbf{x} \neq \mathbf{y}$

$$\limsup_{k \to \infty} \|\mathbf{f}^k(\mathbf{x}) - \mathbf{f}^k(\mathbf{y})\| > 0,$$

(b) for every $\mathbf{x} \in S_p$, and for every periodic point $\mathbf{y}$ of $\mathbf{f}$

$$\liminf_{k \to \infty} \|\mathbf{f}^k(\mathbf{x}) - \mathbf{f}^k(\mathbf{y})\| = 0.$$

The following basic result of Li and Yorke gives a condition for chaos to exist in one-dimensional maps.

**Theorem 3.22** *Let $I$ be an interval in $\mathbf{R}$ and let $f : I \to I$ be continuous. If the difference equation $x_{n+1} = f(x_n)$ has a period three orbit then it is chaotic.*

A simple extension of this result is not available for continuous maps in higher dimensions. Perhaps one of the simplest ways of showing chaos in higher dimensional maps is via a result of Marotto [1979] which we now describe.

**Definition.** The fixed point $\mathbf{x}_0$ of the differentiable map $\mathbf{f} : \mathbf{R}^d \to \mathbf{R}^d$ is called a *snap-back repeller* if for some neighborbood $B$ of $\mathbf{x}_0$ the eigenvalues of the Jacobian $J = D\mathbf{f}(\mathbf{x})$ have norm greater than one for all $\mathbf{x} \in B$ and there exists a point $\mathbf{z} \in B$, $\mathbf{z} \neq \mathbf{x}_0$ obeying $\det(D\mathbf{f}^m(\mathbf{z})) \neq 0$, and $\mathbf{f}^m(\mathbf{z}) = \mathbf{x}_0$ for some positive integer $m$.

The theorem of Marotto is now easy to state.

**Theorem 3.23** *Let* $x_0$ *be a snap-back repeller of the differentiable map* **f** : $\mathbf{R}^d \to \mathbf{R}^d$. *Then* **f** *is chaotic.*

An additional property of chaotic maps with snap-back repellers which we have used is that small perturbations of such maps also remain chaotic. This result is due to Rogers and Marotto [1983].

At first sight, the complicated dynamics and the sensitivity of the orbits to small changes in the initial data of chaotic models appear to negate the predictive value of these deterministic models. This, however, is not the case since there is an underlying order of a statistical nature which allows analytical conclusions and predictions to be made. What essentially happens is that nearby initial data can lead to very different orbits, however, there often is a specific distribution of the frequency with which the points on these orbits return to any particular region. This distribution can sometimes be analytically determined, but more often is computable numerically. Once it is known, it can be used to make predictions, albeit of a statistical nature, about the future average behavior of the system. We shall not go into the details of the theory which supports these conclusions but refer the reader to the book of Lasota and Mackey [1985] for a lucid presentation.

We note in conclusion that the topic of bifurcation and chaos in nonlinear equations is being intensively studied by a large number of research workers, and that new results are being constantly developed. What we have given here is a bare introduction that should allow the reader to follow the particular chaotic models presented in this chapter, and there are many aspects of this area that we leave to the reader to begin exploring in the papers and monographs that we have cited.

# 4 Delay Differential Equations Models

## 4.1 The Role of Delays in Epidemic Models

Time delays are used to model several different mechanisms in the dynamics of epidemics. Incubation periods, maturation times, age structure, seasonal or diurnal variations, interactions across spatial distances or through complicated paths, as well as other mechanisms have been modeled by the introduction of time delays in dynamic models. In fact, all models that employ difference equations, that is, where time or age is discretized, introduce a delay in a fundamental way, since the state of such a system at time $t$ is determined, at least in part, by the state at time $t - \Delta t$, where $\Delta t$ is the discrete time step of the difference equation. This represents a delayed effect in the dynamics which may be justified by the situation that is being modeled. Chapter 3 is devoted to the study of such difference equations models. In this chapter, we consider models which use differential equations with delays in order to account for one or more of the mechanisms we have described above. Even though it is relatively easy to justify the introduction of delays in particular models, the resulting equations often present new mathematical phenomena and difficulties which often require rather complicated tools for their analysis. These mathematical complications are justified by the resulting realism of the models, and by the additional biological phenomena that can be described through the use of time delays.

The overall objective in studying delay differential equation models should be to assess the qualitative or quantitative differences that arise from including the time delays in an explicit way, and also to compare the qualitative or quantitative results for models with delays representing different biological mechanisms. Since these questions are largely unexplored for the dynamics of epidemic models with vertical transmission at this date, we can only present partial results. In Sections 4.2, 4.3 and 4.5 we consider some delay differential equation models due to Busenberg, Cooke and Pozio [1983] which are obtained by including temporary immunity and maturation delays in the classical differential equation model that was discussed in detail in Chapter 2. Here we show that, in some cases, the qualitative dynamics of the disease transmission is not affected by the inclusion of delayed effects, while in other cases new phenomena, such as the appearance of oscillatory solutions, can be caused by the inclusion of delays. Periodic oscillations in the incidence rates of diseases occur frequently, and there has been a considerable amount of work devoted to dynamical mechanisms that can lead to such oscillations. We refer to the work of London and Yorke [1973], Hethcote, Stech and van den Driessche [1981, 1983], and Schwartz [1985] for examples of epidemic models with such oscillations. In Section 4.4 we consider a model with a delay due to an incubation period and present results due to Grabiner [1988] showing that the endemic equilibrium is stable at least for small delays. In Section 4.5 we return to the model of Section 4.2 and discuss a variant which takes into account spatial diffusion due to random dispersion of the population. The details of the mathematical analysis of this type of model are quite involved, and we only provide an outline of the key ideas and discuss some of the implications of spatial diffusion in such models. In Section 4.6 we discuss a model which involves delays due to long subclinical periods of an infection. This is a new model for the transmission of the HIV virus which causes AIDS. The disease can be vertically transmitted during this subclinical period. A similar situation occurs in a model for the transmission of Chagas' disease which is due to Busenberg and Vargas [1991]. The detailed analysis of these models has not yet been completed. We present them here because they serve to illustrate an important epidemiological phenomenon which affects the dynamics of the transmission of a number of different diseases. The final section is devoted to a brief exposition of the mathematical methods that are needed in this chapter in order to study the effects of delays.

## 4.2 A Model with Maturation Delays

In this section we describe a model of a vertically transmitted disease with maturation delays which was introduced and studied by Busenberg, Cooke and Pozio [1983]. This model differs from the model of Section 2.10 because of the introduction of an explicit maturation time $T$ instead of a maturation rate.

Consider a disease that can be propagated through contact between infected and susceptible individuals and through the possibility of infected parents giving birth to infected newborn individuals. Assume that the population is asexual or that it suffices to consider only one sex, and separate the population into two epidemiological classes which interact with each other, the susceptibles (denoted by $S$), and the infectives (denoted by $I$). The model allows for a removed class composed of individuals who have recovered from the infection, and are permanently immune to the disease, provided births from members of this class are negligible in number or are immune. This class does not play a role in the dynamics of the disease. Within each epidemiological class, there is also a possible segregation according to age groups. Assume that there is a maturation period of length $T \geq 0$, during which the newborn do not participate in the horizontal transmission of the disease. After this maturation time $T$, those newborn who survive become involved in the horizontal transfer of the disease. One mechanism that leads to the existence of such a maturation period occurs in egg laying populations where newborn individuals have to undergo a hatching time $T$ before actively interacting with the mature population.

The above assumptions lead to a model involving the number $I(t)$ of mature infectives at time $t$, the number $S(t)$ of mature susceptible individuals at time $t$, and these same functions evaluated at time $t - T$. In order to arrive at explicit dynamical relations, we make the following hypotheses:

(a) Mature infectives and susceptibles are removed (due to death or passage into the immune class) at the constant rates $r'$ and $r$, respectively. The immature individuals are removed at the respective rates $r^{*'}$ and $r^*$. All these rates are non-negative.

(b) The mature susceptibles have a constant non-negative birth rate denoted by $\tilde{b}$, while the mature infectives have a constant non-negative birth rate denoted by $\tilde{b}'$. Thus, the rate of addition of individuals to the mature susceptible class at time $t$, due to births to susceptible parents at time $t - T$, is $\tilde{b}e^{-r^*T}S(t - T) = bS(t - T)$, where $b = \tilde{b}e^{-r^*T}$.

We assume that a proportion $p$, $0 \le p \le 1$, of the offspring of infective parents are susceptible, while the complementary proportion $q = 1 - p$ are infective. Hence, the rate of addition of individuals to the infective class at time $t$, due to births to infective parents at time $t - T$, is $qb'I(t - T) = q\tilde{b}'e^{-r^{*'}T}I(t - T)$ where $\tilde{b}'e^{-r^{*'}T} = b'$. The total addition of individuals to the susceptible class at time $t$, due to births to both susceptible and infective parents at time $t - T$, is $pb'I(t - T) + bS(t - T)$. The parameter $p$ incorporates the notion of vertical transmission into our model. In the special case where $p = 1$, we have a model with only horizontal transmission, while if $p = 0$, the model assumes complete vertical transmission of the disease to all the offspring of infective individuals.

(c) The rate at which susceptibles become infected at time $t$ is assumed to be a function $g$ of $S(t)$ and $I(t)$. So, no incubation period is assumed between the time of exposure and the time of infectivity. If the population is mixing uniformly, we can take $g(S, I) = kSI$, where $k$ is a constant. We will use this latter form, even though a number of our results extend to more general functions $g$. The structure of the model is indicated schematically in Fig. 4.1.

The above assumptions lead to the following equations for $t > 0$:

$$dS(t)/dt = -rS(t) + bS(t - T) + pb'I(t - T) - kS(t)I(t),$$
$$dI(t)/dt = -r'I(t) + qb'I(t - T) + kS(t)I(t),$$

(4.1)

and

$$S(t) = S_0(t), \quad I(t) = I_0(t), \quad -T \le t \le 0,$$

(4.2)

where $b = \tilde{b}e^{-r^*T}$, $b' = \tilde{b}'e^{-r^{*'}T}$, and the initial functions $S_0$ and $I_0$: $[-T, 0] \to [0, \infty)$ are assumed to be known continuous non-negative functions which specify the number of mature susceptibles and infectives on the time interval $[-T, 0]$.

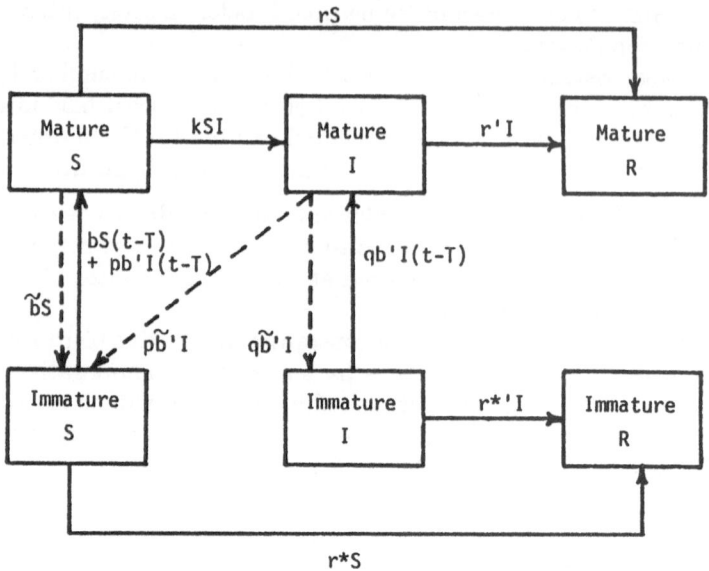

**Fig. 4.1.** Structure of the model with maturation delay

We shall analyze some special cases of this model here and in Section 5 we will consider a generalization that allows for spatial diffusion. We first note that the problem (4.1)-(4.2) is correctly posed in the sense that, if the initial data $S_0$ and $I_0$ are non-negative, then the problem has a unique non-negative solution which exists for all $t \geq 0$. For the arguments which support these conclusions see Section 4.7 and the references given there.

The equations (4.1)-(4.2) have the following finite isolated equilibrium solutions:

$$(0,0) \quad \text{and} \quad (S^*, I^*) = \left( \frac{r' - qb'}{k}, \frac{(b-r)(r'-qb')}{k(r'-b')} \right). \qquad (4.3)$$

The equilibrium solution $(S^*, I^*)$ is of interest only when it is feasible, that is, only when $r' - qb' \geq 0$ and $(b-r)/(r'-b') \geq 0$. If special relationships hold among the parameters of the model, there may exist entire continua of equilibrium solutions. However, these special cases are not important in the biological situation that we are considering because small variations in the parameters destroy the circumstances under which they can exist.

For this model with a maturation period $(T > 0)$, we treat in detail the special case where $r = b = r' = b'$. This restricts the model to a closed population, since the effective birth and removal rates are equal in each subpopulation. Also, there is the added restriction that the susceptible and infected portions of the population have the same maturation and removal rates.

If we let

$$C(t) = S(t) + I(t) + r \int_{t-T}^{t} [S(s) + I(s)]ds, \ t > 0,$$

it is easily shown, using (4.1), that $dC/dt = 0$, and thus $C(t) = C_0$ is a constant. That is, the differential equation system (4.1) has a "first integral". These considerations lead to the following result.

**Theorem 4.1 (A special case with maturation period.)** *Suppose that in the problem (4.1)-(4.2), $r = r' = b = b'$, $T > 0$, and $I_0 \geq 0$, $S_0 \geq 0$ for $-T \leq t \leq 0$. Let*

$$C_0 = S_0(0) + I_0(0) + r \int_{-T}^{0} [S_0(s) + I_0(s)]ds, \tag{4.4}$$

$$P^* = C_0/(1 + rT). \tag{4.5}$$

*Then, if $I_0 \not\equiv 0$ for $t \in [-T, 0]$, the following asymptotic behavior occurs:*

  *Case i.   If $R_0 = kP^*/pr \leq 1$, $(S(t), I(t)) \rightarrow (P^*, 0)$ as $t \rightarrow \infty$.*
  *Case ii.  If $R_0 > 1$, $(S(t), I(t)) \rightarrow (pr/k, P^* - pr/k)$ as $t \rightarrow \infty$.*

Note that the limiting behavior in this case is determined by the initial data and by the delay $T$ in a fairly simple manner. Specifically, if all other parameters are held constant, and the initial population $P_0 = S_0 + I_0$ is increased, then $C_0$ given by (4.4) increases, and so does $P^*$. There is a sharp threshold for $P^*$, namely $pr/k$, below which the infection dies out in time, and above which the infection becomes endemic. This threshold value is directly proportional to the probability $p$ of an infective parent having susceptible offspring. Finally, from (4.4) and (4.5) we see that an increase in the maturation period $T$ does not have a simple stabilizing or destabilizing effect, since $C_0$ typically increases [5] with $T$ while $P^*$ depends on $T$ via (4.5). In fact, $P^*$ increases with $T$ if and only if

$$\frac{P_0(-T)(1 + rT)}{P_0(0) + r \int_{-T}^{0} P(s)ds} > 1,$$

a condition which is easily obtained by computing $\partial P^*/\partial T$, and requiring that it be greater than zero. We also note that, if $T = 0$, then $C_0 = S_0 + I_0 = P_0$ and $P^* = P_0$, hence, the result in Theorem 4.1 agrees with that in Case iii of Theorem 2.1 of Chapter 2. In particular, the maturation delay affects the values of the equilibrium population levels and of the endemic threshold $R_0$. However, regardless of the size of this delay, it does not lead to a destabilization of the endemic equilibrium and to the appearance of oscillatory population levels. We note that the problem (4.1)-(4.2) has not been analyzed, so far as we know, when the condition $r = r' = b = b'$ is not assumed, and we leave this as an open problem.

---

[5] Another interpretation is that the same size initial population is distributed over a longer time, hence, $C_0$ would be independent of $T$.

Because pathogens can reproduce and increase their concentration in an infective, it is often the case that the ages of the infective parent and offspring play a role in the dynamics of vertical transmission. This is a situation that we modeled and studied in Section 3.3, but which we consider only partly here. However, the age-dependent effects are quite important in models of vertical transmission and will be studied in further detail in Chapter 5. In this chapter, we treat such effects only by considering the delay differential equation models of Theorems 4.1, 4.2 and 4.3.

In Theorem 4.1, we introduced a maturation period before newborn carriers become infective. There are several vertically transmitted diseases where such a phenomenon occurs, the most obvious cases being those of egg-laying vector species. However, this phenomenon can also occur in live-bearing species, because the concentration of pathogen that is transmitted from mother to child (often via the infected cytoplasm of the female egg) can be low, and an aging period must elapse before the offspring has a high enough concentration of pathogen to be infective. In the special cases treated in Theorem 4.1, the effect of this age-dependent phenomenon is to make the endemicity threshold value of the initial population dependent on the maturation period (via (4.4) and (4.5)), in addition to its dependence on the removal rates and the horizontal and vertical transmission rates. The endemicity threshold condition can be written as

$$q > 1 - \frac{k}{r(1+rT)} \left[ P_0(0) + r \int_{-T}^0 P_0(s)ds \right].$$

If $P_0(0)$, $r$ and $T$ are fixed, it is seen that the survival of the pathogen requires an increase of the vertical transmission rate $q$ as the horizontal transmission rate $k$ decreases. We note that if

$$k < \frac{r(1+rT)}{P_0(0) + r \int_{-T}^0 P_0(s)ds},$$

then vertical transmission must necessarily be present in order that the endemic condition (that is, survival of the pathogen) occur.

## 4.3 Delays Due to Partial Immunity

The delay $T$, introduced by the presence of the maturation period, does not induce any periodic solutions in the special case considered above where $r = r' = b = b'$. We now address the question of whether or not oscillatory solutions can be induced by other mechanisms that introduce delays. We assume that no maturation period is present (hence, $T = 0$, $r = r^*$, $r' = r^{*'}$), but a proportion $p$, $0 \leq p \leq 1$, of the offspring of infective parents are immune to the disease for a period $T_0$, after which they become susceptible; while the complementary proportion, $q = 1 - p$, become infective after an incubation period $T_1$. The structure of this model is shown in the Fig. 4.2. This situation occurs in diseases where there is a temporary immunity that is conferred by a mother to the offspring.

Taking, for the sake of simplifying the mathematics, $T_0 = T_1 = \tau$, we obtain the following equations for our model

$$dS(t)/dt = (b - r)S(t) + pb'I(t - \tau) - kS(t)I(t), \quad t > 0,$$
$$dI(t)/dt = -r'I(t) + qb'I(t - \tau) + kS(t)I(t) \quad t > 0. \tag{4.6}$$

$$S(0) = S_0, \quad I(t) = I_0(t), \quad -\tau \le t \le 0. \tag{4.7}$$

Note that the initial condition for $S$ needs to be specified only at $t = 0$ since the dependence on this variable is instantaneous and not subject to any delay. Our result, in this case where incubation and immunity periods are present, does not give a complete description of the dynamics of (4.6). However, it does show that, under certain circumstances, periodic solutions can occur in this model. This may be surprising, since the model structure is that of an $S \to I$ type, with the only feedback from $I$ to $S$ being that due to vertical transmission. The details are given in Theorem 4.2.

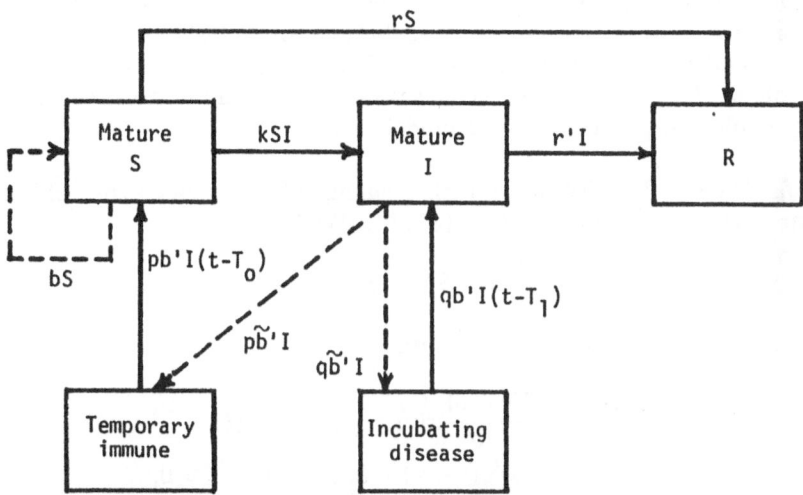

**Fig. 4.2.** Structure of the model with immunity delays

**Theorem 4.2 (A case with an immunity period).** *Suppose that in the problem (4.6)-(4.7), $\tau > 0$, $p > 0$, $S_0 \ge 0$, $I_0 \ge 0$ and $r < b$, $b' < r'$. If $\tau$ is small enough, or else, if*

$$0 < q^*(r', b') = \frac{3r' - b' - \sqrt{(9r' - b')(r' - b')}}{2b'} \le q < 1, \tag{4.8}$$

*or*

$$\xi(r', b', q) < (b - r)/(r' - b'), \tag{4.9}$$

*where*

$$\xi(r', b', q) = \frac{2}{p^2 b'^2} \left[ (r' - qb')^2 - \{ (r' - qb')^4 \right.$$
$$\left. + 2qpb'^2 (r' - qb')^2 - p^2 b'^2 (r'^2 - q^2 b'^2) \}^{1/2} \right], \tag{4.10}$$

*(which is positive if* $0 \leq q < q^*(r', b')$*), then the equilibrium solution* $(S^*, I^*) = ((r' - qb')/k, (b - r)(r' - qb')/k(r' - b'))$*, is feasible and locally asymptotically stable. On the other hand, suppose that* $0 \leq q < q^*(r', b')$ *and*

$$0 < (b - r)/(r' - b') < \xi(r', b', q). \tag{4.11}$$

*Then, as* $\tau$ *increases from zero, there is a value* $\tau^*$ *such that, for* $\tau > \tau^*$ *and* $\tau$ *close to* $\tau^*$*, the system (4.6) has a positive periodic solution near* $(S^*, I^*)$*, and* $(S^*, I^*)$ *is unstable.*

The model that we consider in this theorem incorporates the possibility of an inherited temporary immunity. The case $m = b - r > 0$, $m' = b' - r' < 0$, represents a situation where the pathogen has a net adverse effect on its carriers. We encounter a complicated bifurcation threshold that leads to a possible endemic level that varies periodically with time. This serves as an example of the possibility of vertical transmission leading to such nonlinear periodic phenomena in an $S \to I$ model.

*Proof.* (Theorem 4.2) We start with a change of coordinates that places the origin at the equilibrium solution $(S^*, I^*)$. We let

$$x = S - S^*, \qquad y = I - I^*,$$

and note that (4.6) is transformed into

$$\frac{dx(t)}{dt} = \frac{pb'(r - b)}{r' - b'} x(t) + (qb' - r')y(t)$$
$$+ pb'y(t - \tau) - kx(t)y(t), \qquad t > 0,$$
$$\frac{dy(t)}{dt} = \frac{(b - r)(r' - qb')}{r' - b'} x(t) - qb'y(t)$$
$$+ qb'y(t - \tau) + kx(t)y(t), \qquad t > 0. \tag{4.12}$$

The local asymptotic stability results of the theorem are obtained by using the linearization techniques described in Section 4.7.2. It is clear that the conditions needed in order to apply these results to (4.12) are met, and we need to show that the roots of the characteristic equation of the linearization of (4.12) have negative real parts, if $\tau$ is small enough, or if $\tau$ is arbitrary but either (4.8) or (4.9) hold. This characteristic equation is

$$z^2 + b' \left[ q + p\frac{b-r}{r'-b'} \right] z - qb'ze^{-z\tau} - pb'r'\frac{b-r}{r'-b'}e^{-z\tau}$$

$$+(b-r)\frac{pqb'^2 + (r'-qb')^2}{r'-b'} = 0. \tag{4.13}$$

For $\tau = 0$, this equation reduces to a quadratic equation whose roots have negative real parts. See (1) of the Appendix of the original article by Busenberg, Cooke and Pozio [1983]. Since the roots of (4.13) are continuous functions of $\tau \geq 0$, and since those roots of (4.13) with $0 \leq \mathrm{Re}(z)$ are uniformly bounded for $\tau \in [0,\infty)$, then the roots of (4.13) have negative real parts when $\tau$ is small. Moreover, if (4.9) holds, no root of (4.13) can cross the imaginary axis as $\tau$ increases from zero. The details of the calculations needed to verify this are given in Busenberg, Cooke and Pozio [1983]. So, if (4.9) holds, the roots of the characteristic equation (4.13) have negative real parts for all $\tau \geq 0$, and $(S^*, I^*)$ is locally asymptotically stable. If (4.8) holds, then (4.9) must also hold since $\xi(r', b', q) \leq 0$ and $(b-r)/(r'-b') > 0$. So, all the local asymptotic stability claims in Theorem 4.2 are proved.

If $0 \leq q < q^*(r', b')$ and (4.11) holds, there exists $\tau^* > 0$ such that a pair of complex conjugate pure imaginary roots of (4.13) exists at $\tau = \tau^*$, and all the other roots of (4.13) have negative real parts. Moreover, there exists a neighborhood $N$ of $\tau^*$, and a continuously differentiable function $z: N \to \mathbf{C}$, with $z(\tau^*)$ pure imaginary, $d\mathrm{Re}(z(\tau))/d\tau\big|_{\tau=\tau^*} > 0$, and $z(\tau)$ is a root of (4.13) for all $\tau \in N$. From this, and from the Hopf bifurcation result which is discussed in Section 4.7.4, we see that, for $\tau > \tau^*$ and $\tau$ close to $\tau^*$, there exists a periodic solution of (4.6) near $(S^*, I^*)$ and $(S^*, I^*)$ is unstable. This completes the proof of Theorem 4.2.

The question of whether the bifurcating periodic solution of Theorem 4.2 continues to exist and is stable for all $\tau > \tau^*$ has not been investigated. Also, no work has been done to date on the model with $T_0 \neq T_1$.

## 4.4 Delay Due to an Incubation Period

In the preceding sections, we have considered models that take account of delays due to maturation or to partial immunity, and we now want to construct models that incorporate an incubation period. We, therefore, introduce a class $E$ of individuals who have been infected, but in whom the disease is latent. The equations will be similar to those in (2.31), but instead of assuming that there is a rate of removal of individuals from latency to infectiousness, we now assume that individuals who are infected by horizontal transmission remain in the latent class for a fixed length of time, $T$. We assume that the offspring of susceptible or latent individuals are susceptible, and that offspring of infectious individuals are either susceptible or infectious, not latent. The model equations are then as follows.

$$\frac{dS(t)}{dt} = (b-r)S(t) + bE(t) + pb'I(t) - kS(t)I(t),$$

$$E(t) = e^{-rt}C + k \int_{t-T}^{t} e^{-r(t-t')}S(t')I(t')dt',$$

$$\frac{dI(t)}{dt} = (qb' - r')I(t) + k'S(t-T)I(t-T), \quad t > 0.$$

Here $k'/k = e^{-rT}$ is the fraction of individuals who survive the incubation period. The equation for the exposed class $E$ can be interpreted as saying that the total number of exposed individuals consists of those in that class at time $t = 0$,

$$E(0) = C + k \int_{-T}^{0} e^{rt}S(t)I(t)dt,$$

who have survived to time $t$, plus those who have entered this class during the time interval $[t-T, t]$ and have not left via either loss of immunity or death. The constant $C$ is determined from this balance condition, and remains undefined if one uses the differential equation form of the equation

$$dE(t)/dt = -rE(t) + kS(t)I(t) - k'S(t-T)I(t-T).$$

The use of this latter form of the equation for $E$ can lead to misinterpretations of the model, and the interested reader can consult Section 4.7.5 and the paper of Busenberg and Cooke [1980] for a discussion of this type of equations and their proper integral reformulations.

Since it is difficult to analyze the above model, we shall consider a simplification. Suppose that individuals in the latent class are sterile, or that the length $T$ of the latent period is so short that births to these individuals may be considered negligible. Then the equation for $E$ is decoupled from the others, and we may consider the system

$$dS(t)/dt = (b-r)S(t) + pb'I(t) - kS(t)I(t), \quad t > 0,$$
$$dI(t)/dt = (qb' - r')I(t) + k'S(t-T)I(t-T), \quad t > 0, \tag{4.14}$$

with the initial conditions

$$S(t) = S_0(t), \quad I(t) = I_0(t), \quad -T \le t \le 0. \tag{4.15}$$

A second interpretation also leads to (4.14). Suppose that all offspring of individuals in the latent class are in the same stage of the latent period as their parents. Then newly infected individuals move into the $E$ class, where they are subject to giving birth or dying, and hence, their effective death rate is $r - b$. In this case, we obtain (4.14) with $k' = ke^{(b-r)T}$. Thus by removing the explicit dependent variable $E$, we have introduced a degree of ambiguity in the interpretation of the model.

The system (4.14)-(4.15) has been studied by Grabiner [1988], and we present his results in the following theorem. We first note that, in the absence of the disease, the population will decay to the trivial equilibrium $(0, 0)$ if $r \geq b$, and will increase without bound if $r < b$. If the disease is present, then we have the following result:

**Theorem 4.3** *The system* (4.14) *has the endemic equilibrium* $(S^*, I^*)$, *with*

$$S^* = \frac{r' - qb'}{k'}, \quad I^* = \frac{(b - r)S^*}{kS^* - pb'}.$$

*When* $b > r$ *and this endemic equilibrium is feasible, it is stable if the delay satisfies*

$$T \leq \frac{pb'}{k'S^*|kS^* - 2pb'|}.$$

*The equilibrium is unstable when it is feasible and* $b \leq r$.

Note that this result gives only a sufficient condition for stability of the endemic equilibrium but does not provide a condition which is both necessary and sufficient. Consequently, the model is only partly explained here, however, the result does provide an indication of the interplay between the vertical and horizontal transmission modes of passing the disease.

*Proof.* The proof relies on a method for determining the local stability of delay-differential equations which is due to Stépán [1989] and which is useful in studying equations of this type. Linearizing the system (4.14) about the equilibrium we obtain the system

$$\dot{x} = A_1 x(t) + A_2 x(t - T),$$

where

$$x = \begin{pmatrix} S - S^* \\ I - I^* \end{pmatrix}, \quad A_1 = \begin{pmatrix} b - kI^* - r & pb' - kS^* \\ 0 & qb' - r' \end{pmatrix}, \quad A_2 = \begin{pmatrix} 0 & 0 \\ k'I^* & k'S^* \end{pmatrix}.$$

Here, and in the rest of this chapter, we do not use bold face letters to denote vector valued functions. The characteristic function is

$$\Delta(\lambda) = det(\lambda I - A_1 - e^{-\lambda T} A_2)$$

$$= \lambda^2 + (\frac{pb'I^*}{S^*} + k'S^*)\lambda - k'S^*\lambda e^{-T\lambda}$$

$$+ [(kS^* - pb')k'I^* - pb'I^*k']e^{-T\lambda} + pb'k'I^*,$$

and so

$$\Delta(0) = k'(b - r)S^*.$$

If $b \leq r$ then $\Delta(0) \leq 0$ and since $\Delta(\lambda) \to +\infty$ as $\lambda \to +\infty$, there is a non-negative root of $\Delta(\lambda) = 0$. Consequently, the equilibrium $(S^*, I^*)$ is not asymptotically stable. Now suppose that $b > r$, and apply Stépán's Theorem, presented in Section 4.7.2. We let

$$R(y) = \mathrm{Re}\triangle(iy), \quad S(y) = \mathrm{Im}\triangle(iy),$$

and obtain

$$R(y) = -y^2 - k'S^*y \, \sin Ty + (kS^* - 2pb')k'I^* \cos Ty + pb'k'I^*,$$

$$S(y) = (\frac{pb'I^*}{S^*} + k'S^*)y - k'S^*y \, \cos Ty - (kS^* - 2pb')k'I^* \sin Ty.$$

Since $n = 2$, $m = 1$, we shall now apply part (i) of Stépán's Theorem (see Section 4.7.2). Observing that $R(0) = (kS^* - pb')k'I^* = \triangle(0) = k'(b - r)S^*$, which is positive when $S^* > 0$, and that $R(y)$ is negative for all sufficiently large $y$, we see that $R$ has an odd number of non-negative zeros. If we can show that $S(y)$ is positive for all $y > 0$, we shall have

$$\sum_{k=1}^{r}(-1)^k \, \mathrm{sign} \, S(\rho_k) = -1 = (-1)^m m,$$

and the theorem will guarantee exponential asymptotic stability. Now, for $y > 0, S^* > 0, I^* > 0$, we have

$$S(y) = pb'I^*y/S^* + k'S^*y(1 - \cos \, Ty) - (kS^* - 2pb')k'I^* \sin Ty$$
$$> pb'I^*y/S^* - |kS^* - 2pb'|k'I^*Ty.$$

Thus when

$$T \le \frac{pb'}{k'S^*|kS^* - 2pb'|},$$

we have $S(y) > 0$ for all $y > 0$, and the theorem is proved.

Note that, if $pb' > 0$, the theorem gives a range for the value of the delay $T$ for which the endemic equilibrium, when it exists, remains locally asymptotically stable. Of course, from the general theory of delay differential equations, we can assert that there will always be such a range, however, this result goes further by providing a computable estimate of a lower bound to this range.

## 4.5 A Model with Spatial Diffusion

We now turn to a model which includes the possibility of spatial spread of the population. We consider the same situation as in Section 4.2, and assume, for simplicity, that $r = r' = b = b'$. Let $S(t, x)$ and $I(t, x)$ represent the population densities of susceptible and infected individuals at time $t$ and at point $x \in \mathbf{R}^n$. $S$ and $I$ have units of numbers of individuals per unit volume of $\mathbf{R}^n$. Let $\triangle$ denote the Laplace operator in $\mathbf{R}^n$ and consider the situation studied in Theorem 4.1 with the added possibility that the population diffuses (due to random motion) in a simple Fickian manner. That is, there is a tendency of individuals in the population to move in a random direction which is independent of their past history. A good discussion of these notions can be found in the book of Okubo [1980] which is an excellent source of information on diffusion of biological populations.

We introduce the following formal notation in order to mathematically describe the situation we are modeling. Let $\Omega \subset \mathbf{R}^n$ denote the spatial domain that the population is inhabiting. We assume that $\Omega$ is a bounded, connected, and open set with sufficiently smooth boundary, and that $n \geq 1$ is an integer ($n = 1, 2$, and $3$ are the interesting cases). Assuming that the population cannot leave or enter through the boundary of $\Omega$, we have the following equations for our model.

$$
\begin{aligned}
\partial S(t,x)/\partial t =& rS(t-T,x) + rpI(t-T,x) - rS(t,x) \\
& - kS(t,x)I(t,x) + d\Delta S(t,x), \\
\partial I(t,x)/\partial t =& r(1-p)I(t-T,x) - rI(t,x) \\
& + kS(t,x)I(t,x) + d\Delta I(t,x),
\end{aligned}
\tag{4.16}
$$

valid for $(t,x) \in \mathbf{R}^+ \times \Omega$, $\mathbf{R}^+ = (0,\infty)$, and

$$
S(t,x) = S_0(t,x), \quad I(t,x) = I_0(t,x), \quad (t,x) \in [-T,0] \times \overline{\Omega}, \tag{4.17}
$$

$$
\partial S(t,x)/\partial\eta = \partial I(t,x)/\partial\eta = 0, \quad (t,x) \in [0,\infty) \times \partial\Omega, \tag{4.18}
$$

where $\partial\Omega$ is the boundary of $\Omega$, $\overline{\Omega}$ is its closure, and $\eta$ is the outward unit normal to $\partial\Omega$. Our results on this model are contained in the following theorem, which is a generalization of Theorem 4.1.

**Theorem 4.4 (A case with maturation period and spatial diffusion.)**
*Consider the problem* (4.16)-(4.18) *and define*

$$
C_0 = \frac{1}{|\Omega|} \int_\Omega \left[ S_0(0,x) + I_0(0,x) + r \int_{-T}^0 \{S_0(s,x) + I_0(s,x)\}ds \right] dx \tag{4.19}
$$

*and*

$$
P^* = C_0/(1+rT), \tag{4.20}
$$

*where* $|\Omega| = \int_\Omega dx$. *Then, the following asymptotic behavior occurs as* $t \to \infty$:
*(i) If either* $R_0 = kP^*/pr \leq 1$ *or else* $I_0(t,x) \equiv 0$, $(S(t,x), I(t,x)) \to (P^*, 0)$.
*(ii) If* $R_0 > 1$, *and* $I_0(t,x) \not\equiv 0$, $(S(t,x), I(t,x)) \to (pr/k, P^* - pr/k)$.

The limiting distribution of $S$ and $I$ is not space dependent and is essentially the same as in Theorem 4.1. Also, the threshold criterion depends on the initial size of the total population, but it does not depend on how this initial population is distributed in $\Omega$. So, in this situation, spatial diffusion due to random motion does not affect the asymptotic behavior of the population. We do note that this result depends on the fact that the two subpopulations diffuse with the same velocity. This might not be true if the infection affected mobility of individuals. The proof of the theorem requires considerable technical details which can be found in the original paper by Busenberg, Cooke and Pozio [1983], and which we do not describe here.

Note that if $S_0$, $I_0$ in (4.16)-(4.18) are space independent, the solution $(S(t), I(t))$ of this problem is also space independent and satisfies (4.1)-(4.2) for $r = r' = b = b'$. So, Theorem 4.1 is a particular case of Theorem 4.4 when this restriction is placed on the birth and removal rates.

## 4.6 Diseases with Long Subclinical Periods

One of the characteristics of some vertically transmitted diseases, such as Chagas' disease which was discussed in Section 2.13 of Chapter 2, is the presence of a chronic form of the infection which is of long duration. Infection with the HIV virus which leads to AIDS (Bacchetti and Moss [1989]) also has a long period of infectivity during which the affected individual shows no readily observable symptoms. This subclinical period can last for several years, averaging about ten years for AIDS and fifteen for Chagas' disease (García and Bruckner [1988], Garham [1980]), and significantly affects the population dynamics of the infection. Studies of this effect for the AIDS case have been done by Castillo-Chavez, Cooke, Huang and Levin [1989] and Thieme and Castillo-Chavez [1991] in models that do not take the vertical transmission of the disease into account. Velasco-Hernandez [1991a,b] has developed and analyzed models of Chagas' disease in some of which vertical transmission and delays have been included.

We shall now formulate a simple model of the transmission of HIV, the human immunodeficiency virus, and then extend it to include the long subclinical period. This is based on a previous model of Busenberg, Cooke and Thieme [1991], but extends the previous model by including vertical transmission. The demographic consequences of HIV/AIDS are also studied in Anderson, May and McLean [1988], and May, Anderson and McLean [1989]. HIV is unfortunately very commonly transmitted from human mothers to children, and recent statistics from New York City (see Novick *et al.* [1989]) show that 0.66% of the newborn children are HIV seropositive and may be infected. Sadly, these children are likely to develop AIDS, and their life expectancy is severely reduced.

From the point of view of modeling, one would like to know how the dynamics of the epidemic are affected by vertical transmission. In one sense, there is no effect, since very few, if any, infected children will reach sexual maturity, and therefore they will not pass the virus to other persons. On the other hand, the fact that they will not reach sexual maturity may have an important influence on the age-structure of the population, and the overall rate of growth of the population, and through these on the profile of the epidemic. The model presented here does not permit addressing the question of age structure in a realistic way, because it contains only two age classes, juvenile and adult. However, it is designed to provide information on growth rates and prevalence of the virus in the population, and it may form a basis for future consideration of age structured models.

The basic epidemiological classes in our model are the juveniles and the adults (that is, sexually active). The juvenile population is divided into infected and not infected (susceptible) groups. We assume that infected juveniles do not reach sexual maturity and therefore do not reproduce. The adults may therefore be subdivided into a group of non-core individuals, who do not participate in transmitting the disease, and core adults. The core adults may consist of some homosexuals, needle-sharing addicts and others at high risk of contracting the infection. Thus some of the core adults will be infected and others will be susceptible but not infected. We assume a constant sex ratio in the population, in order to avoid introducing separate groups for the males and females. We can now introduce the following variables.

$S_0(t) = $ The number of uninfected juveniles at time $t$.
$I_0(t) = $ The number of infected juveniles at time $t$.
$N_1(t) = $ The number of non-core adults at time $t$.
$N_2(t) = $ The number of core adults at time $t$.
$I_2(t) = $ The number of infected core adults at time $t$.

We also introduce the following parameters.

$\beta_1 = $ The non-core adult per capita birth rate.
$\beta_2 = $ The core adult per capita birth rate.
$\mu_0 = $ The juvenile death rate from non-AIDS causes (per capita).
$\mu_1 = $ The non-core adult death rate (per capita).
$\mu_2 = $ The core adult death rate (per capita).
$q = $ The proportion of newborn from infected core adults who are infected.
$r_1 = $ The recruitment rate of juveniles into the non-core adult class.
$r_2 = $ The recruitment rate of juveniles into the core adult class.
$k = $ The rate of infection due to effective contacts between infective and non-infective core adults.

The removal of infected adults due to the appearance of severe symptoms will be modeled in two ways. In the first, we introduce a parameter $\gamma$ representing a rate of removal. Thus $1/\gamma$ is the mean length of the period between initial infection and the appearance of symptoms. In the second, we introduce a time delay between the point of initial infection and the appearance of symptoms. The first results in a set of ordinary differential equations, whereas in the second there are both ordinary and delay differential equations. The equations for the first type of model are as follows.

$$\begin{aligned}
S_0' &= \beta_1 N_1 + \beta_2(N_2 - qI_2) - (\mu_0 + r_1 + r_2)S_0, \\
N_1' &= r_1 S_0 - \mu_1 N_1, \\
N_2' &= r_2 S_0 - \mu_2 N_2 - \gamma I_2, \\
I_2' &= k(N_2 - I_2)I_2/N_2 - (\mu_2 + \gamma)I_2.
\end{aligned} \tag{4.21}$$

Since the infected juveniles do not play a role in the dynamics of the disease, the corresponding governing equation

$$I_0' = \beta_2 qI_2 - \mu_3 I_0,$$

where $\mu_3$ is their death rate, need not be included in the system of equations
(4.21). If there were no vertical transmission, $q = 0$, then $I_0(t)$ would be identically zero, and the four equations (4.21) would reduce to the four equations
analyzed in the paper of Busenberg, Cooke and Thieme [1991]. Although the
case $q \neq 0$ is more difficult to analyze, we believe that some aspects of the
analysis can be carried over to it. In particular, since the functions on the right
sides of the equations are homogeneous of degree one, one expects exponentially increasing or decreasing populations. Therefore, it is useful to introduce
new variables such as

$$x = \frac{N_1}{S_0}, \quad y = \frac{N_2}{S_0}, \quad z = \frac{I_2}{N_2}.$$

One can then look for equilibrium values of these ratios. Since

$$x' = \frac{N_1' - xS_0'}{S_0},$$

with similar forms for $y'$ and $z'$, then defining

$$\alpha = \mu_0 + r_1 + r_2,$$

we have the following system in these new variables

$$
\begin{aligned}
x' &= r_1 + x(\alpha - \mu_1) - x(\beta_1 x + \beta_2 y(1 - qz)), \\
y' &= r_2 + y(\alpha - \mu_2) - y(\beta_1 x + \beta_2 y(1 - qz) + \gamma z), \\
z' &= (k - \gamma)z(1 - z) - \frac{r_2 z}{y}.
\end{aligned}
\tag{4.22}
$$

Any steady state of the system (4.22) corresponds to an exponentially growing
or decreasing $S_0$. Clearly, one such steady state is given by setting $z = 0$ and
obtaining the following system for $x$ and $y$:

$$
\begin{aligned}
0 &= r_1 + x(\alpha - \mu_1) - x(\beta_1 x + \beta_2 y), \\
0 &= r_2 + y(\alpha - \mu_2) - y(\beta_1 x + \beta_2 y).
\end{aligned}
$$

This system has a unique solution which represents a *disease-free equilibrium*.
Any endemic equilibrium of (4.22) must satisfy

$$
\begin{aligned}
0 &= r_1 + x(\alpha - \mu_1) - x(\beta_1 x + \beta_2 y(1 - qz)), \\
0 &= r_2 + y(\alpha - \mu_2) - y(\beta_1 x + \beta_2 y(1 - qz) + \gamma z), \\
0 &= (k - \gamma)z(1 - z) - \frac{r_2 z}{y}.
\end{aligned}
\tag{4.23}
$$

There are several basic questions concerning the existence and stability
of endemic equilibria which have not been addressed, and the analysis of this
model and interpretation of the results is left for the interested reader. We
note that the contact patterns of the members of the various subpopulations
have important effects on the progress of the disease. For a discussion see, for
example, Jacquez *et al* [1988].

We now turn to a modified model including an explicit time delay $T$, the time between infection and development of severe symptoms. The differential equations for $S_0$, $I_0$, and $N_1$ are unchanged. The equation for $I_2$ is the following delay integral equation.

$$I_2(t) = \int_{t-T}^{t} kI_2(s)e^{-\mu_2(t-s)}\frac{N_2(s) - I_2(s)}{N_2(s)}ds.$$

The quantity under the integral sign represents the number of individuals who were infected at time $s$, did not die prior to time $t$, and have been infected for no longer than time $T$. If this equation is differentiated, one obtains

$$I_2'(t) = kI_2(t)\frac{N_2(t) - I_2(t)}{N_2(t)} - kI_2(t-T)e^{-\mu_2 T}\frac{N_2(t-T) - I_2(t-T)}{N_2(t-T)} - \mu_2 I_2(t).$$

This equation is not equivalent to the integral equation, however, because its general solution satisfies an equation which differs from that of the integral equation by $C\exp(-\mu_2 t)$, where $C$ is an arbitrary constant. Such situations commonly occur in epidemic models where there is an incubation period between exposure to a disease and entry into the infective class (see Busenberg and Cooke [1980]), and we further discuss such cases in Section 4.7.5.

To complete this model, we note that an equation for $S_2(t)$, the number of susceptible uninfected individuals in the adult core, is

$$S_2' = r_2 S_0 - \mu_2 S_2 - \frac{k(N_2 - I_2)I_2}{N_2}.$$

From this, we see that $N_2 = S_2 + I_2$ satisfies the equation

$$N_2' = r_2 S_0 - \mu_2 N_2 - k\frac{(N_2(t-T) - I_2(t-T))I_2(t-T)e^{-\mu_2 T}}{N_2(t-T)}.$$

The analysis of this model is left as an open problem.

## 4.7 Mathematical Background

This section, like similar sections in preceding chapters, provides a brief explanation of the principal mathematical methods that are used in the analysis of the models of this chapter. We do not attempt to provide a thorough or complete exposition of this material, but rather aim to give a convenient synopsis of a few pertinent topics. Since the mathematical theory of delay differential equations is more complicated than the theory of ordinary differential equations, we can accomplish our task only by assuming more mathematical sophistication from the reader. Consequently, a number of users of this section may desire sources of more detailed expositions, which they can find in the books by Bellman and Cooke [1963], El'sgolt's and Norkin [1973], Halanay [1966], and Hale [1977].

There are subsections dealing with 1) Positivity and Invariant Regions, 2) Equilibria and Stability Analysis, 3) Liapunov Stability Theory, 4) Existence and Bifurcation of Periodic Solutions, and 5) Invariant integral conditions.

### 4.7.1 Positivity and Invariant Regions

The models in this chapter have been formulated in terms of systems of delay differential equations. A *delay differential equation* (DDE) with bounded delay is an equation in which the rate of change at time $t$ of a variable $x$ with values in $\mathbf{R}^n$, depends on values of that variable over an interval $[t - r, t]$, where $r > 0$. An example is the equation

$$\frac{dx(t)}{dt} = f\left(x(t), x(g_1(t)), ..., x(g_m(t))\right),$$

where $f$ is a given function of $m + 1$ variables and

$$t - r \leq g_j(t) \leq t \quad (j = 1, ..., m).$$

The quantities $t - g_j(t)$ are called the *delays* or *lags*. An important special case is that in which the delays are constants, $t - g_j(t) = r_j$. In that case, the equation takes the form

$$\frac{dx(t)}{dt} = f\left(x(t), x(t - r_1), ..., x(t - r_m)\right),$$

and it is frequently called a *differential-difference equation*. More general forms are possible. For example, consider the equation

$$\frac{dx(t)}{dt} = f\left(\int_0^r k(\theta)x(t - \theta)d\theta\right),$$

where $k$ is an integrable function. In this equation, the rate of change of $x$ at time $t$ depends on the previous values of $x$ on the interval $[t - r, t]$, weighted according to the function $k$. This equation is an example of what is called a *functional differential equation* (FDE), or an *integro-differential delay equation*.

Since the models of this chapter are equations with constant delays, we restrict our attention here to equations of that type. For information on more general types of delays, consult the references. Consider a system of the form

$$\frac{dx(t)}{dt} = f\left(x(t), x(t - r_1), ..., x(t - r_m)\right), \quad t > 0, \tag{4.24}$$

where $x$ and $f$ are vectors with components $x_i$ and $f_i$, respectively, $1 \leq i \leq n$, and where

$$0 < r_1 < r_2 < \cdots < r_m.$$

Letting $r = r_m$, the initial value problem for (4.24) has the initial condition

$$x(t) = \phi(t), \quad -r \le t \le 0, \tag{4.25}$$

where $\phi$ is a given vector function. Usually it is asumed that $\phi$ is a continuous function, that is $\phi \in C = C([-r, 0], \mathbf{R}^n)$, and then a solution of the initial value problem is a continuous function $x$ for $t \in [-r, t_1]$, for some $t_1 > 0$, which satisfies (4.25) for $-r \le t \le 0$ and which is differentiable and satisfies (4.24) for $0 \le t < t_1$. We assume here that $f$ satisfies conditions sufficient to guarantee existence and uniqueness of the solution of the initial value problem. We note that if $f$ is continuous and a solution to (4.24) exists for $t > 0$, and $\phi \in C$, then $x$ will be $C^1$ (that is, continuously differentiable) on $(0, \infty)$, $C^2$ on $(r, \infty)$, and so on, with the smoothness of the solution increasing with every step of size $r$.

As in previous chapters, we often want all components of a solution to satisfy $x_i(t) \ge 0$ for $T > 0$. Define the non-negative *cone* or *orthant* by

$$\mathbf{R}^n_+ = \{(x_1, ..., x_n): \; x_j \ge 0, \; j = 1, ..., n)\}.$$

Positive invariance of $\mathbf{R}^n_+$ for a solution $x(t)$ will be assured if the trajectory cannot leave $\mathbf{R}^n_+$ by crossing one of its faces. Suppose that $x_i(t) > 0$ for $0 \le t < t^*$, but the trajectory hits one of the faces, say the face $x_1 = 0$, at $t = t^*$. Then $x_1(t^*) = 0$ and

$$\frac{dx_i(t^*)}{dt} = f_i\left(x(t^*), x(t^* - r_1), \cdots, x(t^* - r_m)\right).$$

If it can be shown that the quantity on the right hand side of this equation is positive, then $x_i$ is increasing at $t = t^*$, which is a contradiction, and it follows that the trajectory cannot leave through this face. The general argument for invariance is thus along the following lines. One has to show that if all $x_i(t)$ are positive for $[t^* - r, t^*)$, $t^* \in (0, \infty)$ then on each face $x_i = 0$, $f_i$ is positive when evaluated at $t^*$.

For example, consider (4.1). On the face $S = 0$, if $S(t^*) = 0$, then

$$\frac{dS(t^*)}{dt} = bS(t^* - T) + pb'I(t^* - T),$$

and this is positive under the assumption that $S(t^* - t)$ and $I(t^* - t)$ are positive. Likewise, if $I(t^*) = 0$, then

$$\frac{dI(t^*)}{dt} = qb'I(t^* - T) > 0.$$

Therefore, if $S(t) > 0$, $I(t) > 0$ for $t \in [-T, 0]$, then $S(t)$ and $I(t)$ are positive for $t > 0$.

### 4.7.2 Equilibria and Stability Analysis

An *equilibrium point* or *steady state* for (4.24) is a constant function that satisfies the equation. That is, $x(t) = \bar{x}$ for $t \ge -r$. If such a solution exists, then

$$f(\bar{x}, ..., \bar{x}) = 0.$$

This is a system of $n$ equations for the $n$ components of $\bar{x} = (\bar{x}_1, \bar{x}_2, ..., \bar{x}_n)$ each of whose solutions represents a constant solution of (4.24). However, note the following. For an ordinary differential system $dx/dt = f(x)$, if $f(c) = 0$, for a constant vector $c$, and if $x(t) = c$ for one value of $t$, then this is true for all $t$, and then $x(t) = c$ is an equilibrium. However, if for one value of $t$

$$x(t) = x(t - r_1) = \cdots = x(t - r_m) = c,$$

with $f(c, ..., c) = 0$, then $x(t)$ may not be the equilibrium $x(t) \equiv c$ of (4.24).

Now, let us discuss the concept of stability of an equilibrium. By a change of coordinates, we can suppose that the equilibrium is at $x = 0$. In stating the definitions that follow, it will be convenient to introduce the following notation. If $x(t)$ is a continuous function, and if $t \geq 0$, we let $x_t$ denote the function in $C = C([-r, 0], \mathbf{R}^n)$ defined by $x_t(s) = x(t + s)$, $-r \leq s \leq 0$. Further, if we let $|| \cdot ||$ denote the supremum norm in $C$, then

$$||\phi|| = \sup \{|\phi(s)| : -r \leq s \leq 0\},$$

where $|\phi|$ denotes a norm of $\phi$ in $\mathbf{R}^n$. We can now make the following definitions. Suppose that $f(0, \cdots, 0) = 0$. The solution $x(t) = 0$ for $t \geq -r$ of (4.24) is said to be *stable* if, for any $\epsilon > 0$, there exists $\delta = \delta(\epsilon)$ such that $||\phi|| < \delta$ implies $||x_t|| < \epsilon$ for all $t \geq 0$. It is said to be *asymptotically stable* if it is stable and, in addition, there is a $b > 0$ such that $||\phi|| < b$ implies that the solution with initial function $\phi$ satisfies

$$x(t) \to 0 \text{ as } t \to \infty.$$

We now describe the method of *linearization* for determining asymptotic stability of the zero equilibrium of (4.24). As was the case with ordinary differential equations, we can always make a simple change of variables which carries any equilibrium to zero, hence, this method works for all equilibria. For ease of exposition, we consider the case of a differential-difference equation with $m = 1$, that is with one fixed delay, and we also take $n = 2$. Then the system has the form

$$\frac{dx_1}{dt} = f_1(x_1(t), x_2(t), x_1(t - r), x_2(t - r)),$$

$$\frac{dx_2}{dt} = f_2(x_1(t), x_2(t), x_1(t - r), x_2(t - r)).$$

We assume that the functions $f_i$ are twice continuously differentiable, even though the results that we shall give also hold under weaker hypotheses. Since we are interested in small perturbations, and since $f_1(0,0,0,0) = f_2(0,0,0,0) = 0$, we may expand $f_1$ and $f_2$ in Taylor series near the origin. Doing this and discarding all terms other than the linear ones, we obtain the following linear system.

$$\frac{dx_1}{dt} = a_{11}x_1(t) + a_{12}x_2(t) + b_{11}x_1(t-r) + b_{12}x_2(t-r),$$

$$\frac{dx_2}{dt} = a_{21}x_1(t) + a_{22}x_2(t) + b_{21}x_1(t-r) + b_{22}x_2(t-r). \tag{4.26}$$

where

$$a_{11} = D_1 f_1(0,0,0,0), a_{12} = D_2 f_1(0,0,0,0),$$
$$a_{21} = D_1 f_2(0,0,0,0), a_{22} = D_2 f_2(0,0,0,0),$$
$$b_{11} = D_3 f_1(0,0,0,0), b_{12} = D_4 f_1(0,0,0,0),$$
$$b_{21} = D_3 f_2(0,0,0,0), b_{22} = D_4 f_2(0,0,0,0), \tag{4.27}$$

and where $D_j f_i$ is the partial derivative of $f_i$ with respect to the $j$th variable $(i = 1,2; j = 1,2,3,4)$. The linear system may be written in matrix notation as

$$\frac{dx}{dt} = Ax(t) + Bx(t-r),$$

$$A = (a_{ij}), \quad B = (b_{ij}). \tag{4.28}$$

The system (4.26) or (4.28) is the linear approximation to (4.24). It is known that the zero solution of (4.24) is asymptotically stable if and only if the zero solution of the linearization (4.28) is asymptotically stable.

We therefore turn to a discussion of (4.28). If $x(t) = e^{\lambda t}u$ is a solution of (4.28), where $u$ is a constant vector, then

$$(\lambda I - A - Be^{-\lambda r})u = 0.$$

Consequently, such solutions exist if and only if $\lambda$ is a root of the characteristic equation

$$\det \Delta(\lambda) = 0, \quad \Delta(\lambda) = \lambda I - A - Be^{-\lambda r}. \tag{4.29}$$

The following facts are known when $r > 0$.

(i) If all characteristic roots $\lambda$ have negative real parts, then all solutions of (4.28) tend to 0 as $t \to \infty$, and the zero solution of (4.24) is asymptotically stable.

(ii) The equation $\det \Delta(\lambda) = 0$ always has a root. In any vertical strip $-\infty < c_1 \le \text{Re}(\lambda) \le c_2 < \infty$, there are at most a finite number of roots. There exists $c_2$ such that there are no roots in the half-plane $\text{Re}(\lambda) > c_2$.

(iii) If all roots satisfy $\text{Re}(\lambda) \le 0$, then a sufficient condition for stability of the zero solution of (4.28) is that all roots with zero real parts be simple roots. For a statement of the necessary and sufficient condition for stability, see Bellman and Cooke [1963] or Hale [1977].

(iv) The characteristic roots, which are the zeros of the entire function $\det \Delta(\lambda)$, depend continuously on $r$ for $r > 0$. For $r = 0$, there are finitely many roots and for $r > 0$, there may be infinitely many. The infinitely many roots that arise at $r = 0$ appear with real parts at $\infty$.

(v) It is not easy to give necessary and sufficient conditions, directly in terms of $A$, $B$ and $r$, for asymptotic stability. Much research has been devoted to this problem for various special cases and applications. The books by

MacDonald [1989] and Stépán [1989] treat this problem. It is worth noting that the natural state space for a differential-difference or functional differential equation is infinite-dimensional. The space that is often chosen is $C$, the continuous functions on $[-r, 0]$ or on $[0, r]$. The concepts of stable and unstable manifold that we encountered in the differential equations models can also be defined in this context. For example, the equilibrium $x = 0$ of the linear equation (4.28) has a stable manifold, which is the set of all functions $\phi$ in $C$ such that the solution $x_t \rightarrow 0$ as $t \rightarrow \infty$. We shall not present any discussion of these concepts, which are described in detail in the book of Hale [1977]. However, we note that they do have an important bearing on the correct interpretation of several results obtained from models which use functional differential equations.

We now give a brief description of the method of Stépán [1989] that we used in Section 4.4. This method is applicable for linear autonomous functional differential (or integro-differential) equations of the form

$$\frac{dx(t)}{dt} = \int_{-\infty}^{0} [d\eta(\theta)]x(t + \theta), \quad t > 0, \tag{4.30}$$

where $\eta(\theta)$ is an $n \times n$ matrix $(\eta_{ij}(\theta))$ of functions of bounded variation on $[-\infty, 0]$. In this equation, the rate of change of $x$ at $t$ depends on values of $x$ in the infinite past, so the equation is said to be an equation with unbounded delay. In our uses, we have assumed bounded delay, which may be included in (4.30) by assuming $\eta(\theta)$ constant for $\theta < -r$, $r > 0$. For some general comments about functional differential equations, refer to Section 4.7.3. Note that (4.28) is the special case of (4.30) obtained when

$$\eta(\theta) = \begin{cases} 0, & -\infty \leq \theta < -r, \\ B, & -r \leq \theta < 0, \\ B + A, & 0 \leq \theta. \end{cases} \tag{4.31}$$

The stability of the zero solution of (4.30) is related to the location of the roots of the characteristic equation

$$\Delta(\lambda) = 0, \quad \Delta(\lambda) = \det(\lambda I - \int_{-\infty}^{0} e^{\lambda\theta} d\eta(\theta)). \tag{4.32}$$

Stépán proves that if there exists a positive number $v$ such that

$$\int_{-\infty}^{0} e^{-v\theta} |d\eta_{jk}(\theta)| < \infty, \quad j, k = 1, ..., n, \tag{4.33}$$

then if all roots of $\Delta(\lambda) = 0$ have negative real parts, it follows that the zero solution of (4.30) is exponentially asymptotically stable. When $\eta(\theta)$ is constant for $[-\infty, -r]$, that is, when the equation has bounded delay, the condition (4.33) automatically holds. Stépán's general theorem is stated as follows.

is satisfied for $t \in [t_0, t_0 + A)$. The derivative $dx(t_0)/dt$ is to be understood as a right-hand derivative. In order to make a well-defined initial value problem, an initial function $\phi \in D$ must be given, and the initial condition is

$$x_0 = \phi, \text{ that is, } x_0(\theta) = \phi(\theta), \quad -r \leq \theta \leq 0. \tag{4.31}$$

The differential-difference system (4.24) may be seen to be a special case by defining

$$f(\phi) = f(\phi(0), \phi(-r_1), \cdots, \phi(-r_m)), \quad \phi \in C.$$

For the general theory of existence and uniqueness of solutions, and the continuous dependence of solutions on the initial data $t_0$, $\phi$, the reader should consult the book of Hale. By an equilibrium of (4.30), we mean a constant vector function $c$, such that $f(c) = 0 \in \mathbf{R}^n$. By the change of variable $\tilde{x} = x - c$, an equilibrium can be moved to the origin, hence, we shall assume that $c = 0$ and $f(0) = 0$. The definitions of stability and asymptotic stability are those given previously.

Instead of the Liapunov functions used for ordinary differential equations that we encountered in Chapter 2, Krasovskii [1963] proposed the use of functionals $V(\phi)$ where $V : C \to \mathbf{R}$, is continuous. In analogy to the idea of the derivative of $V$ along a solution, define

$$\dot{V}(\phi) = \limsup_{h \to 0+} \frac{1}{h} \left[ V(x_h(\phi)) - V(\phi) \right], \tag{4.32}$$

for $\phi \in C$, where $x_h(\phi)$ denotes the segment $x_h$ of the solution starting from the initial function $\phi$ at $t_0 = 0$, that is, $x_0(\phi) = \phi$.

**Definition.** $V : C \to \mathbf{R}$ is called a Liapunov functional on a set $G$ in $C$ for equation (4.30) if $V$ is continuous on the closure of $G$ and $\dot{V}(\phi) \leq 0$ for $\phi \in G$. Let

$$E = \{\phi \in \overline{G} : \dot{V}(\phi) = 0\},$$

where $\overline{G}$ denotes the closure of $G$. A set $S \subset C$ is said to be invariant with respect to the functional differential equation if for any $\phi \in S$, $\phi$ is part of a "complete orbit" in $S$. That is, the solution $x_t(\phi)$ exists for all $t \geq 0$. Moreover, there is a backward continuation of $\phi$ for $t < 0$, so that $x(t)$ exists and is a solution on $-\infty < t < \infty$, and $x_0 = \phi$. This backward continuation of the solution on $-\infty < t$ need not be unique. It is equivalent to saying that $\{x_t(\phi) : \phi \in S\} = \{\phi \in S\}$, for each $t \geq 0$.

We can now state the following results, which are proved in Hale's book.

**Theorem 4.5** *Let $V$ be a Liapunov functional on $G$ and let $x_t(\phi)$ be a bounded solution that remains in $G$ for $t \geq 0$. If $M$ is the largest subset of $E$ that is invariant with respect to (4.30), then $x_t(\phi) \to M$ as $t \to \infty$.*

**Theorem 4.5** *Assume that condition* (4.33) *holds. Let* $\rho_1 \geq ... \geq \rho$, $\sigma_1 \geq ... \geq \sigma_s = 0$ *denote the non-negative real zeros of* $R$ *and* $S$ *re. where*

$$R(y) = Re\Delta(iy), \ S(y) = Im\Delta(iy).$$

*The trivial solution* $x = 0$ *of* (4.30) *is exponentially asymptoticall, and only if one of the following conditions holds.*

$$(i) \quad n \text{ is even, } n = 2m,$$

$$S(\rho_k) \neq 0, \ k = 1, \ ..., \ r,$$

$$\sum_{k=1}^{r}(-1)^k \text{ sign } S(\rho_k) = (-1)^m m,$$

$$(ii) \quad n \text{ is odd, } n = 2m + 1,$$

$$R(\sigma_k) \neq 0, \quad k = 1, \ ..., \ s - 1,$$

$$R(0) > 0,$$

$$\sum_{k=1}^{s-1}(-1)^k \text{ sign } R(\sigma_k) + \frac{1}{2}[(-1)^s + (-1)^m] + (-1)^m \ m = 0$$

The proof of this result can be found in Stépán [1989].

### 4.7.3 Liapunov Stability Theory

The ideas of Liapunov's second method, which we explained for or ferential equations in Section 2.16.4, have been extended to delay tional differential equations by a number of mathematicians workir past thirty years. Here we shall explain some of these extensions needed in the analysis of the models in this chapter. We formulat is customary, for functional differential equations, a class of equa includes (4.24) as a special case. To do this, we use some notation above.

Let $C = C([-r, 0], \mathbf{R}^n)$ be the Banach space of all continuou from the interval $[-r, 0]$ into $\mathbf{R}^n$, with the supremum norm

$$\|f\| = \sup\{|f(\theta)| : -r \leq \theta \leq 0\}.$$

If $x(t)$ is a continous function with domain $[t_0 - r, t_0 + A]$, $A > 0$, a. $\mathbf{R}^n$, then for $t \in [t_0, t_0 + A]$ we let $x_t \in C$ be defined by $x_t(\theta) = x(t \cdot \theta \leq 0$. Now, if $D$ is a subset of $C$, and $f : D \to \mathbf{R}^n$ is a given fu. equation

$$\frac{dx(t)}{dt} = f(x_t)$$

is called an *autonomous functional differential equation*. A function be a solution of (4.30) on $(t_0 - r, t_0 + A)$ if $x$ is continuous, $x_t \in D$,

**Theorem 4.6** *Suppose that $V$ is a Liapunov functional on the set $G_l = \{\phi \in C : V(\phi) < l\}$, and there is a constant $K = K(l)$ such that if $\phi$ is in $G_l$ then $|\phi(0)| < K$. Then any solution $x_t(\phi)$ with $\phi$ in $G_l$ tends to $M$ as $t \to \infty$.*

**Corollary 4.7** *Suppose that $V : C \to \mathbf{R}$ is continuous and there exist non-negative functions $a(r)$ and $b(r)$ such that $a(r) \to \infty$ as $r \to \infty$,*

$$a(|\phi(0)|) \leq V(\phi), \quad \dot{V}(\phi) \leq -b(|\phi(0)|), \quad \text{for } \phi \in C.$$

*Then the solution $x = 0$ of (4.30) is stable and every solution is bounded. If in addition, $b(r)$ is positive definite, then every solution approaches zero as $t \to \infty$.*

### 4.7.4 Existence and Bifurcation of Periodic Solutions

In Section 2.16.6 it was pointed out that periodic fluctuations in the dynamics of populations may arise either because of periodicity in the environment or because of the nonlinear interaction of subpopulations. Also, the Hopf bifurcation theorem was stated for ordinary differential equations. The theorem indicated that when the equations contain a parameter, $\mu$, it can sometimes happen that at a certain value of the parameter, a stable equilibrium becomes unstable, and a small periodic solution appears near the equilibrium point. The same kind of phenomenon can occur for functional differential equations, as we shall now explain.

We consider a one-parameter family of equations

$$\frac{dx(t)}{dt} = L(\mu)x_t + h(\mu, x_t), \tag{4.33}$$

and we make the following assumptions.

We assume that $\mu$ is a real parameter, $L(\mu)$ is a linear operator on $C$ into $\mathbf{R}^n$. Also, $h(\mu, \phi)$ is a (nonlinear) map from $\mathbf{R} \times C$ into $\mathbf{R}^n$, and $h$ has continuous derivatives of orders one to five with respect to $\mu$ and $\phi$ and $h(\mu, 0) = 0$ for all $\mu$. The assumptions on $L$ imply that it can be represented in the form

$$L(\mu)\phi = \int_{-r}^{0} d\eta(\mu, \theta)\phi(\theta),$$

for $\phi$ in $C$, where $\eta$ is a matrix of functions of bounded variation in $\theta$.

The characteristic equation of the linear equation

$$\frac{dx(t)}{dt} = L(\mu)x_t \tag{4.34}$$

has the form

$$\det \Delta(\lambda, \mu) = 0, \quad \Delta(\lambda, \mu) = \lambda I - \int_{-r}^{0} d\eta(\mu, \theta)e^{\lambda\theta}. \tag{4.35}$$

(Compare the form of the characteristic equation in Section 2.16.2). Assume that for $\mu = \mu_0$, the characteristic roots, $\pm i\omega$, are simple, purely imaginary, and not zero. Also assume that no other characteristic roots are integer multiples of these.

Suppose that the function $\lambda(\mu)$ which is a characteristic root of (4.35) satisfying $\lambda(\mu_0) = i\omega$, obeys $d\mathrm{Re}(\lambda)(\mu_0)/d\mu > 0$. That is, the root $\lambda(\mu)$ crosses the imaginary axis with nonzero speed at $\mu = \mu_0$.

The Hopf Bifurcation Theorem states that there are nonconstant periodic solutions of the nonlinear equation (4.33) for small $|\mu - \mu_0| > 0$ which have period close to $\frac{2\pi}{\omega}$. In order to state the result more precisely, we point out that the exponential solutions of the linear equation (4.34) are of the form $x(t) = \xi e^{\lambda t}$ where $\lambda$ is a root of the characteristic equation and $\xi$ is an eigenvector, that is, $\Delta(\mu, \lambda)\xi = 0$. The following result holds.

**Theorem 4.8** *Assume the above hypotheses. Then there exists a positive constant $\epsilon$, and there exist functions $G(\mu, c, \nu)$ and $x(t, \mu, c, \nu)$ defined for real $c$, $|c| < \epsilon$, $|\nu - \omega| < \epsilon$, and $|\mu| < \epsilon$, such that (4.33) has a periodic solution $x(t)$ with period $2\pi/\nu$ with $|x| < \epsilon$, $|\nu - \omega| < \epsilon$ and $|\mu| < \epsilon$, if and only if $x(t)$ is equal to $x(t, \mu, c, \nu)$ (up to phase shift) and $\mu$, $c$, $\nu$ solve the equation $G(\mu, c, \nu) = 0$. Moreover, $x(t, \mu, c, \nu)$ has the form*

$$x(t, \mu, c, \nu) = 2\mathrm{Re}\left[\xi(\mu)e^{\nu i t}\right] c + O(c^2).$$

The calculation of $G(\mu, c, \nu)$ and of $x(t, \mu, c, \nu)$ is difficult in the systems that arise in modeling, and it is even more difficult to determine whether the bifurcating periodic solution is stable or unstable. Information on these calculations may be found in Chow and Mallet-Paret [1977], and Stech [1979, 1985a,b]. In practice one often relies on computer simulations to investigate the stability of these periodic solutions.

### 4.7.5 Invariant Integral Conditions

When an exposed class is present, it often occurs in epidemic models that individuals who enter this class remain in it for a fixed period of time before becoming infective. Thus, the exposed class can be viewed as a holding compartment for a fixed period of time during which individuals do not participate in disease transmission interactions. We saw such a situation in the $S \to E \to I \to S$ model of Section 4.4. A similar situation occurs when there is a fixed period of infectivity at the end of which individuals move into an immune class or else relapse to the susceptible class. Fixed periods of immunity also occur, as is the case, for example, with immunity of newborns due to maternal antibodies. More generally, the time interval that is spent in any of these classes may not be fixed but may be governed by a probability distribution. In all of these circumstances the dynamic equation which describes the evolution of the number of exposed individuals has a first integral, and hence, an arbitrary constant of integration. However, the arbitrariness of this constant is only a mathematical problem, since a closer reflection of the origins of the model typically severely restricts, or else totally specifies, the constant. When this fact is not recognized the formal mathematical analysis may lead to conclusions that are mathematically correct but which are totally inapplicable to the situation that is being modeled. This situation has been discussed in detail by Busenberg and Cooke [1980] but here we shall limit ourselves to describing one example.

In order to fix ideas, let us consider the $S \to I \to R \to S$ epidemic model in a constant total population where the infectious period is $T_1 > 0$, and the duration of acquired immunity is a fixed time $\tau = T - T_1 > 0$.

$$\frac{dS(t)}{dt} = r\left[I(t-T)S(t-T) - I(t)S(t)\right]$$

$$\frac{dI(t)}{dt} = r\left[I(t)S(t) - I(t-T_1)S(t-T_1)\right], \ 0 < T_1 < T. \tag{4.36}$$

The removed class does not play a role here because it simply acts as a holding compartment for a fixed time $\tau > 0$. Clearly, for any pair of constants $(a, b)$ we obtain a solution of (4.36) by setting $S(t) = a$, $I(t) = b$, and one may proceed to study the stability of any such equilibrium. In fact, for this system, Green [1978] has shown that when $r = 0.2$, $T_1 = 1$ and $(a, b)$ and $\tau$ are used as parameters, there are values at which the equilibrium destabilizes and a Hopf bifurcation to periodic solutions occurs.

Returning to the model, we note that the infective class is simply a compartment which holds those who enter it for a fixed time $T_1$, hence, in the steady state, the solutions which are of interest are those that obey the integrated form of the equations for $I$ and $S$,

$$I(t) = r \int_{t-T_1}^{t} I(s)S(s)ds,$$

$$S(t) + I(t) = a - r \int_{t-T}^{t-T_1} I(s)S(s)ds, \tag{4.37}$$

where $a$ is a constant of integration. These equations define a manifold $M$ which is invariant under the flow induced by the system (4.36), and hence, is determined by the initial data

$$\hat{a} = S(t) + I(t) + r \int_{t-T}^{t-T_1} I(s)S(s)ds,$$

with

$$\hat{a} = S_0(0) + I_0(0) + r \int_{-T}^{-T_1} I_0(s)S_0(s)ds.$$

This and condition (4.37) now restrict the steady states to be one of

$$(\hat{S}, 0) = (\hat{a}, 0), \quad \text{or} \quad (\overline{S}, \overline{I}) = \left(\frac{1}{rT_1}, \frac{arT_1 - 1}{rT}\right), \tag{4.38}$$

and not arbitrary constants. It is the stability of these particular steady states that needs to be studied in the context of the model. In fact, the asymptotic stability and instability of the steady states needs to be considered on this manifold $M$, since, when one considers the system (4.36) on the entire space, the steady states are not isolated, hence, they can never be asymptotically stable. Details on the analysis of situations similar to this can be found in the above cited article of Busenberg and Cooke and in Hale [1974].

# 5  Age and Internal Structure

## 5.1  Age Structure and Vertical Transmission

Age plays an important role in the dynamics of disease transmission. Often the degree of susceptibility of an individual to a pathogen is dependent on the individual's age, and contact rates among various parts of the population which may lead to the transfer of infections also depend on age. However, for horizontally transferred diseases it is often a valid approximation to neglect age as an independent parameter and to treat the population as being uniform in age. In fact, Ludwig and Walters [1985] argue that, in certain population models, it is possible that the added requirements for information in an age-structured model may lead to a degradation in the estimation of parameters from available data. In contrast, age enters as a fundamental parameter in vertically transmitted diseases, and it is always necessary to take age into account in one way or another in order to produce a valid model. There are at least two reasons for this. First, it is only the newborn, that is individuals of age zero, that are susceptible to this mode of disease transmission. Consequently, the newborn must be taken into account in some way that distinguishes them from the rest of the population. Second, in a number of cases of vertically transmitted diseases, the pathogenic agent builds up in an infected female as time goes by, and hence, so does the probability of transferring the infection to her offspring. Other effects of the infection, such as increased mortality or decreased fertility, can also depend on the length of the infection, hence on age. So, some means of tracking the internal state of infected fertile individuals needs to be incorporated in the model. Age is the simplest such internal variable. As we shall see later, other variables describing the internal structure of the population may need to be introduced. For an example of estimation of parameters from age-specific data, see Dietz and Schenzle [1985].

In this chapter we shall describe some basic methods for including age and other internal structure variables in models of vertically transmitted diseases. Even though this type of model is necessary for the analysis and understanding of the main questions concerning vertical transmission, the literature on such models is very recent and essentially limited to the studies of Busenberg and Cooke [1982], Cooke and Busenberg [1982], El Doma [1985,1987], Busenberg, Cooke and Iannelli [1988, 1989], Iannelli, Milner and Pugliese [1992], Busenberg, Iannelli and Thieme [1991 a,b], Langlais [1991], Inaba [1989], and Kubo and Langlais [1991]. In addition to describing the results in these papers, we develop a general model with age structure and discuss in some detail the various pertinent epidemiological issues and how they enter in the formulation of the model.

The plan of the chapter is as follows. In the next section we first describe the ways in which vertical transmission and age are coupled in the dynamics of the disease. We give examples of specific vertically transmitted diseases in order to illustrate these couplings and to describe the different physical and chemical processes by which they are realized. We then show the means by which each of these effects can be incorporated in an appropriate age-structured epidemic model.

The standard shorthand notation for distinguishing the dynamic interactions in epidemic models ($S \rightarrow I \rightarrow S$, $S \rightarrow E \rightarrow I \rightarrow R$, etc.) is too crude to be able to separate epidemiologically distinct age-structured models. Consequently, we use the alternate notation developed in Chapter 1 that enables us to give a rapid classification of the dynamics of age-dependent vertically transmitted diseases.

In Section 5.3 we develop and discuss a general age-dependent model for disease transmission where the possibility of vertical transmission is included. We have selected a variation of the classical McKendrick-von Foerster description of age dependent populations in our model (see, McKendrick [1926], von Foerster [1959]), because it allows us to include all of the major effects of vertical transmission and its interactions with age-structure. Moreover, this type of population model has been extensively studied in recent years, and the mathematical techniques for its analysis are highly developed. We note that the first age-dependent disease model (albeit with no vertical transmission) since the work of McKendrick was in the basic paper by Hoppensteadt [1974]. There has been considerable further work in this area, of which we mention that of Webb [1980, 1982], and the recent theses of Andreasen [1988], Inaba [1989], and Velasco-Hernandez [1991a].

Section 5.4 is devoted to describing the results of Busenberg, Cooke and Iannelli [1988, 1989] concerning the relation between age-dependent models and the "catalytic curve" method which is discussed in the book of Muench [1959]. In particular, we investigate the possibility of determining the force of infection term and the presence of vertical transmission from the catalytic curve data.

Sections 5.5 through 5.10 are devoted to the study of specific special cases of the model that we formulate. In some of these cases we can present detailed conclusions that illustrate fundamental aspects of vertically transmitted disease dynamics. Section 5.11 is devoted to a discussion and interpretation of the threshold results that have been obtained for age-dependent epidemic models. In Section 5.12 we describe the work that has been done to date on age-structured models with vertical transmission and spatial diffusion. In Section 5.13 we describe recent results on the possible functional forms of the force of infection terms. These nonlinear terms are very difficult to measure and have been traditionally derived via heuristic reasoning which has, at times, led to questions concerning their validity. In this section we present a particular axiomatic formulation for such terms, and describe the results of Busenberg and Castillo-Chavez [1989, 1991] giving all the possible forms of the force of infection terms that satisfy these axioms and the implications that they have on the identification of the force of infection terms on the basis of disease incidence data.

Because of the considerable array of mathematical tools that are needed in the analysis of models with internal structure, we shall not attempt to provide a synoptic coverage of the mathematical background necessary for the derivation of the results presented in this chapter. We only outline the derivation of the results that we present, and give references to appropriate sources that provide the details of the analysis for each of these results. In a certain sense, the mathematical complications of the current techniques for dealing with population models with internal structure that are formulated in terms of the McKendrick type of equations set a real limit on the general usefulness of these models. However, the added degree of detail and realism that they provide justifies the study of such models. Moreover, the past history of the use of mathematical models in the study of population problems shows a clear trend for continual refinements and simplifications of what initially appear to be complicated mathematical methods. With each generation of researchers, the mathematical methods that are found to be useful are simplified to the point that they can be fairly routinely applied to appropriate models. We believe that the general principles used in analyzing the models in this chapter are of sufficient importance and applicability that they will undergo this process of simplification and general acceptance in the near future.

## 5.2  Modeling Internal Structure

In order to focus our discussion of the interaction between age and vertical transmission we return to a specific example which we encountered already in Chapter 3, the transmission of *Rickettsia rickettsi* in the American dog tick, *Dermacentor andersoni*. Recall that rickettsia is the pathogen that causes Rocky Mountain Spotted Fever and it is transmitted to humans by infected ticks. This is, of course, a case of vector borne horizontal transmission. However, in the ticks, rickettsia is transmitted both horizontally, when ticks feed off an animal that has been infected by another tick, and also vertically from female ticks to their offspring.

There are extensive laboratory and field data (see, for example, Burgdorfer [1975] and Garvie *et al.* [1978]) on this disease, and the following is a brief summary. An infected female tick passes the infection to about fifty percent of its offspring. The load of rickettsia passed on to a newborn depends directly on the load carried by the infected mother and continues to grow throughout the life of the individual. In parts of the eastern U.S., climates are such that the ticks have a one year life cycle, and each generation can be identified with a single year step. Now, a female tick that has acquired the infection by horizontal transmission will have its parasite load increase with its age, and since oviposition occurs soon after a blood meal, the first generation of offspring coming from such a parent will have a light parasite load. The offspring, in turn, will go through the season, overwinter and reproduce the following year, after their parasite load has increased with their aging. Hence, the second generation of vertically infected offspring will start with a higher initial load of rickettsia. This process continues with successive generations from infected lineages starting with increasing loads of rickettsia. By the fifth such generation the parasite load is so high that it can prevent successful oviposition and the process of vertical transmission would end were it not for its coupling with the horizontal transmission mechanism discussed above.

From the above description it is clear that, in order to describe the dynamics of such a disease, one needs to introduce both an age variable and another internal variable, the generation number of vertical transmission inheritance of the rickettsia. So if $i_f$ denoted the density of infected females, one should make $i$ depend on three variables $i_f(t, a, n)$, where $t$ = time, $a$ = age, and $n$ = generation in a vertically transmitted lineage. In the case discussed above, we would take $n \in \{0, 1, 2, \ldots, 5\}$, where $n = 0$ denotes an infected female who obtained the disease via horizontal transmission, $n = 1$ denotes one obtaining the disease from a mother of class $n = 0$, and so on. Clearly, in this example, individuals in class $n = 5$ are involved only in the horizontal transmission of the disease. Here, the internal variable $n$ is an integer, so we are essentially splitting the age-structured female population into six discrete generation classes. In general, there would be several internal variables which play a role in the dynamics of the disease. One of these, which was used in the model of McKendrick [1926], and was introduced by Hoppensteadt [1974] in an age-structured epidemic model, is the period of infectivity, that is, the length of time that the individual has been infected. So, in general, the independent variables would include a multidimensional variable $\mathbf{z}$ which collects all the internal variables other than age. There are two basic types of such internal variables: those that remain fixed with time (such as the generation number) and those that change with time (such as the period of infectivity). These two types of variables will enter differently in the dynamics, and we split the multidimensional vector variable $\mathbf{z}$ into $\mathbf{z} = (\mathbf{u}, \mathbf{v})$, where $\mathbf{u}$ contains all variables of the second type and $\mathbf{v}$ those of the first type.

It is clear that age-specific parameters of the population are dynamically coupled with the process of vertical transmission in the following ways:

(1) The pathogen load carried by an infective parent changes with age, hence, so does the probability that the pathogen be passed to the offspring, thus increasing the likelihood of vertically transmitting the infection. Consequently, changes in maturation times or in the age-specific fertility of the population will affect the degree of vertical transmission.

(2) The probability of acquiring the disease via horizontal transmission mechanisms often depends on age, and possibly on other internal variables. Consequently, in combination with the mechanism in (1) above, horizontal transmission is coupled to both age and vertical transmission.

(3) It is only the newborn who are exposed to the possibility of acquiring the disease via vertical transmission. Moreover, the number of newborn having acquired the disease through vertical transmission depends on the number of infective fertile parents in the total population, hence, on the age-structure of the total population.

(4) Immunity or partial immunity to infection can be transmitted vertically, and this is one special form of vertical transmission.

(5) The pathogen load may increase with age and can adversely affect the fertility and mortality of the infectives, thus reducing the possibility for vertical transmission. This effect may be coupled in complicated ways with that described in (1) above.

From the above, we see that vertical transmission is quite different from horizontal transmission in some very basic ways. One of the differences that we wish to stress is that the pathogen load of the infectives plays a major role in the mechanism of vertical transmission, and cannot be neglected as an internal variable as is often, but not always, done in models of horizontally transmitted diseases. Also, it is not possible to construct valid models for vertical transmission without including the birth dynamics explicitly in the model. The exclusion of birth dynamics from models of horizontally transmitted diseases is a common simplification that is used to reduce their mathematical complexity.

We now return to our shorthand notation, introduced in Chapter 1, for describing vertically transmitted disease dynamics. We separate the population into four basic epidemiological classes: the susceptibles, the exposed, the infective and the removed. We denote the densities per unit age of individuals in these classes by the symbols, $s$, $e$, $i$, and $r$, respectively. As noted above, we use the dynamic variables consisting of time, age, and an internal variable $\mathbf{u}$; and also a labeling internal variable $\mathbf{v}$. The internal variables $\mathbf{u}$ and $\mathbf{v}$ may be vector valued and each may describe more than one epidemiologically distinct scalar internal variable. For example, the variable $\mathbf{v}$ may be a two dimensional vector whose first component can take the values $m$ (for male) or $f$ (female) and whose second component may range over the integers $(0, 1, \ldots 5)$, and denote the generation of vertical inheritance of the disease. It is clear from this notation that we can include the case where there are several subclasses of infectives by introducing an appropriate label in the internal variable $\mathbf{v}$. For example, asymptomatic infectives can be introduced in this way without having to add to our basic four epidemiological classes.

In the next section, we derive a general model with age structure for vertically transmitted diseases. In Section 5.4, we look at two *sirs* models and show the relationship, derived by Busenberg, Cooke and Iannelli [1988, 1989] between the McKendrick and the catalytic curve formulations of age-dependent epidemics. In particular, we show that the catalytic curve formulation contains sufficient information to determine whether or not a disease of this type is vertically transmitted.

In Section 5.5 we describe in some detail a model without recovery of the simple type

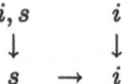

which has been analyzed by El Doma [1985, 1987]. We use this to give examples of the types of complications and effects that can occur because of age dependence and vertical transmission. In Sections 5.6 and 5.7 we discuss a model of the type

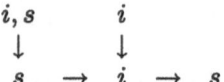

which has been analyzed in great detail by Busenberg, Cooke and Iannelli [1988, 1989], Iannelli, Milner and Pugliese [1992], Busenberg, Iannelli and Thieme [1991, a,b], and Langlais [1991]. This is the only general age-structured epidemic model for which the global dynamics have been obtained. Consequently, the results that have been obtained in this case serve as a guide to further developments in this field.

It will be clear from this discussion that there are many open questions concerning age-dependent vertically transmitted diseases that still need to be analyzed. In the remaining sections we will discuss some of these questions that appear to us to have serious epidemiological implications and describe various approaches that can be used to study them. One particular result that we shall describe, which is due to Thieme [1991b], shows that in an age-dependent model of the type

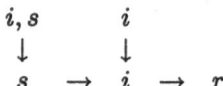

the age-structure of the population can cause an endemic state to become unstable and lead to oscillations in the levels of the prevalence of a disease.

## 5.3 Derivation of the Model Equations

Our aim is to derive model equations which are mathematically tractable yet general enough to include the main types of vertically transmitted diseases. We choose a method which shows the age variable explicitly because age is a fundamental parameter in vertical transmission. The independent variables we use are time $t$, age $a$, a vector $\mathbf{u}$ of dynamic variables that describe internal structure, and a vector $\mathbf{v}$ of variables that describe membership in a particular epidemiological subclass. The four dependent variables we use are age-specific concentrations of susceptibles, exposed, infective and removed individuals and we denote these by

$$s(a, t, \mathbf{u}, \mathbf{v}), \ e(a, t, \mathbf{u}, \mathbf{v}), \ i(a, t, \mathbf{u}, \mathbf{v}) \text{ and } r(a, t, \mathbf{u}, \mathbf{v}).$$

These quantities represent densities in the sense that the number of susceptible individuals of class $\mathbf{v}$ who have ages between $a_1$ and $a_2$ and are in epidemiologic categories between $\mathbf{u}_1$ and $\mathbf{u}_2$ is given by

$$\int_{\mathbf{u}_1}^{\mathbf{u}_2} \int_{a_1}^{a_2} s(a, t, \mathbf{u}, \mathbf{v}) da\, d\mathbf{u}.$$

Here the vector interval $(\mathbf{u}_1, \mathbf{u}_2)$ denotes the set of vectors $\mathbf{u}$ whose coordinates range between the corresponding ones of $\mathbf{u}_1$ and $\mathbf{u}_2$. The densities may be either real valued or vector valued depending on whether we are dealing with a single population or several interacting populations. The total population density is given by $p = s + e + i + r$.

Since age and time increase at the same rate, the basic time derivative is obtained by taking the limit

$$\lim_{h \to 0} \frac{1}{h}[f(a + h, t + h) - f(a, t)] = \frac{\partial f}{\partial a}(a, t) + \frac{\partial f}{\partial t}(a, t)$$

when the function $f$ is differentiable. The time rate of change of a density is due to several causes: removal via death, entry or removal from an epidemiological class due to innoculation, healing, infection, immigration into or out of the population; and finally, entry via birth. However, this last mode of changing membership of a given class affects only the individuals of age zero. So, the basic balance laws take the form, for $t > 0$, and $a > 0$,

$$
\begin{aligned}
\frac{\partial s}{\partial t} + \frac{\partial s}{\partial a} + \frac{\partial}{\partial \mathbf{u}}(g_s) &= -\mu_s + f_s, \\
\frac{\partial e}{\partial t} + \frac{\partial e}{\partial a} + \frac{\partial}{\partial \mathbf{u}}(g_e) &= -\mu_e + f_e, \\
\frac{\partial i}{\partial t} + \frac{\partial i}{\partial a} + \frac{\partial}{\partial \mathbf{u}}(g_i) &= -\mu_i + f_i, \\
\frac{\partial r}{\partial t} + \frac{\partial r}{\partial a} + \frac{\partial}{\partial \mathbf{u}}(g_r) &= -\mu_r + f_r.
\end{aligned}
\tag{5.1}
$$

The birth laws, valid for $t > 0$ and $a = 0$, take the form

$$
\begin{aligned}
s(0, t, \mathbf{u}, \mathbf{v}) &= F_s(s, e, i, r), \\
e(0, t, \mathbf{u}, \mathbf{v}) &= F_e(s, e, i, r), \\
i(0, t, \mathbf{u}, \mathbf{v}) &= F_i(s, e, i, r), \\
r(0, t, \mathbf{u}, \mathbf{v}) &= F_r(s, e, i, r),
\end{aligned}
\tag{5.2}
$$

and the initial conditions are

$$s(a, 0, \mathbf{u}, \mathbf{v}) = s_0(a, \mathbf{u}, \mathbf{v}), \cdots, r(a, 0, \mathbf{u}, \mathbf{v}) = r_0(a, \mathbf{u}, \mathbf{v}). \tag{5.3}$$

The terms $\mu_s, \ldots, \mu_r$ describe the natural mortality rates and are usually taken to be linear, $\mu_s = \mu(a, t, \mathbf{u}, \mathbf{v})s$, etc. However, they can also include effects such as those due to crowding which may make such terms nonlinear. The terms $f_s, \ldots, f_r$ describe the basic dynamic interactions of the epidemiological classes and can include such factors as horizontal transmission, innoculation and cure rates. The terms $F_s, \ldots, F_r$ are the birth laws which include vertical transmission when $F_i \neq 0$, and maternally induced immunity when $F_r \neq 0$. Finally, the terms $\frac{\partial}{\partial u}(g_s), \ldots, \frac{\partial}{\partial u}(g_r)$ represent the evolution of the dynamic internal structure variables. For example, if the period of infection $\tau$ is the only such internal dynamic variable, then $s = s(a, t, \tau)$ and the dynamic equation for $s$ could take the form:

$$\frac{\partial s}{\partial t} + \frac{\partial s}{\partial a} + \frac{\partial s}{\partial \tau} = -\mu s + f_s,$$

because the period of infectivity increases at the same rate as time and age. In this example, which is essentially the model of Hoppensteadt [1974], we have chosen a mortality rate which is age-dependent but linear. In the above formulation we have not included the possibility of individuals switching from one subclass **v** to another but this formulation can be easily generalized to include this type of interclass migration terms.

The form of the interaction terms $f$ and the birth terms $F$ is very important in determining the dynamic behavior of the model. We shall discuss several versions of these terms. Certain forms of the interaction terms that can cover a number of situations were introduced by Cooke and Busenberg [1982] and are:

$$f_s = -s(a, t, \mathbf{u}, \mathbf{v}) \int_0^\infty k(a, a', t) i(a', t, \mathbf{u}, \mathbf{v}) da' + h_s,$$

$$f_i = s(a, t, \mathbf{u}, \mathbf{v}) \int_0^\infty k(a, a', t) i(a', t, \mathbf{u}, \mathbf{v}) da' + h_i.$$

Here, the terms $h_s$ and $h_i$ could include the recovery, loss of immunity, immunization and other rates of transfer between classes that do not involve transmission of the disease via contact between individuals. The kernel $k(a, a', t)$ in the horizontal transmission term measures the infective contacts between infectives of age $a'$ and susceptibles of age $a$. This type of kernel can be used to model the strong intra-cohort horizontal infective interactions that often occur with certain diseases, in particular with school-age childhood diseases, and some hospital infections where the disease transmission is largely restricted to individuals belonging to the same age group.

The birth terms $F$, when they can be taken to be linear, can have the form:

$$F_s = \int_0^\infty \beta(a)[p(a, t, \mathbf{u}, \mathbf{v}) - (q_1 + q_2) i(a, t, \mathbf{u}, \mathbf{v}) - q_3 r(a, t, \mathbf{u}, \mathbf{v})] da,$$

$$F_i = \int_0^\infty \beta(a) q_1 i(a, t, \mathbf{u}, \mathbf{v}) da,$$

$$F_r = \int_0^\infty \beta(a)[q_2 i(a, t, \mathbf{u}, \mathbf{v}) + q_3 r(a, t, \mathbf{u}, \mathbf{v})] da,$$

where $q_1$ is the proportion of offspring of infectives that are infective, $q_2$ is the proportion of offspring of infectives that are immune (maternally induced immunity), and $q_3$ is the proportion of offspring of immune individuals that are immune. Here $0 \leq q_j \leq 1$, $j = 1, 2, 3$, and if $q_1 > 0$, then the disease is vertically transmitted. We have taken $F_e \equiv 0$ here.

The models of age-dependent vertically transmitted diseases that we will treat in subsequent sections will be particular cases of the general model we have given here.

Under appropriate restrictions on the functions $f$, $F$, $g$ and $h$, one can establish existence and uniqueness results for the solutions of the model equations (5.1), (5.2) and (5.3). Examples of such results are in Hoppensteadt [1974], Cooke and Busenberg [1982], Elderkin [1985], Webb [1985], and Busenberg, Iannelli and Thieme [1991]. We shall not treat the mathematical details of these results but rather use this general model as the basis for our discussion of special forms of age-dependent disease transmission mechanisms. We shall see that, even in the simplest possible cases, there are new phenomena associated with vertical transmission that need to be taken into account when dealing with such diseases. We now proceed by first looking in some detail at the relationship between two specific age-structured models and the catalytic curve method of describing epidemics.

## 5.4 Age Structure and the Catalytic Curve

Muench [1959] called attention to the usefulness of the so-called catalytic curve in the study of epidemics. In a steady state population, this is the curve that shows the fraction of individuals who show evidence of having had the infection, as a function of the age of the individuals. Muench formulated simple ordinary differential equations, analogous to those used to model chemical reaction rates, to simulate the observed data for several diseases. These equations generally contained one or two parameters, which he was able to estimate by curve-fitting methods. The question of estimating the age-dependent rates of infection from the catalytic curve has also been addressed by Grenfeld and Anderson [1985].

Our purpose here is to derive an expression for the catalytic curve, starting from age-dependent model equations, and to show that the catalytic curve contains enough information to determine whether or not a disease is vertically transmitted. By doing this, we demonstrate that the catalytic curve follows directly from the assumptions underlying the age-dependent model. We assume, as did Muench, that the population has reached a steady state, that mortality due to disease is negligible, and that there is no migration in or out of the population. The results that we report here are due to Busenberg, Cooke and Iannelli [1988, 1989].

We shall consider two basic models, the first being the $s \rightarrow i$

$$\begin{matrix} & & \nearrow r \\ & & \\ & & \searrow s \end{matrix}$$

model described by

$$\begin{aligned}
\frac{\partial s}{\partial t} + \frac{\partial s}{\partial a} + \mu s &= -\lambda s + \gamma i, \\
\frac{\partial i}{\partial t} + \frac{\partial i}{\partial a} + \mu i &= \lambda s - (\gamma + \delta)i, \\
\frac{\partial r}{\partial t} + \frac{\partial r}{\partial a} + \mu r &= \delta i,
\end{aligned} \tag{5.4}$$

with the renewal conditions

$$i(0, t) = b_1(t), \quad s(0, t) = b_2(t), \quad r(0, t) = 0,$$

and initial data

$$i(a, 0) = i_0(a), \quad s(a, 0) = s_0(a), \quad r(a, 0) = r_0(a),$$

where $\lambda$ denotes the force of infection term. The second model has the diagram

$$s \rightarrow i \quad \begin{matrix} \nearrow r \\ \downarrow \\ \searrow \tilde{s} \rightarrow i \end{matrix}$$

where $\tilde{s}$ denotes "tagged" susceptibles who are counted either through antibody tests or in some other manner as having had the disease. The results in these two cases have basic similarities but also some differences. Consequently, we will discuss them separately. In the first case, the steady state form of (5.4) gives the following system of ordinary differential equations with initial data.

$$\begin{aligned}
\frac{ds}{da} + \mu s &= -\lambda s + \gamma i, \\
\frac{di}{da} + \mu i &= \lambda s - \delta i - \gamma i, \\
\frac{dr}{da} + \mu r &= \delta i, \\
s(0) &= \int_0^\infty \beta(a)[s(a) + (1 - q)i(a) + r(a)]da \\
&= \int_0^\infty \beta(a)[p(a) - qi(a)]da, \\
i(0) &= q \int_0^\infty \beta(a)i(a)da, \quad r(0) = 0.
\end{aligned} \tag{5.5}$$

We have assumed in these equations that all offspring of susceptible or immune parents are susceptible. The steady state assumption requires that the births and removals due to deaths are in a state of balance. This can be shown to be equivalent to the requirement that the net reproduction coefficient $R$ of the population satisfies $R = 1$, where

$$R = \int_0^\infty \beta(a)e^{-\int_0^a \mu(\sigma)d\sigma}da. \tag{5.6}$$

This expression for $R$ has the following intuitive explanation:

$$\Pi(a) = e^{-\int_0^a \mu(\sigma)d\sigma}$$

is the probability that an individual survive to age $a$, hence, $\beta(a)\Delta a$ times this expression is the expected number of offspring born to an individual during the age interval $(a, a + \Delta a)$. The integral over all possible ages of this product, which is the expression for $R$, is therefore the total number of expected offspring of each individual. Thus $R = 1$ is the condition that, on the average over a complete lifespan, each individual give birth to a single offspring. The steady state distribution of the population, $p(a)$, is given by:

$$p(a) = b_0 e^{-\int_0^a \mu(\sigma)d\sigma} = b_0 \Pi(a), \tag{5.7}$$

where $b_0 = p(0) = s(0) + i(0)$.

We now integrate the equation for $s$, and obtain

$$s(a) = e^{-\int_0^a [\mu(\sigma)+\lambda(\sigma)]d\sigma}\left[s(0) + \int_0^a \gamma(\tau)i(\tau)e^{\int_0^\tau [\mu(\sigma)+\lambda(\sigma)]d\sigma}d\tau\right].$$

We are interested in the fraction of individuals of age $a$ who have been infected and have recovered into the immune class or who are still infectious. The graph of this fraction as a function of $a$ is the catalytic curve studied by Muench. Calling this $C(a)$, we have

$$C(a) = \frac{i(a) + r(a)}{p(a)} = \frac{p(a) - s(a)}{p(a)} = 1 - \frac{s(a)}{p(a)}.$$

Using the known form of $p(a)$, we may write

$$C(a) = 1 - \frac{W(a)}{b_0}e^{-\int_0^a \lambda(\sigma)d\sigma}, \tag{5.8}$$

where

$$W(a) = s(0) + \int_0^a \gamma(\tau)i(\tau)e^{\int_0^\tau [\mu(\sigma)+\lambda(\sigma)]d\sigma}d\tau. \tag{5.9}$$

Equation (5.8) is valid for any form of the force of infection. For example, for the intracohort form

(i) *Intracohort*: $\lambda(a, t) = \kappa(a)i(a, t)$, where infectives of age $a$ can pass on the infection only to susceptible individuals of their own age, we have

$$C(a) = 1 - \frac{W(a)}{b_0}e^{-\int_0^a \kappa(\sigma)i(\sigma)d\sigma}.$$

For the intercohort form

(ii) *Intercohort:* $\lambda(a, t) = \kappa(a)I(t)$, $I = \int_0^\infty i(a)da$, where the entire pool of infectives has the same contacts with the susceptibles of all ages, we have

$$C(a) = 1 - \frac{W(a)}{b_0} e^{-I \int_0^a \kappa(\sigma)d\sigma}.$$

In order to obtain more explicit forms, it would be necessary to solve the differential equation for $i(a)$ explicitly. If $\gamma(a) = 0$, $C(a)$ is an increasing function with finite limit, as in the catalytic curve of Muench, but this is not necessarily so in the more general case we are considering here. In general $W(0) = s(0) = \int_0^\infty \beta(a)p(a)da - q \int_0^\infty \beta(a)i(a)da = b_0 - q \int_0^\infty \beta(a)i(a)da$, hence,

$$C(0) = 1 - \frac{W(0)}{b_0} = \frac{q}{b_0} \int_0^\infty \beta(a)i(a)da = \frac{i(0)}{b_0}. \qquad (5.10)$$

From (5.10) we see that, if there is no vertical transmission, $C(0)$ is 0, but if $q > 0$ then $C(0) > 0$. Therefore, the model agrees with the intuition that the presence of vertical transmission may be inferred if a measurable fraction of newborn individuals exhibit antibodies to the infectious agent. However, keep in mind that in (5.5) we have assumed that $r(0) = 0$, that is that no newborn are immune, which we may interpret to mean that antibodies in infants signify infection.

On the other hand, knowing the catalytic curve does not provide sufficient information to identify the form of the force of infection. Of course, from (5.8) we obtain

$$\int_0^a \lambda(\sigma)d\sigma = -\log \frac{b_0}{W(a)}[1 - C(a)], \quad \lambda(a) = \frac{C'(a)}{1 - C(a)} + \frac{W'(a)}{W(a)}. \qquad (5.11)$$

However, we cannot determine $\lambda(a)$ from this equation unless $W(a)$ is known. If $\gamma(a) = 0$, so that $W$ is constant, we can compute $\lambda(a)$ from (5.11) once $C(a)$ is known. But, from this information alone it is not possible to tell whether $\lambda$ has the intracohort, the intercohort, or some other form.

Suppose that the rate of reporting of new infectives is known as a function of age. Then $s(a)\lambda(a)$ is known. If the recovery rates $\gamma(a)$ and $\delta(a)$ are known, the equations in (5.5) can be integrated to yield explicit expressions for $i$ and $r$ in terms of known quantities. Then $s$ can be found, because $s + i + r = p$ is known. Thus, the percentages of susceptibles, infectives, and immune will be known as functions of age.

We now consider the $s \;\longrightarrow\; i \begin{smallmatrix} \nearrow\; r \\ \downarrow \\ \searrow\; \tilde{s}\;\longrightarrow\; i \end{smallmatrix}$ model, which has the following steady state form

$$\frac{ds}{da} + \mu s = -\lambda s,$$

$$\frac{di}{da} + \mu i = \lambda s + \tilde{\lambda}\tilde{s} - \delta i - \gamma i,$$

$$\frac{dr}{da} + \mu r = \delta i - \eta r,$$

$$\frac{d\tilde{s}}{da} + \mu\tilde{s} = -\tilde{\lambda}\tilde{s} + \gamma i + \eta r,$$

$$s(0) = \int_0^\infty \beta(a)[s(a) + \tilde{s}(a) + (1 - q)i(a) + r(a)]da, \qquad (5.12)$$

$$= \int_0^\infty \beta(a)[p(a) - qi(a)]da,$$

$$i(0) = q\int_0^\infty \beta(a)i(a)da,$$

$$r(0) = 0,$$

$$\tilde{s}(0) = 0.$$

The equation for the total population $p(a)$ is again given by (5.7), while the equation for $s$ now becomes

$$s(a) = s(0)e^{-\int_0^a [\mu(\sigma) + \lambda(\sigma)]d\sigma}. \qquad (5.13)$$

The fraction $C(a)$ of all individuals who have had the disease is given by

$$C(a) = \frac{i(a) + r(a) + \tilde{s}(a)}{p(a)} = \frac{p(a) - s(a)}{p(a)} = 1 - \frac{s(a)}{p(a)}.$$

Using the expressions (5.7) and (5.13) for $p(a)$ and $s(a)$ we obtain

$$C(a) = 1 - \frac{s(0)}{b_0}e^{-\int_0^a \lambda(\sigma)d\sigma},$$

hence, $C(a)$ is an increasing function of $a$. Also

$$\lambda(a) = \frac{C'(a)}{1 - C(a)},$$

and knowledge of the catalytic curve yields the force of infection $\lambda$ as a function of age. This contrasts with the result for the first model discussed above. However, knowing $\lambda$ as a function of $a$ does not determine its dependence on $i$. Finally, it is worth noting that this result is independent of whether the recovered or immune individuals can lose their immunity ($\eta \neq 0$) or not ($\eta = 0$).

## 5.5 An $s \to i$ Model with Vertical Transmission

One of the simplest situations that can occur where vertical and horizontal transmission mechanisms interact in a significant way is in an $s \to i$ model. The coupling between these two modes of transmission occurs for two basic reasons. First, individuals who acquire the infection via horizontal contacts, if they are still capable of reproducing, may pass the infection vertically to their offspring. Second, newborn individuals who acquire the disease via vertical transmission may pass it on to others during their life-time via horizontal transmission. The form of the age-specific birth, mortality and contact rates will clearly play an important role in mediating the interaction between vertical and horizontal transmission. For example, in the extreme case where only the very young are fertile, the probability of acquiring the disease via horizontal contacts during the reproductive stage would be small, hence, the coupling between horizontal and vertical transmission would be weak. In the other extreme where there is a long maturation period prior to reproduction, there is a larger probability of horizontally acquiring the disease by the time an individual becomes fertile, and hence, a stronger coupling between horizontal and vertical transmission. These heuristic considerations are largely borne out by the analysis of this model which considers age and time as the only independent variables.

The equations for the model are

$$
\begin{aligned}
\frac{\partial s}{\partial t} + \frac{\partial s}{\partial a} + \mu(a)s &= -s \int_0^\infty k(a)i(a,t)da, \\
\frac{\partial i}{\partial t} + \frac{\partial i}{\partial a} + \mu(a)i &= s \int_0^\infty k(a)i(a,t)da,
\end{aligned}
\tag{5.14}
$$

for $a > 0, t > 0$,

$$
\begin{aligned}
s(0,t) &= \int_0^\infty \beta(a)[s(a,t) + (1-q)i(a,t)]da, \\
i(0,t) &= q \int_0^\infty \beta(a)i(a,t)da, \quad t \geq 0,
\end{aligned}
\tag{5.15}
$$

for $t \geq 0, 0 \leq q \leq 1$, and

$$
\text{for } a > 0, \quad i(a,0) = i_0(a), \quad s(a,0) = s_0(a).
\tag{5.16}
$$

Note that the model has linear age-specific birth and mortality moduli, $\beta$ and $\mu$, and that it describes a disease which does not affect either the birth or the death rates. The disease is vertically transmitted when $q > 0$, because a proportion $q$ of the offspring of infective individuals are infective. The model keeps track only of fertile individuals (females). Finally, the horizontal interaction term takes the form

$$
s(a,t) \int_0^\infty k(a)i(a,t)da,
\tag{5.17}
$$

which allows for variation of the contact rate of infectives with age. However, it is assumed that susceptible individuals of all ages, are equally likely to contract the disease via horizontal transmission. This assumption is valid for populations where there is fairly uniform mixing of individuals of all ages and cannot adequately describe diseases which are mainly transmitted among groups of relatively uniform age, such as measles and other childhood diseases which are largely transmitted among school-age individuals.

The form (5.17) of the interaction term allows a fairly complete treatment of this model and we proceed to describe some of the main results. For simplicity, in giving these results we shall set $k(a)$ equal to a constant. Define

$$\Pi(a_1, a_2) = \exp\left[-\int_{a_1}^{a_2} \mu(s)ds\right], \ \Pi(0, a) \overset{\text{def}}{=} \Pi(a),$$

and make the hypothesis that $\beta$ and $\mu$ are bounded, continuous functions which are non-negative and do not vanish identically; while $\mu$, the death rate, is non-decreasing for $a$ large enough. We note that there exists a unique real number $p^*$ such that

$$\int_0^\infty \beta(a)\Pi(a)e^{-p^* a}da = 1. \tag{5.18}$$

$\Pi(a_1, a_2)$ is the probability for an individual of age $a_1$ to survive to age $a_2$ and $\beta(a)\Pi(a)$ is the probability that an individual survives to age $a$ and then reproduces. Consequently, if $p^* = 0$ in (5.18),

$$R = \int_0^\infty \beta(a)\Pi(a)da = 1,$$

and the population has a net reproduction rate of one, that is, on the average, each individual in the population gives birth to one offspring. If $p^* > 0$ then the reproduction rate exceeds one and the population increases with time while, if $p^* < 0$, the reproduction rate is less than one and the population decreases with time. The parameter $p^*$ is the net Malthusian growth rate of the population.

Because of the vertical transmission, there is another growth rate $p_q^*$ that is associated with this population. This is given by the unique real solution of the equation

$$q \int_0^\infty \beta(a)\Pi(a)e^{-p_q^* a}da = 1.$$

Clearly, for $q \neq 0$, we have $p_q^* < p^*$. There is a substantial difference in the long term behavior of the population between the cases where $p^* = 0$ and $p^* \neq 0$. The following results, obtained by El Doma [1985, 1987], use the notation

$$I(t) = \int_0^\infty i(a, t)da, \ \ P(t) = \int_0^\infty [i(a, t) + s(a, t)]da.$$

**Theorem 5.1** *Suppose that $p^* < 0$ (that is, $R < 1$ and the total population is decreasing in size), that $\beta(a)$ vanishes for $a > A = $ maximum reproductive age, and that*

$$\int_0^\infty e^{-(p^* + p_q^*)a} \Pi(a)da < \infty.$$

*Then the age profile of infectives*

$$w(a,t) = \frac{i(a,t)}{I(t)} = \frac{i(a,t)}{\int_0^\infty i(a,t)da},$$

*satisfies*

$$\lim_{t\to\infty} w(a,t) = \frac{e^{-p_q^* a} \Pi(a)}{\int_0^\infty e^{-p_q^* a} \Pi(a)da},$$

*and*

$$\lim_{t\to\infty} i(a,t) = \frac{e^{-p_q^* a} \Pi(a)}{\int_0^\infty e^{-p_q^* a} \Pi(a)da} \lim_{t\to\infty} I(t),$$

*where $I(t)$ solves the ordinary differential equation*

$$\frac{dI(t)}{dt} = I(t) \left[ \int_0^\infty [q\beta(a) - \mu(a)]w(a,t)da + k(P(t) - I(t)) \right]. \tag{5.19}$$

*Moreover,*

$$\lim_{t\to\infty} \frac{i(a,t)}{s(a,t)} = 0. \tag{5.20}$$

The main conclusion of this result is that, in a decreasing population with a vertically transmitted disease of the type described above, the age-specific density of infectives will vanish faster than the density of susceptibles.

The next result describes the case with $p^* > 0$. This case is of interest because in many underdeveloped countries the total population is increasing, hence, the traditional assumption that $p^* = 0$ is invalid except for short duration epidemics.

**Theorem 5.2** *Suppose that $p^* > 0$ (That is, $R > 1$ and the total population is increasing). Then*

$$\lim_{t\to\infty} \frac{I(t)}{P(t)} = \lim_{t\to\infty} \frac{\int_0^\infty i(a,t)da}{\int_0^\infty p(a,t)da} = 1. \tag{5.21}$$

This result implies that, in an exponentially increasing population, a vertically transmitted disease, in the large time limit, saturates the total population. This result does not imply that the number of susceptibles approaches zero, but that the proportion of susceptibles in the population decreases to zero.

The case where $p^* = 0$ is both of special interest and, in a certain sense, unrealistic, since it represents a situation that occurs with zero probability. The generic cases are the ones covered above with $p^* > 0$ or $p^* < 0$ in this model. However, in considering situations where the demographic changes are much slower than the disease transmission dynamics, a number of age-dependent epidemic models, for example, those in Anderson and May [1979, 1982], Katzmann and Dietz [1984], Schenzle [1984], Tudor [1985], and some of those described in Section 5.4 and in the rest of this chapter, start with the hypothesis that $p^* = 0$. Here, the situation is quite complicated, and we shall only give some results that are obtained by numerically integrating the model equations. In particular, if the fertility modulus $\beta$ is chosen to have the form

$$\beta(a) = \begin{cases} 0, & 0 \leq a < m, \\ \alpha(a-m)e^{-\zeta(a-m)}, & m \leq a \leq 1, \end{cases} \tag{5.22}$$

with $\alpha, \zeta$ positive constants, then the maximum attainable age is normalized to be one and $m$ denotes the maturation time of the population. Fertility moduli of this type have graphs of the form shown in Fig. 5.1,

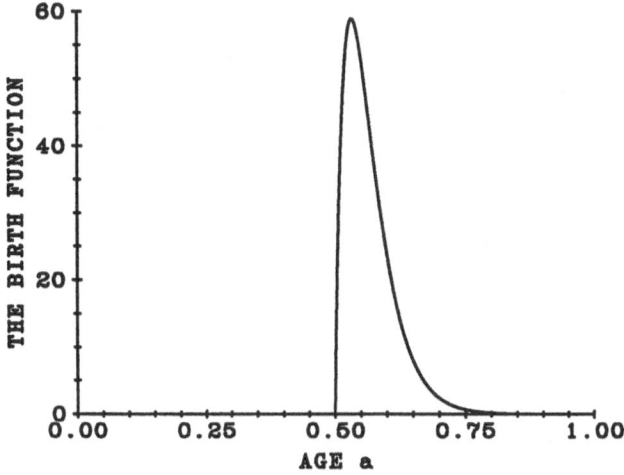

**Fig. 5.1.** Birth rate $\beta(a)$ as a function of age

and reflect a situation where immature individuals $(a < m)$ do not reproduce. As $m$ increases from zero to one, the maturation time increases and, consequently, so does the probability of horizontal infection before entrance into the reproductive age interval. The mortality rate needs to be chosen in a manner that makes $\Pi(a) = 0$ for $a \geq 1$, i.e., the probability of surviving beyond age one is zero. This is accomplished by choosing $\mu$ to have a graph of the form shown in Fig. 5.2 where the integral $\int_0^1 \mu(a)da = \infty$. Now, as $m$ is increased, the proportion of the population that survives to reach the reproductive age decreases, consequently, the fertility rate has to be increased in order to keep

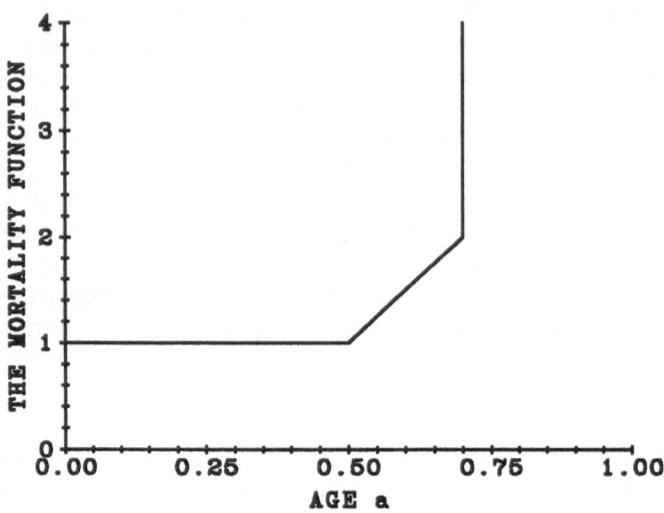

**Fig. 5.2.** Death rate $\mu(a)$ as a function of age

the population in balance. This corresponds to an increase in $\alpha$ in equation (5.22). The graphs in Figs. 5.3–5.5 depict the behavior of the model for three values of $m$ with the parameters $\alpha$ and $\zeta$ chosen so that $p^* = 0$.

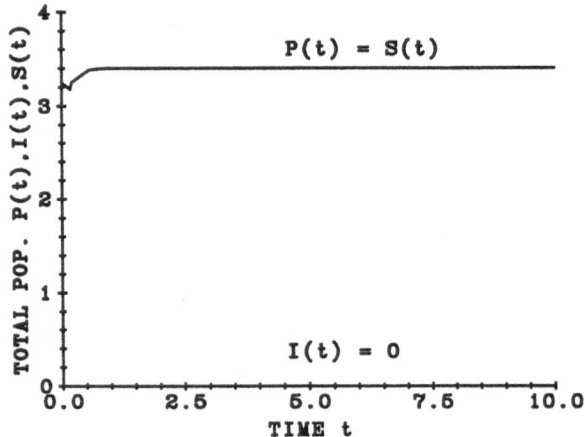

**Fig. 5.3.** Dynamics of the susceptible and infective subpopulations $(m = 0)$

From these graphs we observe that the qualitative behavior of the model shifts as $m$ increases. For $m = 0$, we have $S \to P$ and $I \to 0$ as $t \to \infty$ and this is the type of behavior described by Theorem 5.1 for the case $p^* < 0$. However, when $m = 0.7$, we have $I$ reaching an endemic level close in size to the total population $P$ while $S$ decreases to a small value, and this is analogous to the situation described by Theorem 5.2 for $p^* > 0$. For $m = 0.5$, we have a hybrid case where $I$ and $S$ tend to roughly one half of $P$. So, for the case $p^* = 0$ there is a delicate balance which determines the ultimate asymptotic behavior. It is important to note that, if the population is either increasing $(p^* > 0)$ or decreasing $(p^* < 0)$, no matter how slowly, the behavior described by Theorems 5.1 and 5.2 holds and is generic in the sense that it is invariant under small changes in the parameters of the model.

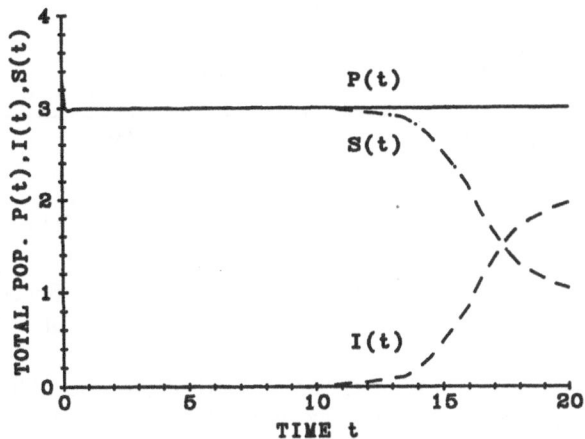

**Fig. 5.4.** Dynamics of the susceptible and infective populations $(m = 0.7)$

The change in the qualitative behavior when the maturation period increases and $p^*$ remains fixed at zero can be explained as follows. For small maturation periods, the probability of horizontal infection prior to reproduction is small, hence most of the newborn individuals are not infected, and the disease cannot establish itself in the population. As $m$ increases, the number of infective parents who have acquired the infection horizontally also increases, hence, so does the number of individuals who acquire the infection via vertical transmission. So, there is a positive mutual reinforcement of the two modes of transmission and the disease becomes established and, in fact, for the longer maturation periods, the infectives become the dominant class in the population.

As mentioned above, the case $p^* = 0$, representing a population in steady state, is improbable and is a critical case in this model where the asymptotic behavior depends on internal variables such as the maturation period of the population. Since the qualitative behavior of the model is quite different in the cases where $p^* > 0$ and $p^* < 0$, it is important in applications of these results to have estimates of the time scales over which the disease is being considered and information on whether the population is increasing or decreasing during

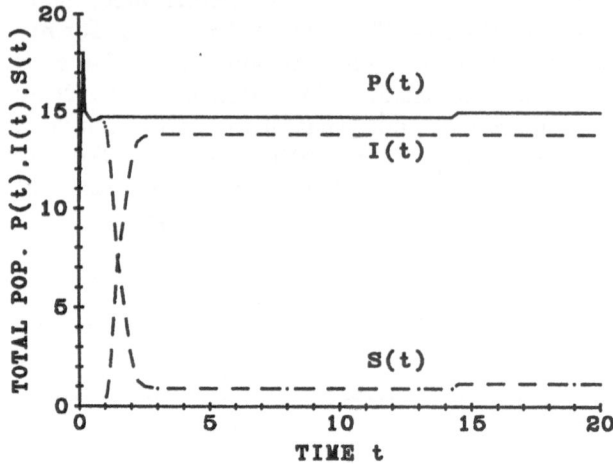

**Fig. 5.5.** Dynamics of the susceptible and infective populations ($m = 0.5$)

the maximal time interval of interest. If the population is fluctuating between a growth and a decay mode, then the above results are not valid and further analysis is needed in that case.

We now present an outline of the method of proof for Theorems 5.1 and 5.2 on which we have based the above discussion. The numerical methods used to obtain the results for the case $p^* = 0$ will also be briefly described.

The main idea of the proofs of Theorem 5.1 and 5.2 is the transformation of the original problem into an equivalent one where the two main variables are the total population $p(a, t)$ and the age profile of the infectives

$$w(a, t) = i(a, t)/I(t).$$

This transformation was introduced in the study of nonlinear age dependent problems by Busenberg and Iannelli [1982], and in the present case it leads to the following problem for $w(a, t)$:

$$\frac{\partial w}{\partial a} + \frac{\partial w}{\partial t} + \mu w = kp + \left\{ -kp + \int_0^\infty [\mu(a) - q\beta(a)w(a, t)]da \right\}w,$$

$$w(0, t) = q \int_0^\infty \beta(a)w(a, t)da,$$

$$w(a, 0) = w_0(a) = \frac{i(a, 0)}{\int_0^\infty i(a, 0)da}, \tag{5.23}$$

$$\int_0^\infty w(a, t)da = 1, \qquad \lim_{a \to \infty} w(a, t) = 0.$$

Here, $p(a, t)$ is the solution of the linear McKendrick-von Foerster equation which describes the dynamics of the total population density. Equation (5.23) has a sufficiently simple nonlinearity that it can be fairly thoroughly analyzed. We shall not describe the rather technical arguments that show that (5.23) has a unique solution. The following nonlinear renewal theorem, however, is a basic result that is used in the analysis of the model. Its proof is again somewhat technical and we refer the reader to Busenberg and Iannelli [1983b] and El Doma [1985, 1987] for the details. We define

$$w_\infty(a) = \frac{e^{-p_q^* a} \Pi(a)}{\int_0^\infty e^{-p_q^*(a)} \Pi(a) da}.$$

**Theorem 5.3** *Suppose that $w_0(a) \neq 0$ for some $a \in$ support($\beta$) and that the equation*

$$\int_0^\infty e^{-\lambda a} \beta(a) \Pi(a) da = 1$$

*has a real solution $\lambda = p^*$ such that*

$$\int_0^\infty e^{-(p^* + p_q^*)a} \Pi(a) da < \infty,$$

*where $p_q^*$ satisfies*

$$q \int_0^\infty e^{-p_q^*} \beta(a) \Pi(a) da = 1.$$

*Then, the solution $w$ of (5.23) has the asymptotic behavior*

$$\lim_{t \to \infty} \int_0^\infty |w(a,t) - w_\infty(a)| da = 0,$$

*whenever one of the following conditions hold:*
  *(i)   $p^* > 0$.*
  *(ii)  $p^* < 0$ and $w_0$ has compact support.*
  *(iii) $p^* < 0$ and $\mu$ is eventually non-decreasing.*

This result is the basis for the study of the asymptotic behavior of the solutions of the system (5.14)-(5.16). We first note that equation (5.19) for $I(t)$ is obtained by integrating the equation for $i(a,t)$ in (5.14) from $a = 0$ to $a = \infty$ and using the birth law in (5.15). The proof of (5.21) is then as follows.
    Defining

$$A(t) = -kP(t) + \int_0^\infty [\mu(a) - q\beta(a)] w(a,t) da,$$

we can write the solution of (5.19) as

$$I(t) = \frac{I(0) \exp[-\int_0^t A(s) ds]}{1 + kI(0) \int_0^t \exp\{-\int_s^t A(s') ds'\} ds}. \tag{5.24}$$

Since $p^* > 0, P(t) \to \infty$ as $t \to \infty$, and noting that

$$\left| \int_0^\infty [\mu(a) - q\beta(a)]w(a,t)da \right| \leq \sup_{a\in[0,\infty]} |\mu(a) - q\beta(a)| < \infty,$$

we see that $A(t) \to -\infty$ as $t \to \infty$, hence, by l'Hôpital's rule

$$\lim_{t\to\infty} I(t) = \lim_{t\to\infty} \left( \frac{-A(t)}{k} \right).$$

From this and a straightforward argument using the properties of $P(t)$, we obtain

$$\lim_{t\to\infty} I(t)/P(t) = 1,$$

and Theorem 5.2 is established.

In order to prove Theorem 5.1, we note that if $p^* < 0$, then $P(t) \to 0$ as $t \to \infty$, and hence,

$$\lim_{t\to\infty} A(t) = \lim_{t\to\infty} \int_0^\infty [\mu(a) - q\beta(a)]w(a,t)da$$
$$= \frac{\int_0^\infty [\mu(a) - q\beta(a)]e^{-p_q^* a}\Pi(a)da}{\int_0^\infty e^{-p^* a}\Pi(a)da}, \tag{5.25}$$

by Theorem 5.3. From (5.25) and the definitions of $p_q^*$ and $\Pi(a)$ it follows that

$$\lim_{t\to\infty} A(t) = -p_q^*.$$

Now, rewrite (5.24) as

$$I(t) = I(0) \Big/ \left[ \exp\left( \int_0^t A(s)ds \right) + kI(0) \int_0^t \exp\left( \int_0^s A(s')ds' \right)ds \right]$$

to see that $I(t) \to 0$ as $t \to \infty$, and in fact, $I(t) \leq Ke^{p_q^* t}$ for $t$ sufficiently large, where $K > 0$ is a constant. This implies that $i(a,t) = I(t)w(a,t) \to 0$ as $t \to \infty$. Since $s(a,t) = p(a,t) - i(a,t)$, it follows that $s(a,t) \to 0$ as $t \to \infty$. Moreover,

$$\lim_{t\to\infty} \frac{i(a,t)}{s(a,t)} = \lim_{t\to\infty} \frac{1}{\frac{p(a,t)}{i(a,t)} - 1},$$

hence,

$$\lim_{t\to\infty} \frac{i(a,t)}{s(a,t)} \leq \lim_{t\to\infty} \frac{1}{Ce^{(t-a)(p^* - p_q^*)} - 1} = 0,$$

since $p_q^* < p^*$. This establishes Theorem 5.1.

The proofs outlined above are given in detail in El Doma [1985, 1987]. The numerical results that were presented earlier in this section are based on a numerical integration of the equations for $w(a,t)$ and $p(a,t)$ using an implicit finite difference scheme. Once $w(a,t)$ is computed, then $I(t)$ can be obtained by solving the ordinary differential equation (5.19), and finally $i(a,t)$ is obtained from $i(a,t) = w(a,t)I(t)$.

The numerical scheme that was used for solving the linear problem for $p$ was developed by Lopez and Trigiante [1982], while that for solving the nonlinear problem for $w(a,t)$ is due to El Doma [1985]. Efficient methods for numerically integrating the equations of age-dependent population dynamics have been developed by Douglas and Milner [1987]. Some examples of the applications of these methods to numerical studies of epidemic models are discussed in Sections 5.7 and 5.8.

## 5.6  Analysis of the Intracohort Model

Here we describe the treatment of the intracohort $s \rightarrow i \rightarrow s$ infection model, and derive an explicit form for the threshold which determines the existence and stability of an endemic steady state. We shall return to this model in Section 5.9 where we will describe the complete global behavior of the solutions of a much more general case which includes the present one. However, the methods of analysis of the general case are considerably more abstract and complicated than the ones with which we can treat the present special case, and require substantial additional analysis in order to lead to the explicit form of the threshold that we obtain here.

We assume that the net demographic reproduction number $R$, defined in Section 5.4, is equal to one, and that the total population $p = i+s$ has reached its equilibrium value $p_\infty$ given by (5.7). This model is more general than that presented in the previous section because it treats the $s \rightarrow i \rightarrow s$ case, but less general in that it restricts the analysis to the case of a constant total population. These results are due to Busenberg, Cooke and Iannelli [1988]. We conclude the section by describing the results of Langlais [1991] for the $s \rightarrow i \rightarrow s$ model where $R > 1$.

The model we consider can be obtained from (5.4) by setting $\delta = 0$, and choosing the intracohort form for the force of infection term $\lambda$. We place the following conditions $(H_1)$-$(H_4)$ on the parameters $\beta(a)$, $\mu(a)$, $\kappa(a)$, $\gamma(a)$:

$(H_1)$  $\beta$, $\mu$ and $p_0$ are non-negative, piecewise continuous functions on $[0, \infty)$.
$(H_2)$  $\beta(a) > 0$ for $a \in (A_0, A)$ and $\beta(a) = 0$ for $a \notin (A_0, A)$.
$(H_3)$  $\int_0^\infty e^{-\int_0^a \mu(\sigma)d\sigma} da < \infty$.
$(H_4)$  $\gamma$ and $\kappa$ are non-negative piecewise continuous functions on $[0, \infty)$ and $\kappa$ is bounded.

Note that $H_3$ implies that $\int_0^\infty \mu(\sigma)d\sigma = \infty$. Setting $s(a,t) = p_\infty(a) - i(a,t)$ we obtain the following problem

a)  $\dfrac{\partial i}{\partial t} + \dfrac{\partial i}{\partial a} + \mu i = \kappa[p_\infty - i]i - \gamma i,$

b)  $i(0,t) = q \displaystyle\int_0^\infty \beta(a)i(a,t)da,$  \hfill (5.26)

c)  $i(a,0) = i_0(a),$

The key threshold parameter is

$$R_0 = \int_0^A q\beta(a)E(a)da = q\int_0^A \beta(a)\Pi(a)e^{\int_0^a [-\gamma(\sigma)+\kappa(\sigma)p_\infty(\sigma)]d\sigma}da, \quad (5.27)$$

and can be interpreted as a net infection reproduction number. In fact, $R_0$ is seen to be the expected number of vertically infected offspring of an infected individual when those offspring who are vertically infected by individuals who have acquired the disease through horizontal transmission from that one infective are taken into account. Note that $R_0$ increases linearly with the vertical transmission probability $q$ and exponentially with the horizontal transmission rate $\kappa$. Thus, control strategies which can reduce the horizontal transmission rate would tend to be more effective in reducing $R_0$ than strategies that bring about an equal amount of reduction of the vertical transmission probability.

We can now give the ultimate behavior of $i(0,t)$ which depends on whether $R_0 \leq 1$ or $R_0 > 1$.

**Theorem 5.4** *If $R_0 \leq 1$, then $\lim_{t\to\infty} i(0,t) = 0$, and if $R_0 > 1$ then $\lim_{t\to\infty} i(0,t) = V_\infty > 0$. Thus, an endemic state persists if and only if the net infection reproduction number $R_0$ is greater than one.*

We proceed to give an outline of the proof of this result. Equation (5.26a) can be explicitly solved along the characteristic lines $t - a = $ constant, leading to the following formula

$$i(a,t) = \begin{cases} \dfrac{i_0(a-t)e^{\int_0^t \alpha(a-t+\sigma)d\sigma}}{1+i_0(a-t)\int_0^t e^{\int_0^\tau \alpha(a-t+\sigma)d\sigma}\kappa(a-t+\tau)d\tau} & \text{if } a > t, \\[2em] \dfrac{i(0,t-a)e^{\int_0^a \alpha(\sigma)d\sigma}}{1+i(0,t-a)\int_0^a e^{\int_0^\tau \alpha(\sigma)d\sigma}\kappa(\tau)d\tau} & \text{if } a < t, \end{cases} \quad (5.28)$$

where

$$\alpha(\sigma) = -\mu(\sigma) - \gamma(\sigma) + \kappa(\sigma)p_\infty(\sigma).$$

Substituting $i(a,t)$ as given by (5.28) into the renewal condition (5.26b) does not determine $i(a,t)$ explicitly except in the special case $q = 0$. In fact, in this case we have

$$i(a,t) = \begin{cases} \dfrac{i_0(a-t)e^{\int_0^t \alpha(a-t+\sigma)d\sigma}}{1+i_0(a-t)\int_0^t e^{\int_0^\tau \alpha(a-t+\sigma)d\sigma}\kappa(a-t+\tau)d\tau} & \text{if } a > t, \\[2em] 0 & \text{if } a < t. \end{cases} \quad (5.29)$$

So the evolution of the disease is explicitly obtained. From (5.29) we can also deduce that, along the characteristic line $a - t = a_0$, we have $i(a_0 + t, t) \to 0$ as $t \to \infty$. That is, the infective cohort which has age $a_0$ at time $t = 0$

eventually vanishes. Thus, when there is no vertical transmission of the disease, the epidemic dies off due to the aging process. For the case $q > 0$ we let $u(t)$ be the infectives' birth rate:

$$u(t) = i(0, t). \tag{5.30}$$

In fact, letting

$$E(a) = e^{\int_0^\infty \alpha(\sigma)d\sigma}$$

and substituting (5.28) into (5.26b) we get an integral equation of the form

$$u(t) = F(t) + \int_0^t G(a, u(t-a))da, \tag{5.31}$$

where

$$F(t) = \int_t^\infty \frac{q\beta(a)E(a)i_0(a-t)da}{E(a-t) + i_0(a-t)\int_{a-t}^a E(\tau)\kappa(\tau)d\tau}, \quad t \geq 0, \tag{5.32}$$

$$G(a, z) = \frac{q\beta(a)E(a)z}{1 + z\int_0^a E(\tau)\kappa(\tau)d\tau}, \quad a \geq 0, \quad z \geq 0. \tag{5.33}$$

Note that, because of the assumptions $(H_1)$-$(H_4)$, we have

$$F(t) = 0 \quad \text{for} \quad t \geq A, \tag{5.34}$$

$$G(a, z) > 0 \quad \text{for} \quad a \in (A_0, A); \quad G(a, z) = 0 \quad \text{for} \quad a \notin (A_0, A). \tag{5.35}$$

Furthermore, setting:

$$G(a, z) = D(a, z)z, \tag{5.36}$$

we note that for $a \in (A_0, A)$ we have

$$z \to G(a, z) \quad \text{is an increasing function,} \tag{5.37}$$

$$z \to D(a, z) \quad \text{is a decreasing function.} \tag{5.38}$$

Equation (5.31) has a unique continuous non-negative solution whose behavior we are going to investigate. Because of the relations (5.34) and (5.35), (5.31) has the following limiting form:

$$v(t) = \int_0^A G(a, v(t-a))da, \quad t \in (-\infty, +\infty). \tag{5.39}$$

The asymptotic behavior of (5.31) is related to the constant solutions $v(t) = V$ of (5.39) which must satisfy

$$V = V \int_0^A D(a, V)da. \tag{5.40}$$

So $V = 0$, or

$$1 = \int_0^A D(a, V)da. \tag{5.41}$$

Now, the function $\Delta(V) = \int_0^A D(a, V)da$ is decreasing with limit zero as $V \to \infty$; thus (5.41) has one and only one solution $V_\infty$, if and only if, the threshold condition:

$$R_0 = \int_0^A D(a, 0) > 1, \tag{5.42}$$

is satisfied. We summarize:

**Proposition.** *Let the net infection reproduction number $R_0$ be defined in (5.27). Then, if $R_0 \leq 1$, (5.40) has only the trivial constant solution $V \equiv 0$. If $R_0 > 1$ then it has also a nontrivial solution $V_\infty > 0$ which is determined by (5.41).*

The proof of the first part of Theorem 5.4 is now obtained by defining

$$M_n = \max\{u(t) : t \in [nA, (n+1)A]\}$$

It can then be shown that

$$M_n < M_{n-1}. \tag{5.44}$$

Thus $M_n$ is decreasing and it can be shown that the limit is zero.

The proof of the second part of this result relies on the same method as above but is a little more complicated. Here, together with $M_n$, we have to consider the behavior of $m_n = \min\{u(t) : t \in [nA, (n+1)A]\}$. We refer the reader to Busenberg, Cooke and Iannelli [1988] for the details.

We emphasize that this is a global result in the sense that if $R_0 > 1$ then for all parameter values and initial functions $i_0(a)$, the birth function $u(t) = i(0, t)$ tends to $V_\infty$. Once this is known, (5.28) gives the asymptotic behavior of $i(a, t)$.

We now turn to a related model which has been recently studied, and where an explicit endemic threshold has been derived. Langlais [1991] has treated the intracohort model in a more general setting where the death and birth rates depend on the total size of the population and represent logistic controls on its demography. In particular, he considers the $s \to i \to s$ model

$$\frac{\partial s}{\partial t} + \frac{\partial s}{\partial a} + [\mu(a) + \mu_e(P(t))]s = -\kappa(a)is + \gamma i,$$

$$\frac{\partial i}{\partial t} + \frac{\partial i}{\partial a} + [\mu(a) + \mu_e(P(t))]i = \kappa(a)is - \gamma i, \tag{5.45}$$

$$i(0, t) = q\beta_e(P(t)) \int_0^\infty \beta(a)i(a, t)da,$$

$$s(0, t) = \beta_e(P(t)) \int_0^\infty \beta(a)[s(a, t) + (1-q)i(a, t)]da,$$

$$i(a, 0) = i_0(a), \quad s(a, 0) = s_0(a), \quad P(t) = \int_0^\infty [i(a, t) + s(a, t)]da.$$

The logistic control birth and death terms are assumed to be monotone nonincreasing and nondecreasing functions, respectively, and to obey

$$\beta_e(0) = 1, \quad \mu_e(0) = 0, \quad 0 \leq \beta_e(P) \to 0, \quad 0 \leq \mu_e(P) \to \infty, \quad \text{as } P \to \infty.$$

The other parameters in the model are assumed to be non-negative and bounded. The vertical transmission probability $q$ obeys $0 \leq q \leq 1$, and $\gamma$ is assumed to be constant.

It immediately follows that the total population, $p = i + s$, satisfies the nonlinear problem

$$
\begin{aligned}
&\frac{\partial p}{\partial t} + \frac{\partial p}{\partial a} + [\mu(a) + \mu_e(P(t))]p = 0, \\
&p(0, t) = \beta_e(P(t)) \int_0^\infty \beta(a) p(a, t) da, \\
&p(a, 0) = p_0(a) = i_0(a) + s_0(a), \\
&P(t) = \int_0^\infty p(a, t) da.
\end{aligned}
\tag{5.46}
$$

It is shown that the total population $p(a, t)$ tends to a nonzero equilibrium whenever the net reproduction number $R$ defined in (5.6) is larger than one. This limiting solution takes the form (compare with (5.7))

$$p_\infty(a) = b_0 e^{-\mu_e(P_\infty)a} \Pi(a), \tag{5.47}$$

where $P_\infty = \int_0^\infty p_\infty(a) da$, $b_0$ is a constant which depends on the initial data, and as before

$$\Pi(a) = e^{-\int_0^a \mu(\sigma) d\sigma}.$$

Langlais [1991] has established the following threshold and stability result for this model.

**Theorem 5.5** *Let*

$$R_0 = q \int_0^\infty \beta_e(P_\infty) \beta(a) \Pi(a) e^{-\mu_e(P_\infty)a} e^{\int_0^\infty \kappa(\sigma) p_\infty(\sigma) d\sigma - \gamma a} da. \tag{5.48}$$

*Then there is a unique nontrivial endemic equilibrium to the system (5.45) if and only if $R_0 > 1$. Moreover, if $R_0 \leq 1$ then $i(a, t) \to 0$ uniformly on any finite age interval $[0, A]$, and if $R_0 > 1$ any solution $i(a, t)$ with $i_0(a) > 0$ converges to the unique nontrivial endemic equilibrium as $t \to \infty$.*

The proof of this result uses a variety of analytical tools including the general stabilization results for nonlinear age-structured problems due to Busenberg and Iannelli [1983, a,b] and Langlais [1985], and new developments in dynamical systems as applied to nonlinear hyperbolic problems. We shall not present the details of the proof which can be found in Langlais [1991] but turn to the discussion of the threshold criteria.

The demographic threshold $R$ given by (5.6) is identical in form to that for the linear McKendrick-von Foerster model because, as the population level $P$ approaches zero, the nonlinear model tends to the linear one due to the hypotheses $\mu_e(0) = 0$ and $\beta_e(0) = 1$. The condition $R > 1$ leads to a bounded population because of the logistic control, whereas in the linear problem this condition leads to an exponentially increasing population. In epidemiological applications of the above result, one needs to verify that the demographic time scale is short enough that the population can attain its equilibrium level during the course of the epidemic. This may be more often the case for diseases that affect animal populations, and probably is only rarely the case for human diseases.

The endemic threshold $R_0$ in (5.48) is analogous to the corresponding threshold given in (5.27), but it is modified by the two logistic control terms $\beta_e(P_\infty)$ and $\mu_e(P_\infty)$ evaluated at the equilibrium total population level. We note that, in both situations, $R_0$ grows linearly with the vertical transmission probability $q$ and exponentially with the horizontal transmission rate $\kappa(a)$. It decreases exponentially with the cure rate $\gamma$. The exponential dependence of this threshold on the horizontal transmission rate is a characteristic of the intracohort mode of transmission and, as we shall see later, may not occur in other age-dependent horizontal transmission mechanisms.

## 5.7 Analysis of the Intercohort $s \to i \to s$ Model

In this section we start by sketching the analysis of the $s \to i \to s$ model with the force of infection term taking the form $\kappa(a)I(t)$ and with the assumption that $R = 1$, and that the total population is at its equilibrium distribution. The main results here yield an explicit form for the endemic threshold $R_0$, establish local stability or instability of equilibria, and show that under certain conditions no periodic solutions can arise from a Hopf bifurcation from an endemic steady state. Our analysis is based on the reduction of the problem to an integral equation whose derivation is described below. The local stability results of this section are special cases of the global results that are given for a more general model in Section 5.10. These results have been used by Iannelli, Milner and Pugliese [1992] to derive explicit threshold criteria for a model with vertical transmission that combines both intercohort and intracohort horizontal transmission. These are presented in Section 5.11. However, the simpler analysis that leads to the explicit form of the threshold that we derive here, gives the present approach, introduced by Busenberg, Cooke and Iannelli [1988], independent value. We conclude this section with a description of the results of Langlais [1991] for a similar model with $R > 1$ that includes vertical transmission and has a logistic control in the birth and death terms. An explicit threshold is again derived under some simplifying hypotheses on the model parameters.

The basic assumptions in this case are that $\lambda(a,t) = \kappa(a)I(t)$, $\delta = 0$, $R = 1$ and $p(a,t) = p_\infty(a)$, where $p_\infty$ is given in (5.7). Setting $s(a,t) = p_\infty(a) - i(a,t)$ in the second equation of (5.4) we obtain the following problem:

$$\frac{\partial i}{\partial t} + \frac{\partial i}{\partial a} + \mu(a)i = \kappa(a)[p_\infty(a) - i(a,t)]I(t) - \gamma(a)i(a,t),$$

$$i(0,t) = q \int_0^\infty \beta(a)i(a,t)da, \tag{5.49}$$

$$i(a,0) = i_0(a).$$

The parameters in this problem satisfy the conditions imposed in the previous section, and in particular, conditions $(H_1) - (H_4)$. Note that if there were no vertical transmission the renewal condition would become $i(0,t) = 0$ which is obtained by setting $q = 0$. Now, setting $u(a,t) = i(a,t)/p_\infty(a)$, we obtain the following problem for $u$.

$$\frac{\partial u}{\partial t} + \frac{\partial u}{\partial a} = \kappa(a)I(t)[1 - u(a,t)] - \gamma(a)u(a,t),$$

$$u(0,t) = \frac{q}{b_0} \int_0^\infty \beta(a)p_\infty(a)u(a,t)da, \tag{5.50}$$

$$u_0(a) = \frac{i_0(a)}{p_\infty(a)}.$$

Note that $0 \le u_0(a) \le 1$ and that (5.50) then implies that $0 \le u(a,t) \le 1$ for all $t \ge 0$.

Assuming that

$$I(t) = \int_0^\infty i(a,t)da = \int_0^\infty p_\infty(a)u(a,t)da$$

has settled to a steady state which we denote by $I$, the stationary form of the system (5.50) can be integrated to yield the expression

$$u(a) = u(0)e^{-\int_0^a [\gamma(\sigma) + \kappa(\sigma)I]d\sigma} + \int_0^a \kappa(\tau)Ie^{-\int_\tau^a [\gamma(\sigma) + \kappa(\sigma)I]d\sigma} d\tau, \tag{5.51}$$

which upon using the second equation in (5.50) implies

$$u(0) = qI \frac{\int_0^\infty \beta(a)p_\infty(a) \int_0^a \kappa(\tau)e^{-\int_\tau^a [\gamma(\sigma)+\kappa(\sigma)I]d\sigma} dad\tau}{b_0 - q \int_0^\infty \beta(a)p_\infty(a)e^{-\int_0^a [\gamma(\sigma)+\kappa(\sigma)I]d\sigma} da} = qIC(q,I), \tag{5.52}$$

with $C(q,I)$ defined to be the fraction in the above equation.

We can now present the basic threshold result for this situation which is due to Iannelli, Milner, Pugliese and Tubaro [1989].

**Theorem 5.6** *Suppose that for the $s \to i \to s$ model described by the system (5.49), $\gamma$ does not vanish identically when $q = 1$, and define the threshold*

$$R_0 = q\frac{\int_0^\infty \beta(a)p_\infty(a) \int_0^a \kappa(\tau)e^{-\int_\tau^a \gamma(\sigma)d\sigma} d\tau da}{b_0 - q \int_0^\infty \beta(a)p_\infty(a)e^{-\int_0^a \gamma(\sigma)d\sigma} da} \left[\int_0^\infty p_\infty(a)e^{-\int_0^a \gamma(\sigma)d\sigma} da\right]$$

$$+ \int_0^\infty p_\infty(a) \int_0^a \kappa(\tau)e^{-\int_\tau^a \gamma(\sigma)d\sigma} d\tau da. \tag{5.53}$$

*Then, if $R_0 \leq 1$ there exists only the trivial equilibrium $i(a) \equiv 0$, and all solutions of the system tend to zero as t tends to $\infty$. If $R_0 > 1$, then there exists a unique endemic nonzero steady state $i^*(a)$ and all initial data $i_0(a)$ which satisfy for some $t \geq 0$*

$$\int_t^\infty \beta(a) i_0(a - t) da > 0$$

*lead to solutions $i(a, t)$ which tend to the endemic equilibrium.*

*If $q = 1$ and $\gamma \equiv 0$, the unique endemic equilibrium is given by $i(a) = p_\infty(a)$.*

*Proof.* We only give an outline of the proof of the threshold criterion since the results on the global convergence of solutions are discussed in Section 5.9. First, note that the denominator in the expression for $C(q, I)$ in (5.52) does not vanish, hence, the threshold $R_0$ is well defined. Now, substituting the expression of $u(0)$ in (5.52) into (5.51) we obtain

$$u(a) = I \left[ qC(q, I) e^{-\int_0^a [\gamma(\sigma) + \kappa(\sigma) I] d\sigma} + \int_0^a \kappa(\tau) e^{-\int_\tau^a [\gamma(\sigma) + \kappa(\sigma) I] d\sigma} d\tau \right],$$

which when multiplied by $p_\infty(a)$ and integrated from 0 to $\infty$ yields

$$1 = F(q, I) = qC(q, I) \int_0^\infty p_\infty(a) e^{-\int_0^a [\gamma(\sigma) + \kappa(\sigma) I] d\sigma} da$$
$$+ \int_0^\infty p_\infty(a) \int_0^a \kappa(\tau) e^{-\int_\tau^a [\gamma(\sigma) d\sigma + \kappa(\sigma) I] d\sigma} d\tau da. \tag{5.54}$$

The dependence of $F(q, I)$ on $I$ can now be used to show that a nontrivial solution $I^*$ to (5.54) exists if and only if $R_0 > 1$. This is done by noting that

$$F(q, I) \leq \frac{P}{I} + \left[ qC(q, I) - \frac{1}{I} \right] \int_0^\infty p_\infty(a) e^{-\int_0^a \kappa(\sigma) I d\sigma} da < PqC(q, I),$$

and from (5.52) $C(q, I) > 1/(qI)$, which implies $F(q, I) < P/I$, hence $F(q, P) < 1$. Noting that $F(q, I)$ is a decreasing function of $I$ whenever $q > 0$, $I > 0$ and $q < 1$, and recalling that $R_0 = F(q, 0)$, we obtain the threshold criterion. The part of the theorem which assumes that $\gamma$ does not vanish identically when $q = 1$ follows from (5.54). When $\gamma \equiv 0$ and $q = 1$, the system (5.50) has the solution $u(a) \equiv 1$, thus $i(a) = p_\infty(a)$ is the endemic steady state solution.

Langlais [1991] considers a special case of the intercohort $s \to i \to s$ model with a logistic control and with the demographic threshold $R > 1$. He assumes that the fertility, mortality and recovery rates take the forms

$$\mu(a, t) = \bar{\mu} + \mu_e(P(t)), \quad \beta(a, t) = \bar{\beta} + \beta_e(P(t)), \quad \gamma(a) = \bar{\gamma}, \tag{5.55}$$

and that the force of infection term is $\bar{\kappa} I(t)$, where all parameters with a bar are taken to be constants. The model equations become

$$\frac{\partial i}{\partial t} + \frac{\partial i}{\partial a} + [\bar{\mu} + \mu_e(P(t))]i = \bar{\kappa}I(p - i) - \bar{\gamma}i, \qquad (5.56)$$

$$i(0, t) = q\bar{\beta}\beta_e(P(t))I(t),$$

$$i(a, 0) = i_0(a), \quad P(t) = \int_0^\infty [i(a, t) + s(a, t)]da, \quad I(t) = \int_0^\infty i(a, t)da.$$

Letting $P_\infty$ be the positive root of the equation

$$\bar{\beta}\beta_e(P_\infty) - \bar{\mu} - \mu_e(P_\infty) = 0, \qquad (5.57)$$

and

$$R_0 = \frac{q\bar{\beta}\beta_e(P_\infty) + \bar{\kappa}P_\infty}{\bar{\mu} + \mu_e(P_\infty) + \bar{\gamma}}, \qquad (5.58)$$

we have the threshold condition: If $R_0 \leq 1$ then $I(t) \to 0$ as $t \to \infty$, while if $R_0 > 1$ there exists a positive endemic level $I_\infty > 0$, and $I(t) \to I_\infty$ as $t \to \infty$. The threshold $R_0$, in this case, can be interpreted as the ratio of the rate at which new infectives are being added due to vertical and horizontal transmission and the rate at which they are removed due to death and recovery. It is interesting to note the difference in complexity in the thresholds given by (5.53) and (5.58). The simplicity of the latter form is due to the fact that the hypotheses (5.55) remove the age specific dependence of a number of the demographic and epidemiological parameters. We shall return to the discussion of such thresholds in Section 5.11.

## 5.8 Numerical Simulations

Here we present some numerical results from Busenberg, Cooke and Iannelli [1989] which illustrate the dynamic behavior of the $s \to i \to s$ model with the intracohort, the intercohort and a more general form of the force of infection. For all cases we take the maximal age $A = 60$ with $\mu(a) = 1/|60 - a|$ and $\beta(a) = 84.66 \sin(\pi a/100)$. All figures show the graphs of $I(t) = \int_0^\infty i(a, t)da$ and $S(t) = \int_0^\infty s(a, t)da$ as $P(t)$ settles to its limiting value.

For the intracohort case we chose $\lambda(a, t) = 1000i(a, t)$, and $\gamma = 0.001$. In Fig. 5.6 we use $q = 0$ (no vertical transmission) and, consequently, $R_0 = 0$, and the graph illustrates the extinction of the infective population that is predicted by the analysis. In Fig. 5.7 we show the same situation, however with $q = 0.6$, and the effect of vertical transmission in raising the level of the total infected population $I(t)$ is clearly seen.

Figures 5.8, 5.9 and 5.10 illustrate the behavior of the intercohort model for which we have discussed some partial stability results. We have taken $\lambda(a, t) = k \exp(-2a^2)I(t)$, $\gamma = 0.01$, and with $k = 1,000$ for Fig. 5.8 and 5.9, and $k = 2,300$ for Fig. 5.10. The graphs show the difference in the effects of changes in both the vertical transmission probability and the force of horizontal transmission. Note that there are no persistent oscillations in these graphs.

As we shall see in the next section, such oscillations can be ruled out in this type of model.

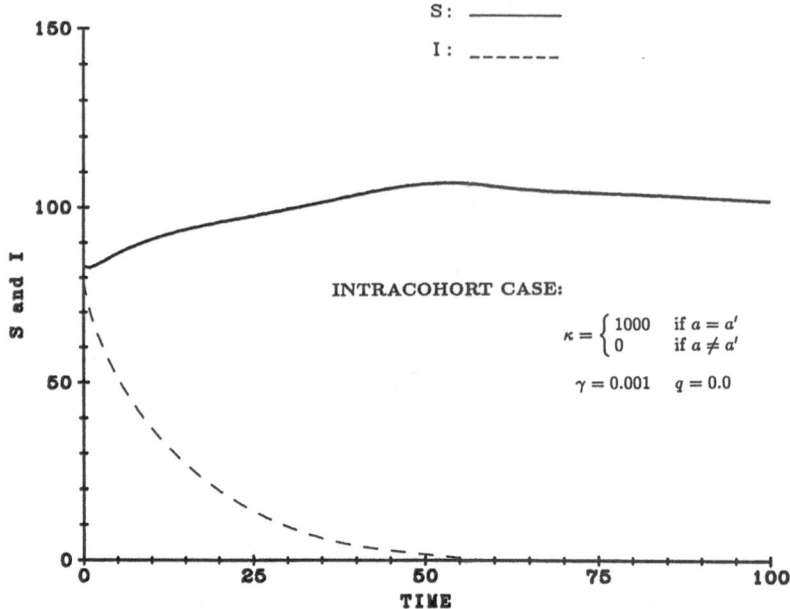

**Fig. 5.6.** Behavior of the intracohort model with no vertical transmission

In Figs. 5.11 and 5.12 we use a general form of the force of horizontal infection and take

$$\kappa(a, a') = \begin{cases} 0, & \text{if } a < \omega/4, \\ ke^{-2(a-a')^2}, & \text{if } \omega/4 < a < 3\omega/4, \\ 0, & \text{if } a > 3\omega/4, \end{cases}$$

with $k = 2000$ and $q = 0.8$ in Fig. 5.11 while $k = 9000$ and $q = 0$ in Fig. 5.12 and $\gamma = 0.01$ in both figures.

In both of these graphs the maximum age of the population is assumed to be $\omega = 60$. The relative influences of changes in the horizontal and vertical transmission coefficients are seen as well as the lack of persistent oscillations. As we shall see in Section 5.9, persistent oscillations in the subpopulation levels can be ruled out in this model. However, the damped oscillations that are observed in certain parameter ranges could have epidemiological significance if influences external to the model as it now stands tend to periodically reset the initial conditions before the oscillations have damped out. Sources of such influences would include migration of infective individuals and possibly seasonal variations in the contact rate, the recovery rate, and the demographic parameters.

These numerical simulations were obtained using a program developed by Busenberg and Tsai based on an extension of a method of discretizing the lin-

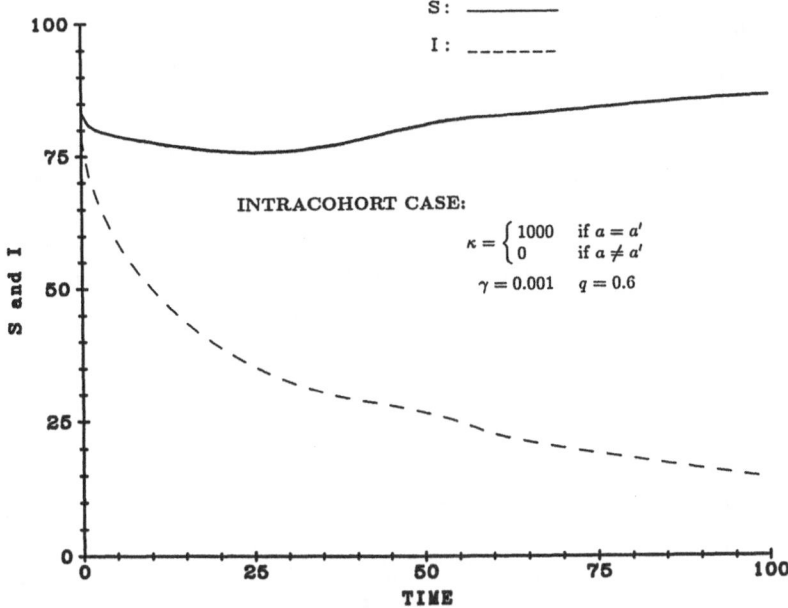

**Fig. 5.7.** Behavior of the intracohort model with vertical transmission

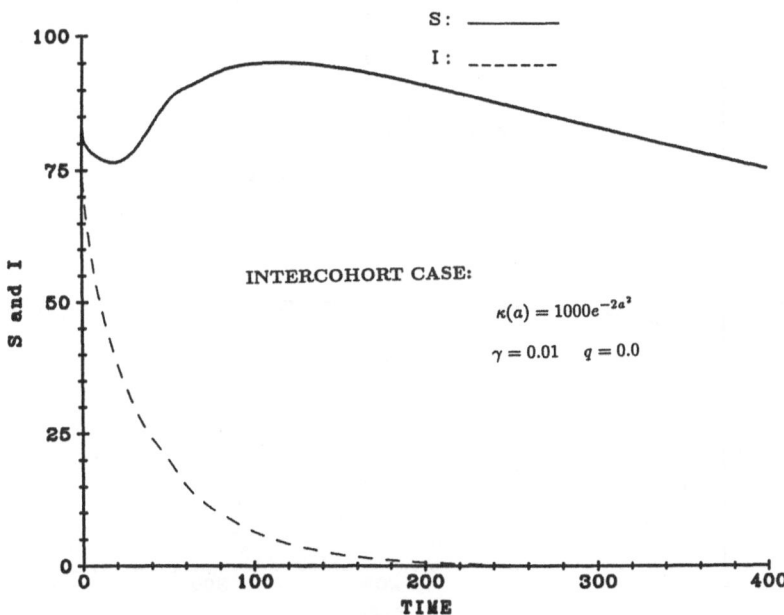

**Fig. 5.8.** Behavior of the intercohort model

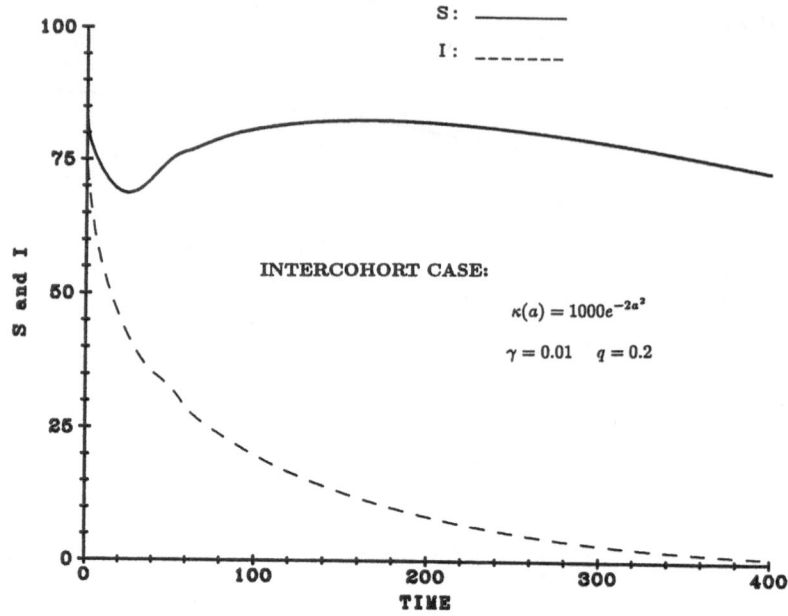

**Fig. 5.9.** Behavior of the intercohort model

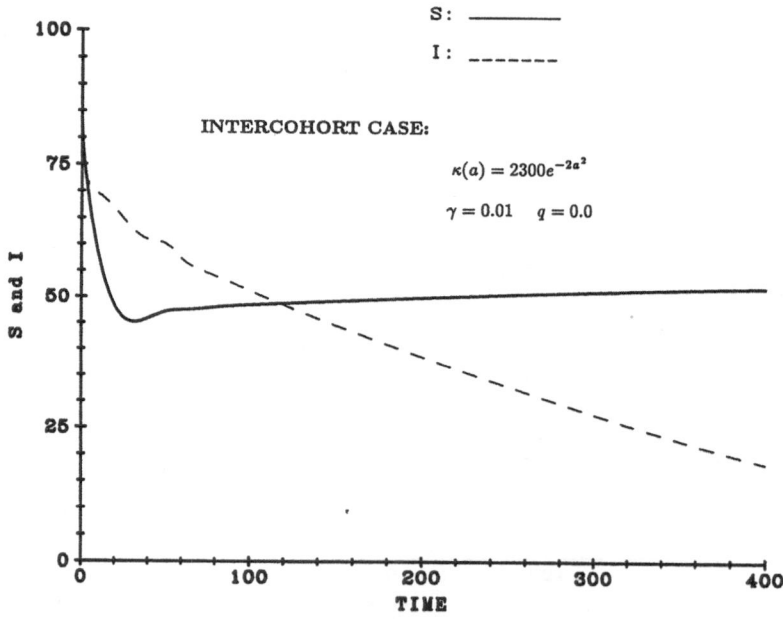

**Fig. 5.10.** Behavior of the intercohort model

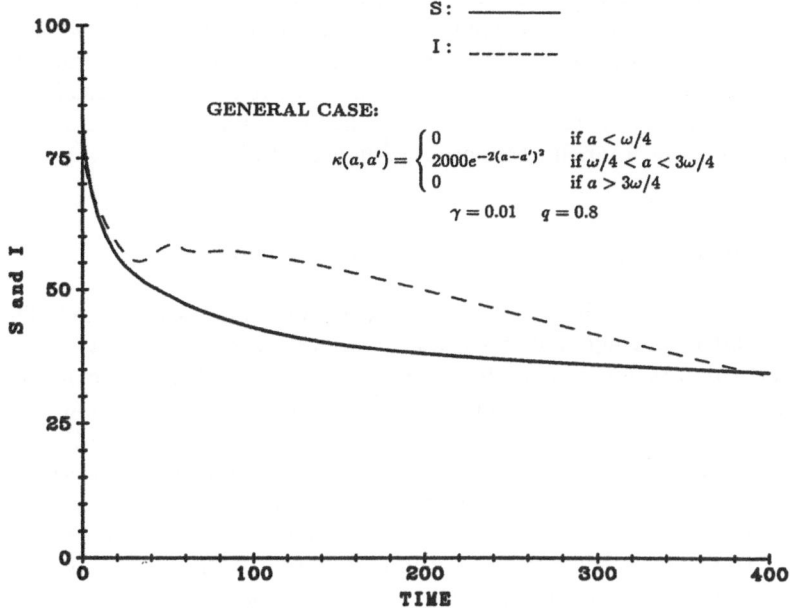

**Fig. 5.11.** General force of infection term

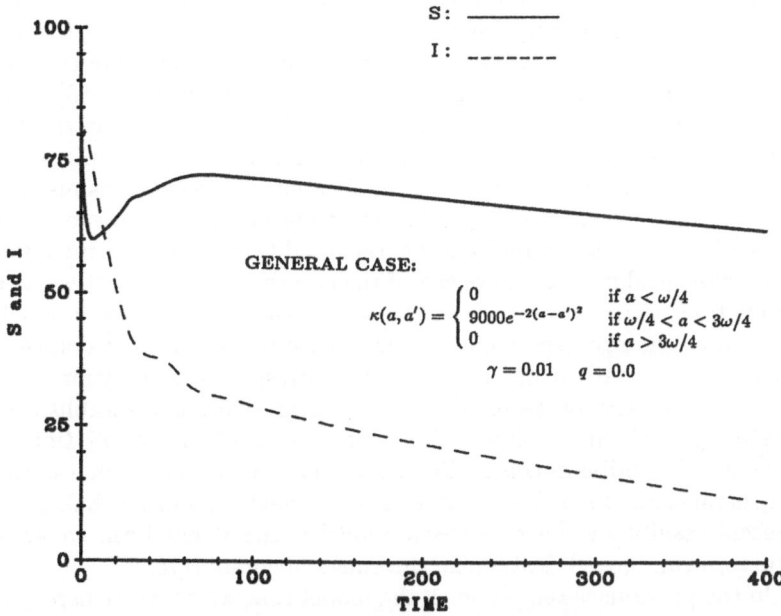

**Fig. 5.12.** General force of infection term

ear McKendrick equations whose convergence and stability is proved in Saints [1987]. Saints also points out some of the difficulties that occur when naive discretizations of these equations are used for either numerical simulation or for generating simpler discrete time Leslie models. Reliable numerical schemes for the integration of such equations have also been developed by Douglas and Milner [1987], and Iannelli, Milner and Pugliese [1992].

## 5.9 Global Behavior of the $s \to i \to s$ Model

In this section we describe the recent results of Busenberg, Iannelli and Thieme [1991a, 1991b] showing that, for the general age-structured $s \to i \to s$ model with vertical transmission of the disease, periodic oscillations do not occur. In fact, a sharp endemic threshold exists and the complete global dynamical behavior for such a model is obtained when the age distribution of the total population has reached equilibrium. The results in this section, in a broad sense, include as special cases those described in Sections 5.6–5.8. However, because of the generality of the criteria that are obtained here, it is not possible to derive explicit forms of the threshold in terms of the parameters entering into the model. Rather, the threshold in this general setting is described in terms of the leading eigenvalue of a specific operator, and can only be computed numerically.

For a number of diseases, the incidence rates of infectives undergo periodic oscillations, and there are several dynamical mechanisms that could be the causes of this oscillatory behavior. For example, there is a pronounced biennial oscillation in the occurrence of measles that is reported in the data of several large cities, see Hethcote, Stech and van den Driessche [1983], London and Yorke [1973], Schenzle [1984]. These have been variously attributed to the incubation delays, to the age-structured seasonal interaction rates that are due to school attendance, and to complicated nonlinear transmission dynamics. The simplest epidemiological interactions occur for diseases which do not impart immunity and which can be described by models that include only two epidemiological classes composed of the susceptible and infective parts of the population, that is, they are of the $s \to i \to s$ type. Since it has been suggested that the age dependence of the transmission rate of a disease may cause oscillations that do not occur in the corresponding situation without age structure, a basic problem in this area is to rigorously establish either the possibility or the impossibility of the occurrence of such oscillations. The results that we describe in this section show that oscillations cannot occur for a very general class of $s \to i \to s$ models. In the next section we shall examine some recent results for the $s \to i \to r$ model where it has been shown that age structure can indeed destabilize the endemic equilibrium.

As in the previous three sections, the model that we consider here divides the affected population into two epidemiologically distinct classes, composed of the susceptible and the infective individuals. The force of infection term that is considered here is as follows. Let $K(a, a')$ denote the rate at which an infective individual of age $a'$ comes into a disease transmitting contact with a susceptible individual of age $a$; let also $K_0(a)$ be the infection rate for pure intracohort interaction. Then the rate at which susceptible individuals of age $a$ are moved over into the infective class is given by

$$s(a,t)\lambda(a,t) = s(a,t)\left[K_0(a)i(a,t) + \int_0^\infty K(a,a')i(a',t)da'\right].$$

Denoting, as before, the age specific mortality, birth rate and cure rate by $\mu(a)$, $\beta(a)$, and $\gamma(a)$, respectively, we obtain the following system of equations that describe the dynamics of this model:

$$\frac{\partial s(a,t)}{\partial t} + \frac{\partial s(a,t)}{\partial a} + \mu(a)s(a,t) = -s(a,t)\lambda(a;t) + \gamma(a)i(a,t),$$

$$\text{(5.59)}$$

$$\frac{\partial i(a,t)}{\partial t} + \frac{\partial i(a,t)}{\partial a} + \mu(a)i(a,t) = s(a,t)\lambda(a,t) - \gamma(a)i(a,t),$$

with initial and boundary conditions

$$s(0,t) = \int_0^\infty \beta(a)[s(a,t) + (1-q)i(a,t)]da,$$

$$i(0,t) = q\int_0^\infty \beta(a)i(a,t)da,$$

$$\text{(5.60)}$$

$$s(a,0) = s_0(a),$$

$$i(a,0) = i_0(a).$$

As usual, $q$ is the probability of vertical transmission of the disease, that is, the probability that an infective parent give birth to an offspring who is also infective; thus $0 < q \leq 1$. We note that in our assumptions the disease does not affect the natural mortality and fertility rates.

We shall be dealing with these equations under the hypothesis that the total population, $p(a,t) = s(a,t) + i(a,t)$, has reached a steady state distribution $p_\infty(a)$. From the classical theory of the linear McKendrick-Von Foerster equation which $p(a,t)$ satisfies, this occurs when the demographic reproduction number, $R$, of the total population is equal to one. That is,

$$R = \int_0^\infty \beta(a)\exp(-\int_0^a \mu(a')da')da = 1. \qquad \text{(5.61)}$$

It is worth noting that, if all the basic parameters in the model, $\beta$, $\mu$, $\gamma$, and $K$ do not depend on age, then since the term $K_0(a)i(a,t)$ represents a force of infection that is concentrated in one age group, the assumption that there be no age dependence requires that $K_0 = 0$. The corresponding equations for the total populations $S(t)$ and $I(t)$ can be obtained by integrating (5.59) from $a = 0$ to $\infty$, and using the conditions (5.60), and $s(\infty,t) = i(\infty,t) = 0$. These last conditions simply mean that no individual in the population can survive to infinite age. The resulting equations are

$$\frac{dS(t)}{dt} = (\beta - \mu)S(t) + [\gamma + (1-q)\beta]I(t) - KS(t)I(t),$$
$$\frac{dI(t)}{dt} = (q\beta - \mu - \gamma)I(t) + KS(t)I(t). \tag{5.62}$$

This is the standard $S \rightarrow I \rightarrow S$ epidemic model with vital dynamics and vertical transmission which we discussed in Chapter 2, and which we showed cannot exhibit time periodic behavior. The main result of this section is to show that the introduction of age-dependent contact rates does not produce a model which has periodic solutions, regardless of the choice of the age-dependent parameters entering in equations (5.59)-(5.60), and to derive a sharp endemic threshold condition.

This is done by transforming the problem (5.59)-(5.60) to one that involves only a single dependent variable $u(a,t) = i(a,t)/p_\infty(a)$. This problem can be viewed as a dynamical system for which one has existence of an appropriate unique solution, under mild restrictions on the parameters appearing in the equations. Exploiting the monotonicity and convexity properties of this formulation of the problem it can be shown that all solutions stabilize to steady states, regardless of their initial data.

The conditions we impose on the contact rate $K(a,a')$ include all epidemiologically significant cases. Thus, for the general $s \rightarrow i \rightarrow s$ age-structured model with vertical transmission and $R = 1$, the global behavior of solutions is settled, and oscillatory solutions do not occur.

Here we shall only outline the analysis of this model that is given in Busenberg, Iannelli and Thieme [1991b] and will concentrate on discussing the main results and their epidemiological implications. Let us first state the assumptions on the demographic parameters $\beta(a)$ and $\mu(a)$; namely, we assume that there is a maximum age $a_\dagger$ for the population so that we can restrict ourselves to the age interval $[0, a_\dagger]$ , and :

$$\beta(a) \quad \text{is non-negative and belongs to} \quad L^\infty(0, a_\dagger), \tag{5.63}$$

$$\mu(a) \quad \text{is non-negative and measurable,} \tag{5.64}$$

$$R = \int_0^{a_\dagger} \beta(a) e^{-\int_0^a \mu(a')da'} da = 1. \tag{5.65}$$

This last parameter $R$ is the demographic reproduction number of the population and represents the mean number of newborns from an individual, during her whole life-span. Thus, by (5.65) we are assuming that the demographic parameters are such that a steady asymptotic state exists:

$$p_\infty(a) = b_0 e^{-\int_0^a \mu(\sigma)d\sigma}, \tag{5.66}$$

where

$$b_0 = \int_0^{a_\dagger} \beta(a)p_\infty(a)da. \tag{5.67}$$

Now, we assume that the total population $p(a, t) = s(a, t) + i(a, t)$, is at the steady state distribution (5.66), thus we have:

$$s(a, t) = p_\infty(a) - i(a, t), \tag{5.68}$$

and the system can be reduced to a single equation for $i(a, t)$. In fact, fitting (5.68) into the second equation in (5.59) we have:

$$\frac{\partial i(a, t)}{\partial t} + \frac{\partial i(a, t)}{\partial a} + \mu(a)i(a, t) = \lambda[a \mid i(., t)][p_\infty(a) - i(a, t)] - \gamma(a)i(a, t),$$

$$\lambda[a \mid i(., t)] = K_0(a)i(a, t) + \int_0^{a_\dagger} K(a, a')i(a', t)da',$$

$$i(0, t) = q \int_0^{a_\dagger} \beta(a)i(a, t)da,$$

$$i(a, 0) = i_0(a).$$

Further we perform the change of variables $u(a, t) = \dfrac{i(a, t)}{p_\infty(a)}$,    so that:

$$\frac{\partial u(a, t)}{\partial t} + \frac{\partial u(a, t)}{\partial a} = \lambda[a \mid u(., t)][1 - u(a, t)] - \gamma(a)u(a, t),$$

$$\lambda[a \mid u(., t)] = K_0(a)p_\infty(a)u(a, t) + \int_0^{a_\dagger} K(a, a')p_\infty(a')u(a', t)da',$$

$$u(0, t) = \frac{q}{b_0} \int_0^{a_\dagger} \beta(a)p_\infty(a)u(a, t)da, \tag{5.69}$$

$$u(a, 0) = \frac{i_0(a)}{p_\infty(a)} = u_0(a).$$

This is the problem that we are going to consider in the following.

Let us now state the assumptions on $\gamma(a)$ and on the contact rates $K_0(a)$ and $K(a, a')$. We assume that:

$$\gamma(a), \ K_0(a) \text{ are non-negative and belong to } L^\infty(0, a_\dagger), \tag{5.70}$$

moreover, $K(a, a')$ is measurable and there exist a positive constant $\epsilon$ and non-negative functions $K_1(a)$, $K_2(a)$ such that :

$$\epsilon \, K_1(a)K_2(a') \ \leq \ K(a, a')p_\infty(a') \ \leq \ K_1(a)K_2(a'), \tag{5.71}$$
$$K_1 \in L^\infty(0, a_\dagger) \, , \ K_2 \in L^1(0, a_\dagger).$$

There are $\ 0 \ \leq \ a_1, \ a_2, \ b_1, \ b_2 \ \leq \ a_\dagger \ $ such that :

$$a_1 \ < \ b_1, \quad a_2 \ < \ b_2, \quad a_1 \ < \ b_2, \tag{5.72}$$

$$K_1(a) > 0 \quad \text{if} \quad a_1 < a < b_1,$$
$$K_2(a) > 0 \quad \text{if} \quad a_2 < a < b_2. \tag{5.73}$$

Also recall that the vertical transmission probability $q$ satisfies $0 < q \le 1$.

The conditions (5.71)-(5.73) do not place any essential restrictions on $K(a, a')$ that go beyond what would be dictated by the biological situation that is being modeled. However, from (5.71) it is seen that if $K(\tilde{a}, \tilde{a}') = 0$ for some fixed $(\tilde{a}, \tilde{a}') \in [0, a_\dagger] \times [0, a_\dagger]$, then either $K_1(\tilde{a}) = 0$, or $K_2(\tilde{a}') = 0$. Hence, we either have $K(\tilde{a}, a) = 0$, or $K(a, \tilde{a}') = 0$ for all $a \in [0, a_\dagger]$. That is, if the disease is never transmitted to any age $\tilde{a}$ individual from every age $\tilde{a}'$ individual, then either it cannot be transmitted from any age group $a \ne \tilde{a}$ to age $\tilde{a}$ individuals, or it cannot be transmitted from any age $\tilde{a}'$ individual to an age $a \ne \tilde{a}'$ individual for all $a \in [0, a_\dagger]$. Since we are dealing with densities which are defined almost everywhere, this represents a real restriction only when there exist two age-class intervals $I_1, I_2 \subset [0, a_\dagger]$, for which $K(a, a') = 0$ for all $(a, a') \subset I_1 \times I_2$. In the epidemiological situation that we are modeling, such complete immunity to disease transmission across two separate age classes is extremely unlikely. Hence, condition (5.71) includes the situations that are of interest from the viewpoint of the epidemiological model. In particular, asymmetric forms of $K$ with $K(a, a') \ne K(a', a)$ are included in our result, as well as cases where individuals from two separate age groups have only limited, but non-vanishing, disease transmitting interactions. Nevertheless, it would be interesting to explore the dynamic implications of any substantial weakening of condition (5.71).

In order to properly state the results in this general setting we need to identify the problem as an abstract differential equation (see, Pazy [1983] and Webb [1985], for an introduction to the mathematical background). To this purpose we consider the Banach space $E = L^1(0, a_\dagger)$ and define $A$ with domain $D_A$ by:

$$D_A = \{f \in E \text{ is absolutely continuous}; f' \in E; \text{ and}$$
$$f(0) = \frac{q}{b_0} \int_0^{a_\dagger} \beta(a) p_\infty(a) f(a) da\},$$
$$(Af)(a) = -f'(a).$$

We also define

$$F(f)(a) = \lambda[a \mid f(\cdot)][1 - f(a)] - \gamma(a) f(a), \tag{5.74}$$

where

$$\lambda[a \mid f(\cdot)] = K_0(a) p_\infty(a) f(a) + \int_0^{a_\dagger} K(a, a') p_\infty(a') f(a') da'.$$

Thus (5.69) can be expressed as the following abstract initial value problem in $E$:

$$\frac{du(t)}{dt} = Au(t) + F(u(t)),$$
(5.75)

$$u(0) = u_0.$$

Due to the meaning of $u(a, t)$, we look for a solution in the closed convex set:

$$C = \{ f \in L^1(0, a_\dagger) : \ 0 \le f(a) \le 1 \ \text{a.e.} \}$$

Now, it is shown in Busenberg, Iannelli and Thieme [1991a] that there exists $\alpha \in (0, 1)$ such that

$$(I - \alpha A)^{-1}(C) \subset C, \quad \text{and} \ (I + \alpha F)(C) \subset C,$$

where $I$ stands for the identity operator on the space. With this notation, it is easy to see that steady states must satisfy the equation

$$u = (I - \alpha A)^{-1}(I + \alpha F)u = Tu,$$

where

$$T = (I - \alpha A)^{-1}(I + \alpha F).$$

Clearly, the steady state equation always has the trivial solution $u = 0$ which represents the disease-free equilibrium. The existence and stability of a non-trivial equilibrium $u_\infty$ is related to the Fréchet derivative of $T$, which we denote by $DT[u]$, and depends on the spectral radius $R_0$ of $DT[0]$. Also, we define an initial state $u_0$ to be nontrivial if

$$\int_t^{a_\dagger} [\beta(a)p_\infty(a) + K_2(a)]u_0(a)(a - t)da > 0 \ \text{for some} \ t \ge 0.$$

With this notation in place, we can state the central result for this model. We first place the following restriction

$$\int_0^{a_\dagger} \left( \beta(a)p_\infty(a) \int_0^a K_1(a')da' \right) da > 0,$$
(5.76)

which prevents the situation where individuals are susceptible only after the end of their reproductive period. As we shall see later in this section, when condition (5.76) does not hold, the dynamics of the disease transmission become complicated.

**Theorem 5.7** *If $R_0 \le 1$, then the disease free equilibrium is the only steady state in $C$, and for all initial data $u_0 \in C$, the unique solution $u(t, a) \to 0$ as $t \to \infty$, where the convergence is in the $L^1$ sense. If $R_0 > 1$ and (5.76) holds, then there exists a unique nontrivial endemic steady-state $u_\infty(a)$, and for all non-trivial initial data $u_0$ the corresponding solution $u(t, a) \to u_\infty(a)$, as $t \to \infty$. If $u_0$ is a trivial initial datum, then $u(t, a) = 0$, for $t \ge a_\dagger$.*

Thus, when (5.76) holds, there is a sharp threshold which governs the existence and global stability of the endemic equilibrium. This threshold $R_0$ has been characterized only as the spectral radius of a specific linear operator and in this general situation it is not given explicitly in terms of the epidemiological parameters. In Sections 5.4–5.8 we took advantage of special forms of the horizontal transmission terms to derive explicit forms of this threshold.

We now turn to the case where (5.76) does not hold, and in particular, we assume throughout the rest of this section that

$$\int_0^{a_\dagger} \left( \beta(a)p_\infty(a) \int_0^a K_1(a')da' \right) da = 0. \qquad (5.77)$$

We shall see below that when (5.77) holds, it is possible for the disease to be maintained through horizontal transmission in the portion of the population which has passed the reproductive age.

Letting $a_0 = \inf\{a \mid \beta = 0 \text{ a.e. in } [a, a_\dagger]\}$, then we note that (5.77) implies

$$K_1(a) = 0 \qquad \text{a.e. in} \quad [0, a_0]. \qquad (5.78)$$

Thus the fertility window lies below the intercohort infectivity window and any nontrivial endemic state $u_\infty$ must satisfy the following problem for $a \in [0, a_0]$:

$$u_\infty'(a) = K_0(a)[1 - u_\infty(a)]p_\infty(a)u_\infty(a) - \gamma(a)u_\infty(a), \quad a \in [0, a_0],$$
$$u_\infty(0) = \frac{q}{b_0} \int_0^{a_0} \beta(a)p_\infty(a)u_\infty(a)da. \qquad (5.79)$$

Actually the existence of solutions to this latter problem implies the existence of endemic steady states. In fact, we have:

**Theorem 5.8** *Let (5.77) be verified. Then any solution of (5.79) can be extended to a stationary solution for $a \in [0, a_\dagger]$.*

*Proof.* The proof is immediate because, if $u_\infty(a)$ solves (5.79) then we only have to perform a second step of looking for existence of solutions to the following problem on $[a_0, a_\dagger]$:

$$v'(a) = \lambda[a \mid v(\cdot)][1 - v(a)] - \gamma(a)v(a), \quad a \in [a_0, a_\dagger],$$
$$v(a) = u_\infty(a), \quad a \in [0, a_0], \qquad (5.80)$$

and for this problem existence of a solution follows by a standard ordinary differential equation argument.

It is shown in Busenberg, Iannelli and Thieme [1991a] that there exists a threshold $\tilde{R}_0$, which is defined in the same manner as $R_0$ above, except that $q$ is taken to be zero, such that the following result holds.

**Theorem 5.9**    *Let (5.77) be satisfied and let $\tilde{R}_0$ be defined as above. Then, if $\tilde{R}_0 \leq 1$, there is no nontrivial endemic steady state vanishing on $[0, a_0]$. If $\tilde{R}_0 > 1$, then there exists one and only one nontrivial endemic steady state vanishing on $[0, a_0]$.*

Thus $\tilde{R}_0$ is the threshold which indicates when the horizontal transmission of the disease is sufficient to maintain an endemic state in the total absence of vertical transmission. Consequently, there is the possibility that the two mechanisms of horizontal and vertical transmission can each by itself maintain the disease at an endemic level. Since condition (5.77) excludes individuals in the age group $[0, a_0]$ from horizontally acquiring the disease, the endemic solution which occurred when $\tilde{R}_0 > 1$ does not affect the population in that age group. To complete our analysis, we must examine the conditions under which we have endemic solutions which do not vanish on $[0, a_0]$, that is, when there exist nontrivial solutions to (5.79). As we will see below, this is governed by a different threshold. Solving the first equation in (5.79) we have:

$$u_\infty(a) = \frac{E(a)u_\infty(0)}{1 + u_\infty(0) \int_0^a K_0(a')E(a')da'},$$

where

$$E(a) = \exp\left(\int_0^a [K_0(\sigma) - \gamma(\sigma)] \, d\sigma\right),$$

and $u_\infty(0)$ has to be determined by the second equation in (5.79). This leads to the following equation for $u_\infty(0)$ :

$$1 = \frac{q}{b_0} \int_0^{a_0} \frac{E(a)\beta(a)p_\infty(a)}{1 + u_\infty(0) \int_0^a K_0(a')E(a')da'} da. \tag{5.81}$$

Now, we replace $u_\infty(0)$ with a positive variable $z$, and note that the function

$$z \rightarrow \frac{q}{b_0} \int_0^{a_0} \frac{E(a)\beta(a)p_\infty(a)}{1 + z \int_0^a K_0(a')E(a')da'} da$$

is strictly decreasing, unless

$$K_0(a) = 0, \qquad \text{a.e. in} \quad [0, a_0], \tag{5.82}$$

in which case it is constant. As a consequence, we have that, unless (5.82) occurs, a nontrivial solution to (5.81) exists if and only if

$$R_1 = \frac{q}{b_0} \int_0^{a_0} E(a)\beta(a)p_\infty(a)da > 1.$$

If, instead, (5.82) is verified, then (5.81) has either no solution or it is satisfied by any $u_\infty(0)$. This latter case occurs if and only if

$$\frac{q}{b_0} \int_0^{a_0} e^{-\int_0^a \gamma(\sigma)d\sigma} \beta(a)p_\infty(a)da = 1, \tag{5.83}$$

that is, if and only if $q = 1$ and $\gamma = 0$ a.e. on the set $\{a : \beta(a) > 0\}$. We collect these observations in the following theorem.

**Theorem 5.10** *Let (5.77) be verified. If (5.82) does not occur, then (5.79) has a nontrivial solution if and only if $R_1 > 1$ and, moreover, this solution is unique.*

The previous result shows that, if $R_1 > 1$, there exists an endemic equilibrium solution which does not vanish on $[0, a_0]$, and that when (5.82) does not hold this equilibrium is unique. We now turn to the cases where this kind of solution may no longer be unique, that is when (5.82) holds.

**Theorem 5.11** *Let (5.77) be satisfied and let $R_1$ be defined as above. If (5.82) holds, and $R_1 \neq 1$ then an endemic equilibrium solution which does not vanish on $[0, a_0]$ does not exist. If $R_1 = 1$ then there are an infinite number of nontrivial endemic equilibrium solutions.*

The results stated in the above theorems refer to two disease transmission processes which behave independently from each other, so that it is possible to have different situations. In particular, we may have existence of multiple endemic states, namely we have an infinite number of them when (5.82) and $R_1 = 1$ occur simultaneously, while we have two endemic states when (5.82) does not hold and if $\tilde{R}_0 > 1$ and $R_1 > 1$. In this latter case, one of the two endemic equilibria vanishes on $[0, a_0]$ and the other does not. Furthermore, we have a unique endemic state when, in addition to (5.77), one of the following three sets of conditions is satisfied:

$$\tilde{R}_0 \leq 1, \quad R_1 > 1, \quad \text{and (5.82) does not occur, or} \tag{5.84}$$

$$\tilde{R}_0 > 1, \quad R_1 < 1, \quad \text{or} \tag{5.85}$$

$$\tilde{R}_0 > 1, \quad R_1 \neq 1, \quad \text{and (5.82) occurs.} \tag{5.86}$$

When (5.84) holds the unique endemic equilibrium does not vanish on $[0, a_0]$ and it is maintained by the vertical transmission mechanism. When (5.85) or (5.86) hold, the unique endemic equilibrium vanishes on $[0, a_0]$ and the disease is maintained by the horizontal transmission mechanism. In these cases where there is a unique endemic state, one has the same global behavior as before.

We note that condition (5.83) is a very special one because it occurs if and only if

$$q = 1 \quad \text{and} \quad \gamma(a) = 0 \quad \text{a.e. on} \quad S \equiv \{a \mid \beta(a) > 0\}.$$

When (5.77) holds and (5.82) does not hold, and both $\tilde{R}_0$ and $R_1$ are greater than one, there are two endemic equilibria, one which vanishes on $[0, a_0]$ and one which does not. The initial conditions determine which equilibrium is approached as $t \to \infty$. If $u_0(a) = 0$ for $0 \leq a \leq a_0 < a_\dagger$, and $\int_t^{a_\dagger} K_2(a)u_0(a - t)da > 0$, then the endemic equilibrium which is approached is the one which is concentrated on $[a_0, a_\dagger]$. If $\int_0^{a_\dagger} \beta(a)p_\infty(a)u_0(a - t)da > 0$ for some $t > 0$, then the endemic equilibrium which is approached is the one which is strictly positive in $[0, a_\dagger]$. Here, each of the two disease transmission mechanisms is strong enough to maintain the disease at an endemic level, and the initial conditions determine whether or not a certain portion of the population will remain free of the disease.

We note the occurrence of a fine structure to the thresholds which govern the dynamics of disease transmission in realistic models. We encountered a similar situation in quite different settings in the models that we studied in Section 5.5 and earlier in Sections 2.13.1 and 2.14, and we caution against placing too much emphasis on the single threshold $R_0$ which is the only one that is commonly computed in disease transmission models. This threshold can often be computed because it can be viewed as the spectral radius of an appropriate linear operator, as has been noted for a long time in models of epidemics (see, for example, Busenberg and Cooke [1978]) and as has also been recently stressed in the work of Diekmann, Heesterbeck and Metz [1990].

## 5.10  Destabilization Due to Age Structure

The rather complete results that have been obtained for the age-dependent $s \to i \to s$ model and which were described in the previous sections may lead one to the expectation that the $s \to i \to r$ model may also exhibit a dynamic behavior that is similar to that of the comparable model with no age structure. Under certain very restrictive hypotheses this is indeed the case, and results in this direction have been obtained in a model with no vertical transmission by Gripenberg [1983], Greenhalgh [1987, 1988] and Inaba [1989, 1990]. In fact, both Greenhalgh and Inaba conjecture on the basis of their results that the dynamic behavior of the age-dependent model does not lead to oscillatory states. However, this is not the case, and the situation is quite complex as evidenced by the result of Thieme [1991b] which we shall describe here and which gives an example of an $s \to i \to r$ age-dependent model in which the endemic equilibrium can become unstable thus leading to oscillatory, and perhaps more complicated, dynamic behavior. Such behavior had previously been strongly suggested by the numerical studies of Schenzle [1984]. Cushing [1980] discusses the general question of destabilizing effects of delays and maturation periods. We note that these results are for the case where there is no vertical transmission, however, they point to age-dependence as a candidate mechanism for the observed periodic oscillations in the prevalence level of certain diseases (measles is one well documented example), and are of considerable current interest.

Because of the incomplete present state of the results on the age-structured $s \to i \to r$ model, we shall limit our description to an outline of the result of Thieme [1991b]. The equations describing this model are a special case of (5.4) and are as follows:

$$
\begin{aligned}
\frac{\partial s}{\partial t} + \frac{\partial s}{\partial a} + \mu s &= -\lambda s, \\
\frac{\partial i}{\partial t} + \frac{\partial i}{\partial a} + \mu i &= \lambda s - \delta i, \\
\frac{\partial r}{\partial t} + \frac{\partial r}{\partial a} + \mu r &= \delta i,
\end{aligned}
\tag{5.87}
$$

$$s(0,t) = \int_0^\infty \beta(a)p(a,t)da, \quad i(0,t) = r(0,t) = 0,$$

$$i(a,0) = i_0(a), \quad s(a,0) = s_0(a), \quad r(a,0) = r_0(a),$$

$p = i + r + s$, $p_0 = i_0 + r_0 + s_0$, and the force of infection term $\lambda$ takes the special intercohort form

$$\lambda(t) = \int_0^\infty k(a)i(a,t)da.$$

We place the same positivity assumptions on the parameters as we did in the previous sections. Also, the assumption is made that the basic demographic reproduction number $R$ is one, and that the total population $p$ is in the stationary state given by (5.7).

In order to describe the result of Thieme we introduce the endemic threshold

$$R_0 = \kappa \int_0^\infty T(a)(e^{\gamma a} - 1)da,$$

where

$$\kappa = \int_0^\infty \tilde{k}(a)e^{-a}da,$$

$$\tilde{k}(a) = \frac{k(a)\int_0^\infty p(a)da}{\delta^2 \Pi(a)}, \quad \Pi(a) = \int_0^a e^{-\mu(s)}ds,$$

$$T(a) = \frac{\gamma}{\kappa}\tilde{k}(a)e^{-a},$$

$$\gamma = \frac{1}{\kappa}\int_0^\infty ae^{-a}da.$$

We also introduce the parameter $\nu*$ as the solution of the equation

$$1 = \gamma\kappa \int_0^\infty T(a)\int_0^a e^{(\gamma - \nu*)b}dbda. \tag{5.88}$$

It is easy to see that the right hand side of this equation is strictly decreasing as a function of $\nu*$ when $T$ is not identically zero, consequently, there is a unique solution $\nu*$ which satisfies the equation. The following results are proved by Thieme [1991b].

**Theorem 5.12** *Under the above hypotheses, there exists an endemic equilibrium if and only if $R_0 > 1$. Moreover, whenever it exists, the endemic equilibrium is unique.*

**Theorem 5.13** *Suppose that $T$ has compact support in $[0, \alpha_\dagger]$. Then if $\nu* > 0$ is sufficiently small, the endemic equilibrium is locally asymptotically stable. However, if $T$ is a Dirac measure concentrated at 1, and $\nu*$ is sufficiently large, the endemic equilibrium is unstable.*

Theorem 5.13 shows that the endemic equilibrium can lose its stability at certain parameter values even when the force of infection is independent of the age of the susceptible individuals but is highly concentrated in a specific age class. This would happen in situations where the incidence of the disease and the mean age of infectivity are both relatively high. It is important to note that the restrictions placed by the hypotheses of this theorem are due to the mathematical difficulties encountered in the analysis of the characteristic equation which governs the stability of the endemic state. It is very likely that there are much broader classes of parameters than those included in Theorem 5.13 for which the endemic state is unstable.

Note that the instability of the steady state does not in itself imply that the prevalence of the disease oscillates in an undamped periodic fashion. This, however, is likely to be the case, even though more complicated dynamics could also occur. These questions are currently being studied, and more definitive results and conclusions will probably become available in the near future. It is worth noting that this type of destabilization due to the age structure of the population may provide a deterministic mechanism for the complicated dynamics that have been investigated by Olsen, Truty and Schaffer [1989] and which we described in Section 3.5. General surveys of the occurrence of periodic solutions in epidemic models are provided by Hethcote, Stech and van den Driessche [1981] and by Hethcote and Levin [1989].

## 5.11 Thresholds in Age Dependent Models

One of the major goals of deterministic models of epidemics is the derivation of explicit relations between the mechanisms that influence the dynamics of disease transmission and easily computable and understood epidemiological parameters or thresholds that are useful in arriving at disease assessment and control strategies. For example, when an endemic threshold is explicitly represented in terms of the parameters that enter in a dynamic model, then it becomes possible to analyze the effectiveness of a variety of hypothetical control strategies and arrive at one or more that are optimal from the viewpoint of available resources and acceptable controls. In the more general age-structured models that we have presented above, even though the existence of sharp thresholds can at times be demonstrated, the threshold values often cannot be explicitly written in terms of the parameters in the dynamic model. A general result that demonstrates that the endemic threshold $R_0$ is the spectral radius of a particular abstract operator is limited in value when it does not lead to further sufficiently specific relations between the threshold and the epidemiological and demographic parameters that enter in the dynamical model. Perhaps it should be mentioned that the traditional statistical methods that are widely employed in epidemiology suffer from a similar weakness, since the establishment of a correlation between a particular characteristic and the disease seldom leads to a method for estimating the effectiveness of alternate control strategies. Consequently, it is valuable to study particular special cases which, while limiting the generality of the results that can be obtained, also lead to explicit expressions for the thresholds. For age-dependent models, we have done this in Sections 5.6 and 5.7 when we obtained the expressions (5.27) and (5.53) for $R_0$ in the intracohort and the intercohort case, respectively. These explicit forms of the thresholds give considerable insight into the close interplay between the demographics of an age-structured population and the conditions that lead to endemic persistence of a disease. Iannelli, Milner and Pugliese [1992] have derived another explicit, but more complicated, expression for the endemic threshold for a force of infection which allows for a mixing of the intercohort and intracohort types. In particular, they assume that

$$\lambda[a, i(\cdot, t)] = c^1(a)i(a, t) + c^2(a)I(t). \tag{5.89}$$

where the functions $c^1$, $c^2$ are non-negative and continuous on $[0, a_\dagger]$ with $a_\dagger < \infty$ being a maximal age above which the disease is not transmitted. The resulting model equations are

$$\frac{\partial i}{\partial t} + \frac{\partial i}{\partial a} + \mu i = [p_\infty - i][c^1 i + c^2 I] - \gamma i,$$

$$i(0, t) = q \int_0^{a_\dagger} \beta(a)p_\infty(a)i(a, t)da, \tag{5.90}$$

$$i(a, 0) = i_0(a).$$

Define

$$C_1(a) = p_\infty(a)e^{\int_0^a [c^1(\sigma)p_\infty(\sigma) - \gamma(\sigma)]d\sigma},$$

and

$$C_2(a) = p_\infty(a) \int_0^a e^{\int_\sigma^a [c^1(\tau)p_\infty(\tau) - \gamma(\tau)]d\tau} c^2(\sigma)d\sigma.$$

The threshold condition that they obtain is given in the following result.

**Theorem 5.14** *Consider the $s \to i \to s$ model (5.90) with force of infection term given by (5.89), and with the total population distribution at the equilibrium level $p_\infty(a)$. Suppose that $c^2(a)$ is not identically equal to zero. Then the disease free solution with $i(a, t) = 0$ is globally asymptotically stable if and only if both of the conditions $R_0^1 \leq 1$ and $R_0^2 \leq 1$ hold, where*

$$R_0^1 = \frac{q}{b_0} \int_0^{a_\dagger} \beta(a)C_1(a)da,$$

$$R_0^2 = \frac{q \int_0^{a_\dagger} \beta(a)C_2(a)da \int_0^{a_\dagger} C_1(a)da}{b_0 - q \int_0^{a_\dagger} \beta(a)C_1(a)da} + \int_0^{a_\dagger} C_2(a)da. \tag{5.91}$$

We note that when this result is combined with the general global stability results of Section 5.9 we also have the following conclusion.

**Theorem 5.15** *Under the same hypotheses as in Theorem 5.14, if either $R_0^1 > 1$ or $R_0^2 > 1$ then there exists a unique endemic steady state with $I_\infty > 0$, and all solutions with nontrivial initial data tend to it as $t \to \infty$.*

The proof of Theorem 5.14 is obtained by explicitly computing the spectral radius of the linear operator which yields $R_0$. This is possible in this case because of the special form of the force of infection. The reader is referred to the paper of Iannelli, Milner and Pugliese [1992] for the detailed derivation which is based on the results presented in Section 5.9 and on general theorems on nonlinear positive operators.

We now turn to the interpretation of the threshold given by the two inequalities in Theorems 5.14 and 5.15. If the initial population distribution corresponds to trivial initial data in the sense defined above, the disease dies out and the population settles to a disease free state. Henceforth we assume that the initial population data is not trivial. When $c^2 = 0$ the model reduces to the intracohort case that was studied in Section 5.6 and $R_0^2 = 0$. The condition for global stability of the disease-free equilibrium now becomes $R_0^1 \leq 1$ which is the same condition as in Theorem 5.4. When $c^1 = 0$ then $R_0^1 < 1$ as long as either $q < 1$ or $\gamma \neq 0$ (since the demographic net reproduction number $R = 1$). If $\gamma = 0$ and $q = 1$, that is, there is no recovery and also there is a 100% chance of vertical transmission, then the population settles in an endemic state whenever either $c^1$ or $c^2$ is not identically equal to zero. This is so in the case where $c^1$ does not vanish because then $R_0^1 > 1$, and when $c^1$ vanishes and $c^2$ does not, because then $R_0^2 > 1$. If $c^1 = 0$ and $q = 0$ then the threshold reduces to the intercohort case that we described in Section 5.7 where $a_\dagger = \infty$. In order to see this, first note that $R_0^2$ reduces to

$$R_0^2 = \int_0^\infty p_\infty(a) \int_0^a e^{-\int_\sigma^a \gamma(\tau)d\tau} c^2(\sigma) d\sigma da,$$

which is equal to the threshold $R_0$ in (5.53) when $q = 0$. The dependence of this threshold on the death rate is seen more clearly by noting that

$$p_\infty(a)e^{-\int_a^\sigma \mu(\tau)d\tau} = p_\infty(\sigma),$$

and rewriting $R_0^2$ in the form

$$R_0^2 = \int_0^\infty \int_0^a e^{\int_\sigma^a [-\gamma(\tau)-\mu(\tau)]d\tau} p_\infty(\sigma) c^2(\sigma) d\sigma da$$

$$= \int_0^\infty c^2(\sigma) p_\infty(\sigma) \int_\sigma^\infty e^{\int_\sigma^a [-\gamma(\tau)-\mu(\tau)]d\tau} da d\sigma$$

$$= \int_0^\infty \int_0^\infty c^2(\sigma) p_\infty(\sigma) e^{\int_\sigma^{\sigma+a} [-\gamma(\tau)-\mu(\tau)]d\tau} d\sigma da.$$

It is clear from (5.91) that both $R_0^1$ and $R_0^2$ increase exponentially with the intracohort contact rate $c^1$, and linearly with the intercohort horizontal transmission rate $c^2$. They increase in a nonlinear manner with the fertility $\beta$ and the vertical transmission probability $q$. They decrease exponentially with the cure rate $\gamma$. Thus, any changes that enter through the intercohort transmission rate have a linear effect on the threshold, while changes that enter via the intracohort horizontal contact rate $c^1$ and the recovery rate $\gamma$ result in an exponential effect. Thus, when all other things are equal, control strategies that can affect the cure rate and the intracohort transmission rate can be expected to be more efficient than those that influence the vertical transmission rate, the fertility rate and the intercohort transmission rate. The complicated functional form of the thresholds in (5.91) and the difference in the effects of the intercohort and intracohort horizontal transmission rates are quite striking and could not be easily deduced from heuristic grounds that would bypass the analysis that has been employed in deriving the above two theorems.

Figure 5.13 shows graphs which are taken from the work of Iannelli, Milner and Pugliese [1992] and which show the two components $R_0^1$ and $R_0^2$ of the threshold as $c^1$ is varied while $\gamma = 1.5$, $q = 0.111111$, $c^2 = 0.1$ are kept constant. In this figure, the force of infection term has the form

$$\chi[1, \infty)(a)[k_1 T(a)i(a, t) + k_2 l(a)I(t)/P],$$

where $\chi[1, \infty)(a) = 1$ if $a \geq 1$ and equals zero for $0 \leq a < 1$, $P$ is the total population,

$$l(a) = \begin{cases} 0, & a \leq 0, \\ a/15, & 0 < a \leq 15, \\ 1, & 15 < a, \end{cases}$$

and

$$T(a) = \begin{cases} 0, & a \leq 1, \\ a/5, & 1 < a \leq 5, \\ 1, & 5 < a \leq 10, \\ 1 - (a - 10)/5, & 10 < a \leq 15, \\ 0, & 15 < a. \end{cases}$$

The mortality $\mu(a)$ was taken as the actual mortality of the female population of the U.S. in 1980, and the fertility $\beta(a)$ was chosen to be a smooth function supported on the age interval from 15 to 45 years and scaled so that the net demographic reproduction number $R$ was one. The cure rate $\gamma$ was taken to be constant and such that the average infective period $1/\gamma$ was eight months.

It is clear from Fig. 5.13 that for this particular choice of parameters $R_0^1 < 1$ whenever $R_0^2 < 1$, hence, it is this second condition that determines the stability of the disease-free equilibrium. Because the fertility $\beta(a)$ and $T(a)$ have disjoint supports, we obtain

$$R_0^1 = \frac{q}{b_0} e^{k_1 \int_1^{15} T(\sigma)p_\infty(\sigma)d\sigma} \int_{15}^{45} \beta(a)p_\infty(a)e^{-\gamma a}da,$$

and it is independent of $k_2$. On the other hand, the exponential dependence of $R_0^2$ on $k_1$ is easily seen from the figure.

The demographic threshold $R$ and the endemic threshold $R_0$ have a simple mathematical description as the spectral radii of particular positive operators

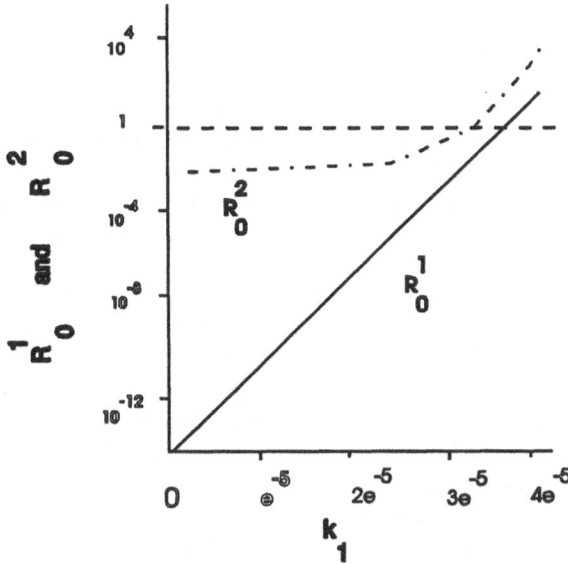

**Fig. 5.13.** Variation of the threshold parameters

because they represent the destabilization of solutions which lie on the boundary of a positive cone in an appropriate function space setting. The observation that this was the case for $R$ harks back to the work of Lotka [1939] and the rigorous proof together with a clear explanation of the implications of positivity is in the basic paper of Feller [1941], who established what is often called the "renewal theorem" for these types of equations. Since that time various elaborations and recastings of this result in the language of functional analysis have been given, and we refer to Bellman and Cooke [1963, Chapter 7], and Webb [1985] for accessible discussions. The fact that $R_0$ is the spectral radius of a positive operator has recently been discussed in detail and used in computing some specific thresholds by Diekmann, Heesterbeck and Metz [1990]. A generalization of the renewal theorem of Feller which extends the applicability of these threshold results to a useful class of nonlinear problems has been given by Busenberg and Iannelli [1983a,b], and applied to a variety of age dependent population problems by Busenberg and Iannelli [1985] and others. An early contribution in this direction which went part way towards showing such a nonlinear renewal result is in the thesis of Simmes [1978] which, unfortunately, was never published, and did not come to light until after the independent and more complete results of Busenberg and Iannelli [1983a,b] became available. The applications of this nonlinear renewal result include the treatment of the $s \to i$ model with vertical transmission discussed in Section 5.5, and the intracohort and intercohort $s \to i \to s$ model with variable population size that have been studied by Langlais [1991] and which were described in Sections 5.6 and 5.7.

## 5.12 Spatial Structure

All of the above models assume that the spatial distribution of the population does not have any effect on the disease transmission dynamics, and hence, averages of the population densities over the spatial domain can be used as adequate approximations. As we saw already in Chapter 4, models of vertically transmitted diseases with some form of spatial structure have been formulated and studied. In the case of age dependent populations, there has only been the one paper of Kubo and Langlais [1991] in which a model with both vertical transmission and spatial structure has been studied. However, spatial diffusion in age structured populations has been studied by Skellam [1951], Marcati and Serafini [1979], Marcati and Pozio [1980], Webb [1980, 1982a,b], Gurtin and MacCamy [1981], MacCamy [1981], Busenberg and Iannelli [1982, 1983a,b, 1984], Busenberg and Travis [1983], Langlais and Phillips [1985], Seck [1986], Langlais [1988, 1991], and Thieme [1991a]. We give a brief discussion of the part of this work which involves disease transmission in age-structured populations since it provides part of the basis of what needs to be done in this area. Before we begin this description we wish to note that, even though there have been several serious studies of spatial structure of populations (see the book of Okubo [1980], and the discussions in Skellam [1951], Gurtin and MacCamy [1981], Busenberg and Travis [1983], and in Levin [1983]), we believe that this is an area of epidemiology where much of the fundamental mathematical formulation of the problem has yet to be addressed, and where detailed field observations are needed before adequate models can be developed.

At the simplest level, one can conceive of the infection as diffusing through the spatial domain with a flux rate that is proportional to the gradient of the density of the infectives. This hypothesis is based on the observation that when a large number of individuals are moving in an uncorrelated random manner, then their average flux is governed by such a rule. As we shall see later, this is probably not the correct form of the diffusion term when the movement is due to population migration rather than local random movements.

We now describe the results of Kubo and Langlais [1991] who assume this kind of random diffusion of the population in the case of an $s \to i \to s$ model with intracohort form for the force of infection. They consider a population $p = i + s$ occupying a spatial domain $\Omega$ with boundary $\partial\Omega$ and denote by $x$ any point in this domain. Assuming an external migration influx given by $f(a, t, x)$ into the interior of the domain $\Omega$ and that the population at the boundary is kept at a predetermined level $g(a, t, x)$ they obtain a system of equations in which $p$ satisfies

$$\text{(a)} \quad \frac{\partial p}{\partial t} + \frac{\partial p}{\partial a} + \mu p = D \triangle p + f,$$

$$\text{(b)} \quad p(0, t, x) = \int_0^\infty \beta(a)p(a, t, x)da, \qquad (5.92)$$

$$\text{(c)} \quad p(a, 0, x) = p_0(a),$$

$$\text{(d)} \quad p(a, t, x) = g(a, t, x), \quad x \in \partial\Omega.$$

Set $s = p - i$, to obtain

(a) $\dfrac{\partial i}{\partial t} + \dfrac{\partial i}{\partial a} + \mu i = D \, \Delta \, i + \kappa[p - i]i - \gamma i + f_i,$

(b) $i(0, t, x) = q \displaystyle\int_0^\infty \beta(a) i(a, t, x) da,$    (5.93)

(c) $i(a, 0, x) = i_0(a),$

(d) $i(a, t, x) = g_i(a, t, x), \quad x \in \partial\Omega.$

Here $D > 0$ is the diffusion rate, and the other parameters have the same interpretations as in Section 5.6. The time dependence of $f, f_i, g, g_i$ is assumed to be periodic with period $T$ to possibly include seasonal or other variations. The results that they obtain require the introduction of the standard Malthusian parameter $p^*$ of exponential change of the total population which is the largest root $p$ of the equation

$$\int_0^\infty \beta(a) e^{-pa - \int_0^a \mu(\sigma) d\sigma} da = 1,$$

and a parameter $\lambda_1$ which describes the spatial domain and which is the first eigenvalue of the problem

$$-\Delta u = \lambda u \quad \text{in} \quad \Omega,$$
$$u = 0 \quad \text{on} \quad \partial\Omega.$$

**Theorem 5.16** *Assume that $f, f_i$ and $g, g_i$ are bounded and periodic of period $T$, and let $0 \le f_i \le f$, $0 \le g_i \le g$. Then*

*(i) If $p^* \lambda_1 < 1$ there is a unique non-negative $T$-periodic solution of the population problem (5.92) and this solution is globally asymptotically stable. Moreover, the epidemic problem (5.93) has at least one non-negative solution.*

*(ii) If $p^* \lambda_1 \ge 1$ any solution of the population problem (5.92) tends to $\infty$ as the time $t$ tends to $\infty$.*

We shall not give the proof of this result and refer the interested reader to the original paper. The result gives only a partial description of the epidemic problem and, in fact, it does not describe the possible endemic thresholds in this case. However, it shows how the spatial diffusion and the shape of the spatial domain enter into the description of the demographic threshold, and points to the way in which they might influence any endemic thresholds that might occur in such a model. Similar results for non-vertically transmitted diseases and for populations with no age structure can be found in the work of Capasso [1978] and Capasso and Maddalena [1981]. The boundary condition which is used in this model is probably not very realistic since it prescribes the population density on the boundary. A condition that is probably more likely to occur is one which prescribes the population flux at the boundary, that is, one that describes the rate at which migrations through the domain boundary occur.

An alternate way of describing the spread of the infection over a spatial domain invokes a force of infection term which is "nonlocal" in space and which in the intracohort case takes the form

$$\int_\Omega k(a, x, x')i(a, t, x')dx',$$

while in the general case it would take the form

$$\int_\Omega \left( \int_0^\infty k(a, a', x, x')i(a, t, x')da' \right) dx'.$$

Such terms, but without age-dependence or vertical transmission, have been studied in a number of epidemic models (see for example, Thieme [1979], Diekmann [1978], De Mottoni, Orlandi and Tesei [1979], Levin [1983], and Busenberg and Travis [1983]). The kernel $k(a, x, x')$ describes the effect that an infected individual located at position $x'$ at time $t$ would have on susceptible individuals who are located at the position $x$ at time $t$. These types of kernels can be chosen to describe situations that go beyond random population movements, and where individuals have strong effects in more than one location, as one would expect in populations whose various habitual activities require them to regularly go to different locations. For example, in human populations, among school-age children, the effects of an infective child would be felt with various degrees of importance at home, at school and in the location of play or social contacts.

The above types of terms describe population movements which do not involve permanent migrations. Mathematical descriptions of migratory terms are also quite important and we here describe a model that has been proposed by Busenberg and Travis [1983] which includes such terms in addition to the type of spatial terms described in the previous paragraph. Here, if one thinks of individuals in the population migrating because of total population pressures, and doing so in groups that contain individuals of all epidemic classes, then one obtains a non-linear diffusion term of the form

$$D\nabla \cdot \left( \frac{i(a, t, x)}{p(a, t, x)} \nabla p(a, t, x) \right),$$

instead of the first term on the right hand side of (5.93). Another important generalization is obtained by having a diffusion term of the form used in (5.92) but with the diffusion coefficient depending on age, $D(a)$, rather than being constant. This certainly occurs in vertically transmitted diseases such as tuberculosis in possums (see Barlow [1990]) where the juveniles at about the age of nine months tend to have a much larger tendency for spatial dispersion than the other age groups which, in fact, are fairly sedentary. Another pertinent example is that of the spatial movement of vector transmitted diseases such as rickettsia and Lyme disease which are vertically transmitted in the tick vectors. These vectors are very sedentary but disperse during specific age stages when they require blood meals and attach themselves to mobile mammals. Models that include such effects are being currently studied, and some initial theoretical results have been obtained by Thieme [1991a], however, much still waits to be done in this important area.

## 5.13 The Force of Infection Terms

As we have seen on several occasions throughout this monograph, the form that the horizontal force of infection terms take has a large influence on the dynamics of the disease transmission and on the endemic thresholds. Consequently, it is important to analyze the basic properties of such terms and obtain a rational foundation for their derivation. This has recently been done for disease transmission due to pairing of individuals in age-dependent populations by Busenberg and Castillo-Chavez [1989, 1991], and we shall describe these results here. Disease transfer via pairwise contact of individuals occurs in sexually transmitted diseases as well as in vector transmitted diseases. The axiomatization of pair formation and its relation to disease transmission is a topic of considerable current research activity. The papers by Hadeler [1989] and Castillo-Chavez and Busenberg [1991], the thesis of Waldstätter [1990], in addition to the above cited papers provide an introduction to the basic ideas in this area. The formulation that we describe here will be restricted to the case of a single population but the extension to multiple populations has also been done, see Castillo-Chavez and Busenberg [1991], and follows the same lines.

We let $a, \tau$, and $t$ stand for age, time since infection, and time, respectively, and introduce a parameter $r$ which labels the risk level of an individual. Thus we may speak of an "$a, \tau, r$ individual" to mean a person who is of age $a$, of risk level $r$ and has had the disease for a length of time $\tau$. Similarly, by an $(r, a)$ individual we mean a person who is of risk level $r$ and of age $a$. In order to fix ideas, we consider a population consisting of susceptible, infective and removed individuals and keep track of the first two classes whose densities we denote, as usual, by $s(a, r, t)$ and $i(a, r, \tau, t)$. Note that only $i$ depends on the internal variable $\tau$. Since we are concerned with disease transmission via contact between pairs of individuals, we introduce the mixing function $\rho$ which is defined as follows:

$\rho(r, a, r'a')$ = the proportion of contacts of an $(r, a)$ individual which are with $(r', a')$ individuals.

We also let $T$ denote the total active population

$$T(r, a, t) = S(r, a, t) + \int_0^\infty i(r, a, \tau, t)d\tau,$$

and define

$C(r, a, T(r, a, t))$ = the expected or average number of contacts per unit time of an $(r, a)$ individual, given that the active population size is $T$.

We shall base our derivation of the force of infection terms on the following properties which we take as reasonable axioms that must be satisfied.

(a) $\rho \geq 0$,
(b) $\int_0^\infty \int_0^\infty \rho(r, a, r', a', t) dr' da' = 1$,
(c) $Q(r, a, r', a', t) = Q(r', a', r, a, t)$, where

$$Q(r, a, r', a', t) = \rho(r, a, r', a', t) C(r, a, T(r, a, t)) T(r, a, t),$$

(d) If $C(r, a, T(r, a, t)) T(r, a, t) C(r', a', T(r', a', t)) T(r', a', t) = 0$,
then $\rho(r, a, r', a', t) \rho(r', a', r, a, t) = 0$.

Conditions (a) and (b) are simply due to the fact that $\rho$ is a proportion. Condition (c) is a balance equation which says that the total number of pairings of $(r, a)$ individuals with $(r', a')$ individuals is equal to the total number of pairings of $(r', a')$ individuals with $(r, a)$ individuals. Condition (d) says that no mixing can occur in the age and risk level groups where there are no active individuals, that is, on the set $S$ consisting of all points $(r, a, r', a', t)$ for which

$$C(r, a, T(r, a, t)) T(r, a, t) C(r', a', T(r', a', t)) T(r', a', t) = 0.$$

In some situations it is convenient to consider mixing functions which involve Dirac distributions, and a generalization of the above formalism can be obtained that covers that case, however, we shall not consider it here.

The force of infection term is obtained from the mixing function as follows. Let $\beta(r, a, \tau, r', a')$ denote the probability that a pairing between an $(r', a', \tau)$ infective individual and an $(r, a)$ susceptible will lead to the passing of the infection, then the force of infection $\lambda$ is given by

$$\lambda(r, a, t) = C(r, a, T(r, a, t)) \int \int \int_0^\infty \beta(r, a, \tau, r', a') \rho(r, a, r', a', t)$$
$$\frac{I(r', a', \tau, t)}{T(r', a', t)} dr' da' d\tau. \tag{5.94}$$

This form of $\lambda$ follows from the reasoning that the contact rate of an $(r, a)$ susceptible is $C(r, a, T(r, a, t))$, and of these contacts

$$C(r, a, T(r, a, t)) \rho(r, a, r', a', t)$$

are with active individuals in the $(r', a')$ class. A proportion

$$I(r', a', \tau, t) / T(r', a', t)$$

of these are with individuals of class $(r', a', \tau)$, hence the total number of contacts per unit time of an $(r, a)$ individual with $(r', a', \tau)$ infectives is

$$C(r, a, T(r, a, t))\rho(r, a, r', a', t)\frac{I(r', a', \tau, t)}{T(r', a', t)}.$$

Consequently, the expected rate of disease transmission due to such contacts with infectives is

$$C(r, a, T(r, a, t))\beta(r, a, \tau, r', a')\rho(r, a, r', a', t)\frac{I(r', a', \tau, t)}{T(r', a', t)}.$$

The integral sums over all possible contacts that the single $(r, a)$ susceptible could have.

We now present the results of Busenberg and Castillo-Chavez [1989] which characterize mixing functions. We first define a mixing function $\rho$ to be *separable* if it can be written in the form

$$\rho(r, a, r', a', t) = \rho_1(r, a, t)\rho_2(r', a', t). \tag{5.95}$$

It turns out that such separable mixing functions are quite special.

**Theorem 5.17** *The only separable mixing function $\rho$ satisfying conditions (a)-(d) is the "total proportionate mixing" function*

$$\bar{\rho}(r', a', t) = \frac{C(r', a', T(r', a', t))T(r', a', t)}{\int_0^\infty \int_0^\infty C(r', a', T(r', a', t))T(r', a', t)da'dr'}. \tag{5.96}$$

*Proof.* Suppose that $\rho$ is separable, then from (b),

$$\rho_1(r, a, t) = \frac{1}{\int_0^\infty \int_0^\infty \rho_2(r', a', t)dr'da'} = k(t).$$

Thus $\rho_1(r, a, t)$ is a function $k(t)$ of $t$ only, and therefore, $\rho(r, a, r', a', t) = k(t)\rho_2(r', a', t)$. Substituting this in (c), integrating over the variables $r', a'$ and using (b), we obtain

$$C(r, a, T(r, a, t))T(r, a, t) = k(t)\rho_2(r, a, t)\int_0^\infty \int_0^\infty C(r', a', T(r', a', t))$$
$$T(r', a', t)dr'da'.$$

Thus, $\rho = k\rho_2$ is given by (5.96). It is an easy direct computation to show that $\bar{\rho}$ given by (5.96) satisfies the hypotheses (a)-(d), and this completes the proof.

The following two results give general formulas for arbitrary mixing functions in terms of the separable mixing function $\bar{\rho}$.

**Theorem 5.18** *Let $\phi(r, a, r', a', t) \geq 0$ be symmetric in the $(r, a)$ and $(r', a')$ variables, $\phi(r, a, r', a', t) = \phi(r', a', r, a, t)$, and let*

$$\int_0^\infty \int_0^\infty \bar{\rho}(r', a', t)\phi(r, a, r', a', t)dr'da' = 1,$$

*where $\bar{\rho}$ is the proportionate mixing function given in (5.96). Then*

$$\rho(r, a, r', a', t) = \bar{\rho}(r', a', t)\phi(r, a, r', a', t), \tag{5.97}$$

*is a mixing function. Conversely, every mixing function $\rho$ is given by the form (5.97) where $\phi$ is symmetric and satisfies the above hypotheses.*

**Theorem 5.19** *Let $\phi(r, a, r', a', t) \geq 0$ be measurable and symmetric in the $(r, a)$ and $(r', a')$ variables, and suppose that*

$$\int_0^\infty \int_0^\infty \bar{\rho}(r', a', t)\phi(r, a, r', a', t)dr'da' \leq 1,$$

*and*

$$\int_0^\infty \int_0^\infty \bar{\rho}(r, a, t)\left(\int_0^\infty \int_0^\infty \bar{\rho}(r', a', t)\phi(r, a, r', a', t)dr'da'\right)drda < 1.$$

*Letting*

$$\rho_1(r, a, t) = 1 - \int_0^\infty \int_0^\infty \bar{\rho}(r', a', t)\phi(r, a, r', a', t)dr'da', \tag{5.98}$$

*then*

$$\rho(r, a, r', a', t) =$$
$$\bar{\rho}(r', a', t)\left[\frac{\rho_1(r, a, t)\rho_1(r', a', t)}{\int_0^\infty \int_0^\infty \bar{\rho}(r', a', t)dr'da'} + \phi(r, a, r', a', t)\right], \tag{5.99}$$

*is a mixing function. Conversely, for every mixing function $\rho$ there exists a $\phi$ that satisfies the above hypotheses and is such that $\rho$ is given by (5.99) with $\rho_1$ defined by (5.98).*

The first of the above two results shows that any arbitrary mixing function can be viewed as a specific multiplicative perturbation of the proportionate mixing function $\bar{\rho}$, while the second result gives $\rho$ as an additive perturbation of $\bar{\rho}$. These results can be used to construct various mixing functions and force of infection terms which have additional specific properties. We refer the reader to the papers of Busenberg and Castillo-Chavez [1989, 1991] for the proofs of these results and for some of their applications; and to the paper of Castillo-Chavez, Busenberg and Gerow [1991] for examples of a variety of special forms of the force of infection term that have been constructed by using these theorems.

An immediate consequence of the above formulation is that any convex combination of mixing functions is again a mixing function. From this one can easily see that the widely used "preferential mixing" function is one of the special cases of the general forms we have obtained above. The importance of these general forms is that they provide the means of approximating the correct mixing function and the corresponding force of infection term by using parameter estimation methods. This is an area that is now starting to be actively pursued (see, Blythe, Castillo-Chavez and Casella [1990], Pugliese[1990], Castillo-Chavez, Busenberg and Gerow [1991], Nussbaum [1992]) and which is promising to lead to more appropriate forms of the force of infection terms for particular diseases.

# References

Anderson, R., and May, R. (1979): Population biology of infectious diseases: Part II. Nature **280**, 455–461.

Anderson, R., and May, R. (1981): The population dynamics of microparasites and their invertebrate hosts. Philos. Trans. R. Soc. Lond. **B 291**, 451–524.

Anderson, R., and May, R. (1982): Directly transmitted infectious diseases: control by vaccination. Science **215**, 1053–1060.

Anderson, R., and May, R. (1991): Infectious Diseases of Humans. Oxford University Press, Oxford-London-Tokyo.

Anderson, R., May, R., and McLean, A. (1988): Possible demographic consequences of AIDS in developing countries. Nature **334**, 228–233.

Andreason, V. (1988): Dynamical models of epidemics in age-structured populations – Analysis and simplification. Ph.D. thesis, Cornell University, Ithaca, New York.

Aron, J., and Schwartz, I. (1984): Seasonality and period-doubling bifurcations in an epidemic model. J. Theor. Biol. **110**, 665–679.

Bacchetti, P., and Moss, A. (1989): Incubation period of AIDS in San Francisco. Nature **338**, 251–253.

Bailey, N. (1975): The Mathematical Theory of Infectious Diseases and its Applications. Second Edition, Hafner Press, New York.

Bartlett, M. (1960): Stochastic Population Models in Ecology and Epidemiology. Methuen, London.

Barlow, N. (1990): A model for endemic bovine Tb in New Zealand's possum population. J. of Applied Ecol., to appear.

Bellman, R., and Cooke, K. (1963): Differential-Difference Equations, Academic Press, New York, London.

Beretta, E., and Capasso, E. (1986): On the general structure of epidemic systems, global asymptotic stability. Comp. and Maths. with Appls. **12A**, 677–694.

Bittencourt, A. (1984): Actual aspects and epidemiological significance of congenital transmission of Chagas' disease. Mem. Inst. Oswaldo Cruz **79**, 133–137.

Black, F., and Singer, B. (1987): Elaboration versus simplification in refining mathematical models of infectious disease. Ann. Rev. Microbiol. **41**, 677–701.

Blythe, S., Castillo-Chavez, C., and Casella, G. (1990): Emperical methods for the estimation of the mixing probabilities for socially structured populations from a single survey sample. preprint.

Brauer, F. (1990): Models for the spread of universally fatal diseases. J. Math. Biol. **28**, 451–462.

Bremermann, H., and Thieme, H. (1989): A competitive exclusion principle for pathogen virulence. J. Math. Biol. **27**, 179–190.

Burgdorfer, W. (1975): Rocky mountain spotted fever. In Diseases Transmitted from Animal to Man. 6th Edition, W. Hubbert, et al, Eds., Charles Thomas, Illinois, Chapter 26.

Busenberg, S., and Castillo-Chavez, C. (1989): Interaction, pair formation and force of infection terms in sexually transmitted diseases. In Mathematical and Statistical Approaches to AIDS Epidemiology, C. Chavez, Ed., Lecture Notes in Biomathematics **83**, Springer-Verlag, Berlin-Heidelberg-New York, 289–300.

Busenberg, S., and Castillo-Chavez, C. (1991): A general solution of the mixing of subpopulations and its application to risk- and age-structured epidemic models of the spread of AIDS, IMA J. Math. Appl. Med. Biol. **8**, 1–29.

Busenberg, S., and Cooke, K. (1978): Periodic solutions of a periodic non-linear delay differential equation. SIAM J. Appl. Math. **35**, 704–721.

Busenberg, S., and Cooke, K. (1980): The effect of integral conditions in certain equations modelling epidemics and population growth. J. Math. Biol. **10**, 13–32.

Busenberg, S., and Cooke, K. (1982): Models of vertically transmitted diseases with sequential-continuous dynamics. In Nonlinear Phenomena in Mathematical Sciences, V. Lakshmikantham, Ed., Academic Press, New York, 179–187.

Busenberg, S., and Cooke, K. (1988): The population dynamics of two vertically transmitted infections. Theor. Pop. Biol. **33**, 181–198.

Busenberg, S., Cooke, K., and Iannelli, M. (1988): Endemic thresholds and stability in a class of age-structured epidemics. SIAM J. Appl. Math. **48**, 1379–1395.

Busenberg, S., Cooke, K., and Iannelli, M. (1989): Stability and thresholds in some age-structured epidemics. Lecture Notes in Biomathematics 81, C. Castillo-Chavez, S. Levin and C. Shoemaker, Ed., Springer-Verlag, Berlin-Heidelberg- New York, 124–141.

Busenberg, S., Cooke, K., and Pozio, A. (1983): Analysis of a model of a vertically transmitted disease. J. Math. Biol. **17**, 305–329.

Busenberg, S., Cooke, K., and Thieme, H. (1991): Demographic change and persistence of HIV/AIDS in a heterogeneous population. SIAM J. Appl. Math. **51**, 1030–1052.

Busenberg, S., and Hadeler, K. (1990): Demography and epidemics. Math. Biosc. **101**, 63–74.

Busenberg, S., and Iannelli, M. (1982): A method for treating a class of nonlinear diffusion problems. Rendiconti Accad. Naz. Lincei, Ser. 8, **72**, 121–127.

Busenberg, S., and Iannelli, M. (1983a): A class of nonlinear diffusion problems in age-dependent population dynamics. Nonlinear Anal. T.M.A. **7**, 501–529.

Busenberg, S., and Iannelli, M. (1983b): A degenerate nonlinear diffusion problem in age-structured population dynamics. Nonlinear Anal. T.M.A. **7**, 1411–1429.

Busenberg, S., and Iannelli, M. (1984): Nonlinear diffusion problems in age-structured population dynamics. In Mathematical Ecology, S.A. Levin and T. Hallam, Eds., Springer Lecture Notes in Biomathematics **54**, 425–440.

Busenberg, S., and Iannelli, M. (1985): Separable models in age-dependent population dynamics. J. Math. Biol. **22**, 145–173.

Busenberg, S., Iannelli, M., and Thieme, H. (1991a): Global behavior of an age-structured S–I–S epidemic model. SIAM J. Math. Analysis **22**, 1065–1080.

Busenberg, S., Iannelli, M., and Thieme, H. (1991b): Dynamics of an age-structured epidemic model. preprint.

Busenberg, S., and Travis, C. (1983): Epidemic models with spatial spread due to population migration. J. Math. Biol. **16**, 181–198.

Busenberg, S., and van den Driessche, P. (1990): Analysis of a disease transmission model in a population with varying size. J. Math. Biol. **28**, 257–270.

Busenberg, S., and Vargas, C. (1991): Modeling Chagas' disease: variable population size and demographic implications. In Mathematical Population Dynamics, O. Arino, D. Axelrod and M. Kimmel, Eds., Marcel Dekker, New York, Basel, Hong Kong, 283–296.

Capasso, E. (1978): Global solution for a diffusive nonlinear deterministic epidemic model. SIAM J. Appl. Math. **35**, 274–284.

Capasso, E., and Maddalena, L. (1981): Convergence to equilibrium states for a reaction-diffusion system modelling the spatial spread of a class of bacterial and viral diseases. J. Math. Biol. **13**, 173–184.

Castillo-Chavez, C., Busenberg, S., and Gerow, K. (1991): Pair formation in structured populations. In Differential Equations with Applications in Biology, Physics and Engineering, J. Goldstein, F. Kappel, and W. Schappacher, Eds., Marcel Dekker, New York-Basel-Hong Kong, 47–65.

Castillo-Chavez, C., and Busenberg, S. (1991): On the solution of the two-sex mixing problem. In Differential Equations Models in Biology, Epidemiology and Ecology, S. Busenberg and M. Martelli, Eds., Springer Lecture Notes in Biomathematics 92, 80–98.

Castillo-Chavez, C., Cooke, K., Huang, W., and Levin, S. (1989): On the role of long incubation periods in the dynamics of acquired immunodeficiency syndrome (AIDS). Part 1: Single population models. J. Math. Biol. 27, 373–398.

Castillo-Chavez, C., Hethcote, H., Andreassen, V., Levin, S., and Liu, W. (1989): Epidemiological models with age structure, proportionate mixing and cross-immunity. J. Math. Biol. 27, 233–258.

Cavalli-Sforza, L., and Feldman, M. (1981): Cultural Transmission and Evolution: A Quantitative Approach. Princeton University Press, Princeton.

Chagas, C. (1909): Nova triponosomiase humana. Estudios sobre a morfología e o ciclo evolutivo do shizotrypanum Cruzai n. gen., s. sp., agente etiologico de nova entidad morbidado homem. Mem. Inst. Oswaldo Cruz 1, 159–218.

Chow, S.N., and Hale, J. (1982): Methods of Bifurcation Theory. Springer-Verlag, Berlin-Heidelberg-New York.

Chow, S.N., and Mallet-Paret, J. (1977): Integral averaging and bifurcation. J. Diff. Eq. 16, 112–159.

Clay, K. (1988): Fungal endophytes of grasses, a defensive mutualism between plants and fungi. Ecology 69, 10–17.

Cooke, K., and Busenberg, S. (1982): Vertically transmitted diseases. In Nonlinear Phenomena in Mathematical Sciences, V. Lakshmikantham, Ed., Academic Press, New York, 189–197.

Coura, J. (1988): Determinantes epidemiológicos da doenca de Chagas no Brazil: a infeccao, a doenca e sua morbi mortalidade. Mem. Inst. Oswaldo Cruz 83, 394–402.

Cushing, J. (1980): Model stability and instability in age structured population dynamics. J. Theor. Biol. 86, 709–730.

De Mottoni, P., Orlandi, P., and Tesei, E. (1979): Asymptotic behavior for a system describing epidemics with migration and spatial spread of infection. Nonlinear Anal. T.M.A. 3, 663–675.

Devaney, R. (1986): An Introduction to Chaotic Dynamics. Benjamin, Menlo Park, California.

Diekmann, O. (1978): Thresholds and travelling waves for the geographical spread of infections. J. Math. Biol. 6, 109–130.

Diekmann, O., Heesterbeck, J., and Metz, H. (1990): On the definition and the computation of the basic reproduction ratio $R_0$ in models for infectious diseases in heterogeneous populations. J. Math. Biol. 28, 365–382.

Dietz, K. (1975): Transmission and control of arbovirus diseases. In Proceedings of SIMS conference on Epidemiology, D. Ludwig and K. Cooke, Eds., SIAM, Philadelphia, 104–121.

Dietz, K. (1976): The incidence of infectious diseases under the influence of seasonal fluctuations. Lecture Notes in Biomathematics 11, S. Levin, Ed., Springer-Verlag, Berlin-Heidelberg-New York, 1–15.

Dietz, K., and Schenzle, D. (1985): Mathematical models for infectious disease statistics. Centenary volume of the International Statistical Institute, A.C. Atkinson and S.E. Fienberg, Eds., Springer-Verlag, Berlin-Heidelberg-New York, 167–204.

Douglas, Jr., J., and Milner, F. (1987): Numerical methods for a model of population dynamics. Calcolo. 24, 247–254.

Edelstein-Keshet, L. (1988): Mathematical Models in Biology. Random House, Birkhauser, New York.

Elderkin, R. (1985): Nonlinear, globally age-dependent population models: some basic theory. J. Math. Anal. Appl. **108**, 546–562.

El Doma, M. (1985): Analysis of nonlinear integro-differential equations arising in age dependent epidemic models. Ph.D. Thesis, Claremont Graduate School, Claremont, CA.

El Doma, M. (1987): Analysis of nonlinear integro-differential equations arising in age dependent epidemic models. Nonlinear Anal. T.M.A. **11**, 913–937.

El'sgol'ts, L., and Norkin, S. (1973): Introduction to the Theory and Application of Differential Equations with Deviating Arguments. Academic Press, New York, London.

Falkow, S. (1975): Infectious Multiple Drug Resistance. Pion, London.

Feller, W. (1941): On the integral equation of renewal theory. Ann. Math. Statistics **12**, 243–267.

Fine, P. (1975): Vectors and vertical transmission, an epidemiologic perspective. Annals N.Y. Acad. Sci. **266**, 173–194.

Fine, P., and Clarkson, J. (1982): Measles in England and Wales. An analysis of factors underlying seasonal patterns. International J. of Epidemiology **11**, 5–14.

Fine, P., and Le Duc, J. (1978): Towards a quantitative understanding of the epidemiology of Keystone virus in the Eastern United States. Amer. J. Trop. Med. Hyg. **27**, 322–388.

Freier, J., Rosen, L. (1987): Vertical transmission of dengue viruses by mosquitoes of the *Aedes Scutellaris* group. Amer. J. Trop. Med. Hyg. **37**, 640–647.

García, L., and Bruckner, D. (1988): Diagnostic Medical Parasitology. Elsevier, New York.

Garham, P. (1980): The significance of inapparent infections in Chagas' disease and forms of trypanosomiasis. Mem. Inst. Oswaldo Cruz. **75**, 181–188.

Garvie, M., McKeil, J., Sonenshine, D. and Campbell, A. (1978): Seasonal dynamics of American dog tick, Dermacentor variabilis (say), population in South Western Nova Scotia. Canad. J. Zool. **65**, 28–39.

Goh, B. (1977): Global stability in many species systems. American Naturalist **111**, 135–143.

Goh, B. (1978): Global stability in a class of predator-prey models. Bull. Math. Biol. **40**, 525–533.

Goh, B. (1980): Management and Analysis of Biological Populations. Elsevier North-Holland, Amsterdam, New York.

Grabiner, D. (1988): Mathematical models for vertically transmitted diseases. Technical Report, Pomona College, Claremont.

Green, D. (1978): Self-oscillations for epidemic models. Math. Biosci. **38**, 91-111.

Greenhalgh, D. (1987): Analytical results on the stability of age-structured recurrent epidemic models. IMA J. Math. Appl. Med. Biol. **4**, 109–144.

Greenhalgh, D. (1988): Threshold and stability results for an epidemic model with an age-structured meeting rate. IMA J. Math. Appl. Med. Biol. **5**, 81–100.

Grenfeld, B., and Anderson, R. (1985): The estimation of age-related rates of infection from case notifications and serological data. J. Hyg. Camb. **95**, 429–436.

Gripenberg, G. (1983): On a nonlinear integral equation modelling an epidemic in an age structured population. J. Reine Angew. Math. **341**, 54–67.

Grossman, Z. (1980): Oscillatory phenomena in a model of infectious diseases. Theor. Pop. Biol. **18**, 204–243.

Grossman, Z., Gumowski, I., and Dietz, K. (1977): The incidence of infectious diseases under the influence of seasonal fluctuations. Analytic approach. In Nonlinear Systems and Applications to Life Sciences, V. Lakshmikantham, Ed., Academic Press. New York, 525–546.

Gurtin, M., and MacCamy, R. (1981): Diffusion models for age-structured populations. Math. Biosc. **54**, 49–59.

Hadeler, K. (1989): Pair formation in age-structured populations. Acta Applic. Math. **14**, 91–102.

Hahn, W. (1967): Stability of Motion. Springer-Verlag, Berlin-Heidelberg-New York.

Halanay, A. (1966): Differential Equations: Stability, Oscillations, Time Lags. Academic Press, New York and London.

Hale, J. (1974): Behavior near constant solutions of functional differential equations. J. Diff. Eq. **15**, 278–294.

Hale, J. (1977): Theory of Functional Differential Equations. Applied Math. Sciences, Vol. 3, Springer-Verlag, Berlin-Heidelberg-New York.

Hassard, B., Kazarinoff, N. and Wan, Y. (1981): Theory and Application of Hopf Bifurcation. Cambridge Univ. Press, Cambridge.

Hassell, M., and May, R. (1973): Stability in insect host-parasite models. J. Anim. Ecol. **42**, 693–726.

Hethcote, H., and Levin, S. (1989): Periodicity in epidemiological models. In Applied Mathematical Ecology, S.A. Levin, T.G. Hallam, L. J. Gross, Eds., Springer-Verlag, Berlin-Heidelberg-New York. 293–211 .

Hethcote, H., Stech, H., and van den Driessche, P. (1981): Nonlinear oscillations in epidemic models. SIAM J. Appl. Math. **40**, 1–9.

Hethcote, H., Stech, H., and van den Driessche, P. (1983): Periodicity and stability in epidemic models: a survey. In Differential Equations and Applications in Ecology, Epidemics and Population Dynamics, S. Busenberg and K.L. Cooke, Eds., Academic Press, New York, 65–82.

Hethcote, H., and van Ark, J. (1987): Epidemiological models for heterogeneous populations: proportionate mixing, parameter estimation and immunization programs. Math. Biosci. **84**, 85-118.

Hethcote, H., and Yorke, J. (1984): Gonorrohea Transmission Dynamics and Control. Lecture Notes in Biomathematics **56**, Springer-Verlag, Berlin-Heidelberg-New York.

Hoppensteadt, F. (1974): An age-dependent epidemic model. J. Franklin Inst. **197**, 325–333.

Hoppensteadt, F. (1975): Mathematical Theories of Populations: Demographics, Genetics and Epidemics. Society for Industrial and Applied Mathematics, Philadelphia.

Huang, W. (1990): Studies in Differential Equations and Applications. Ph.D dissertation. Claremont Graduate School, Claremont, California.

Iannelli, M., Milner, F., and Pugliese, A. (1992): Analytical and numerical results for the age-structured S–I–S epidemic model with mixed inter-intracohort transmission. SIAM J. Appl. Math. **23**, 662–688.

Iannelli, M., Milner, F., Pugliese, A., and Tubaro, L. (1989): A mathematical model for epidemics: the case of diseases that do not impart immunity (S–I–S). Preprint, Center for Applied Mathematics, Purdue University, Technical Report **103**.

Inaba, H. (1989): Functional Analytic Approach to Age-Structured Population Dynamics. Chapter VII: Thresholds and stability results for an age-structured epidemic model. Ph.D dissertation, Leiden.

Inaba, H. (1990): Thresholds and stability results for an age-structured epidemic model. J. Math. Biol. **28**, 411–434.

Ishii, M., Yasuo, S., and Yamaguchi, T. (1970): Epidemiological studies on rice dwarf disease in Kanto-Tosan district Japan. (Japanese with English summary) Journal of Central Agricultural Experiment Station **14**, 1–115.

Jacquez, J., Simon, C., Koopman, J., Sattenspiel, L., and Perry, T. (1988): Modelling and analyzing HIV transmission: the effect of contact patterns. Math. Biosci. **92**, 119–199.

MacCamy, R. (1981): A population model with nonlinear diffusion. J. Diff. Eq. **39**, 57–72.

Macdonald, G. (1957): The Epidemiology and Control of Malaria. Oxford University Press, London.

MacDonald, N. (1989): Biological Delay Systems. Cambridge University Press, Cambridge.

Marcati, P., and Pozio, M. (1980): Global asymptotic stability for a vector disease model with spatial spread. J. Math. Biology **9**, 179–187.

Marcati. P., and Serafini, R. (1979): Asymptotic behaviour in age dependent population dynamics with spatial spread. Bolletino U.M.I. **16**-B, 734–753.

Marotto, F. (1979): Perturbation of stable and chaotic difference equations. J. Math. Anal. Appl. **72**, 716–729.

Marsden, J., and McCracken, M. (1976): The Hopf Bifucation Theorem and its Applications. Springer-Verlag, Berlin-Heidelberg-New York.

May, R., Anderson, R., and McLean, A. (1989): Possible demographic consequences of HIV/AIDS epidemics: II, Assuming HIV infection does not necessarily lead to AIDS. In Mathematical Approaches to Problems in Resource Management and Epidemiology, C. Castillo-Chavez, S. Levin, and C. Showmaker, Eds., Springer Lecture Notes in Biomathematics **81**, 220–248..

McKendrick, A. (1926): Applications of mathematics to medical problems. Proc. Edin. Math. Soc. **44**, 98–130.

Mena-Lorca, J. (1988): Periodicity and stability in epidemiological models with disease-related deaths. Ph.D. thesis, University of Iowa, Iowa City.

Molyneux, D., and Ashford, R. (1983): The biology of *trypanosoma* and *leishmania* parasites of man and domestic animals. International Publication Service, Taylor and Francis, New York.

Muench, H. (1959): Catalytic Models in Epidemiology. Harvard U. Press, Cambridge.

Murray, J. (1989): Mathematical Biology. Springer-Verlag, Berlin-Heidelberg-New York.

Nakasuji, F., Miyai, S., Kawamoto, H., and Kiritani, K. (1985): Mathematical epidemiology of rice dwarf virus transmitted by green rice leafhoppers: a differential equation model. J. Appl. Ecology **22**, 839–847.

Nold, A. (1980): Heterogeneity in disease-transmission modeling. Math. Biosci. **52**, 227–240.

Novick, L., and Hoppensteadt, F. (1978): On plasmid incompatibility. Plasmid **1**, 421-434.

Novick, L., Berns, D., Stricof, R., Stevens, R., Pass, K., Wethers, J. (1989): HIV seroprevalence in newborns in New York state. J. Amer. Med. Assoc. **261**, 1745–1750.

Nowak, M. (1991): The evolution of viruses. Competition between horizontal and vertical transmission of mobile genes. J. Theoret. Biol. **150**, 339–347.

Nussbaum, R. (1992): Entropy minimization, Hilbert's projective metric, and scaling integral kernels. Lefschetz Center for Dynamical Systems report LCDS # 92-3, Brown University, Providence.

Okubo, A. (1980): Diffusion and Ecological Problems: Mathematical Models. Springer-Verlag, Berlin-Heidelberg-New York.

Olsen, L., Truty, G., and Schaffer, W. (1989): Oscillations and chaos in epidemics: a nonlinear dynamics study of six childhood diseases in Copenhagen, Denmark. Theor. Pop. Biol. **33**, 344–370.

Pazy, A. (1983): Semigroups of Linear Operators and Applications to Partial Differential Equations. Applied Mathematical Sciences 44, Springer-Verlag, Berlin-Heidelberg-New York.

Ponce, C., and Zeledon, R. (1973): La enfermedad de Chagas en Honduras. Bol. Of. Sanit. Panam. **75**, 239–248.

Preer, J., Preer, L., and Jurand, A. (1974): Kappa and other endosymbionts in *Paramecium aurelia*. Bacteriol. Rev. **38**, 113–163.

Pugliese, A. (1990): Contact matrices for multipopulation epidemic models: how to build a consistent matrix close to data? Preprint, Dipartimento di Matematica, Università degli Studi di Trento, UTM **338**.

Régnière, J. (1984): Vertical transmission of diseases and population dynamics of insects with discrete generations: a model. J. Theoret. Biol. **107**, 287–301.

Rogers, T., and Marotto, F. (1983): Perturbations of mappings with periodic repellers. Nonlinear Anal. T.M.A. **7**, 97–100.

Ross, R. (1911): The Prevention of Malaria. Second Edition, John Murray, London.

Saints, K. (1987): Discrete and continuous models of age-structured population dynamics. Harvey Mudd College Senior Research Report 1987-1, Claremont.

Salazar, P., de Haro, I., and Uribarren, T. (1988): Chagas's disease in Mexico. Parasitology Today **4**, 348–352.

Schaffer, W. (1985): Can nonlinear dynamics elucidate mechanisms in ecology and epidemiology? IMA J. Math. Appl. Biol. Med. **2**, 221–252.

Schaffer, W., Ellner, S., and Kot, M. (1986): Effects of noise on some dynamical models in ecology. J. Math. Biol. **245**, 479–523.

Schaffer, W., and Kot, M. (1985): Nearly one dimensional dynamics in an epidemic. J. Theoret. Biol. **112**, 403–427.

Scharfstein, J, Luqueti, A., Mureta, A., Senna, M., Renzede, J., Rassi, A. and Mendonca-Previato, L. (1985): Chagas' disease: serodiagnosis with purified Gp25 antigen. Amer. J. Trop. Med. Hyg. **34**, 1153–1160.

Schenzle, D. (1984): An age structured model for pre and post-vaccination measles transmission. IMA J. Math. Appl. Biol. Med. **1**, 169–191.

Schneider, I. (1965): Introduction, translocation and distribution of viruses in plants. Advances in Virus Research **11**, K. Smith and M. Lauffer, Eds., Academic Press, 163–221.

Schwartz, I. (1985): Multiple stable recurrent outbreaks and predictability in seasonally forced nonlinear epidemic models. J. Math. Biol. **21**, 347–361.

Schwartz, I., Smith, H. (1983): Infinite subharmonic bifurcation in an SEIR epidemic model. J. Math. Biol. **18**, 233–253.

Seck, O. (1986): Sur un modele de diffusion non lineaire en dynamique des populations. Doctorat thesis, University of Nancy I.

Simmes, S. (1978): Age dependent population dynamics with nonlinear interactions. Ph.D. Dissertation, Carnegie-Mellon University, Pittsburgh.

Simpson, D. (1972): Arbovirus diseases. Brit. Med. Bull. **27**, 10–15.

Skellam, J. (1951): Random dispersal in theoretical populations. Biometrica **38**, 196–218.

Smith, H. (1983a): Subharmonics bifurcation in an $S - I - R$ epidemic model. J. Math. Biol. **17**, 163-177.

Smith, H. (1983b): Multiple stable subharmonics for a periodic epidemic model. J. Math. Biol. **17**, 179–190.

Sonenshine, D. (1971): Ecology of the American Dog Tick, *Dermacentor variabilis* in a study area in Virginia. 1. Studies on population dynamics using radiological methods. Ann. Entom. Soc. Amer. **65**, 1164–1175.

Stech, H. (1979): The Hopf bifurcation: a stability result and application. J. Math. Anal. Appl. **71**, 525–546.

Stech, H. (1985a): Hopf bifurcation calculations for functional differential equations. J. Math. Anal. Appl. **109**, 472–491.

Stech, H. (1985b): Hopf bifurcation analysis on a class of scalar functional differential equations. In Physical Mathematics and Nonlinear Partial Differential Equations, J. Lightbourne, III, and S. Rankin, III, Eds., Marcel Dekker, New York, 175–185.

Stépán, G. (1989): Retarded Dynamical Systems: Stability and Characteristic Function. Pitman Lecture Notes in Mathematics **210**, Longman Scientific and Technical and John Wiley Press, New York.

Stewart, F., and Levin, B. (1984): The population biology of bacterial viruses: why be temperate. Theor. Pop. Biol. **26**, 93–117.

Takens, F. (1980): Detecting strange attractors in turbulence. In Dynamical Systems and Turbulence, D. Rand and L. Young eds., Springer Lecture Notes in Mathematics **898**, 366–381.

Theis, J., Tibayrenc, M., Mason, D., and Ault, S. (1987): Exotic stock of *Trypanosoma Cruzi (Schisotrypanum)* capable of development in and transmission by *Triatoma Protracta Protracta* from California: public health implications. Amer. J. Trop. Med. Hyg. **36**. 523–528.

Thieme, H. (1979): Asymptotic estimates of the solutions of nonlinear integral equations and asymptotic speeds for the spread of populations. J. Reine Angew. Math. **306**, 94–121.

Thieme, H. (1991a): Analysis of age-structured population models with an additional structure. In Mathematical Population Dynamics, O. Arino, D. Axelrod and M. Kimmel, Eds., Marcel Dekker, New York, Basel, Hong Kong, 115–126.

Thieme, H. (1991b): Stability change of the endemic equilibrium in age-structured models for the spread of S–I–R type infectious diseases. In Differential Equations Models in Biology, Epidemiology and Ecology, S. Busenberg and M. Martelli, Eds., Springer Lecture Notes in Biomathematics **92**, 139–158.

Thieme, H., and Castillo-Chavez, C. (1991): How may infection-age dependent infectivity affect the dynamics of HIV/AIDS? SIAM J. Appl. Math., to appear.

Tudor, D. (1985): An age dependent epidemic model with application to measles. Math. Biosci. **73**, 131–147.

Varga, R. (1962): Matrix Iterative Analysis. Prentice-Hall, Englewood Cliffs, New Jersey.

Velasco-Hernandez, J. (1991a): Models of Chagas' disease, stability, thresholds and asymptotic analysis. Ph. D. thesis, Claremont Graduate School, Claremont, California.

Velasco-Hernandez, J. (1991b): Models for the population dynamics of Chagas' disease. preprint.

Velasco-Hernandez, J. (1991c): An epidemiological model for the dynamics of Chagas' disease. preprint.

Von Foerster, H. (1959): Some remarks on changing populations. In The Kinetics of Cellular Proliferation, F. Stohlman, Ed., Grunne & Stratton, New York, 382–407.

Waldstätter, R. (1990): Models for pair formation with applications to demography and epidemiology. Ph.D. Thesis, University of Tübingen.

Waltman, P. (1974): Deterministic Threshold Models in the Theory of Epidemics. Lecture Notes in Biomathematics 1. Springer-Verlag, Berlin-Heidelberg-New York.

Webb, G. (1980): An age-dependent epidemic model with spatial diffusion. Arch. Ration. Mech. Anal. **75**, 91–102.

Webb, G. (1982a): A recovery-relapse epidemic model with spatial diffusion. J. Math. Biol. **14**, 177-194.

Webb, G. (1982b): A genetics model with age-dependence and spatial diffusion. In Differential Equations and Applications in Ecology, Epidemics and Population Dynamics, S. Busenberg and K.L. Cooke, Eds., Academic Press, New York, 29–40.

Webb, G. (1985): Theory of Nonlinear Age-Dependent Population Dynamics. Marcel Dekker, New York and Basel.

Wilson, E., and Worcester, J. (1945a): The law of mass-action in epidemiology. Proc. Nat. Acad. Sci. **31**, 24–34.

Wilson, E., and Worcester, J. (1945b): The law of mass-action in epidemiology II. Proc. Nat. Acad. Sci. **31**, 109–116.

Woodson, T. (1987): A discrete time population model for ticks. Technical Report, Harvey Mudd College, Claremont.

# Author Index

# Subject Index